HEREDITARY DISEASES AND BLOOD TRANSFUSION

DEVELOPMENTS IN HEMATOLOGY AND IMMUNOLOGY

Volume 30

The titles published in this series are listed at the end of this volume.

Hereditary Diseases and Blood Transfusion

Proceedings of the Nineteenth International Symposium on Blood Transfusion, Groningen 1994, organized by the Red Cross Blood Bank Groningen-Drenthe

edited by

C. Th. SMIT SIBINGA and P. C. DAS

Red Cross Blood Bank Groningen-Drenthe, The Netherlands

and

E. BRIËT

Leiden, The Netherlands

Kluwer Academic Publishers

Dordrecht / Boston / London

A C.I.P. Catalogue record for this book is available from the Library of Congress.

ISBN 0-7923-3694-1

Published by Kluwer Academic Publishers,
P.O. Box 17, 3300 AA Dordrecht, The Netherlands.

Kluwer Academic Publishers incorporates
the publishing programmes of
D. Reidel, Martinus Nijhoff, Dr W. Junk and MTP Press.

Sold and distributed in the U.S.A. and Canada
by Kluwer Academic Publishers,
101 Philip Drive, Norwell, MA 02061, U.S.A.

In all other countries, sold and distributed
by Kluwer Academic Publishers Group,
P.O. Box 322, 3300 AH Dordrecht, The Netherlands.

Printed on acid-free paper

Printed in the Netherlands

Baxter

Acknowledgement

This publication has been made possible through the support of Baxter, which is gratefully acknowledged.

CONTENTS

III. White Cells and Malignancies

IV. Gene Technology, Ethics and the Future

MODERATORS AND SPEAKERS

Moderators

E. Briët (chairman)	– Academic Hospital Leiden, Leiden, NL
P.C. Das	– Red Cross Blood Bank Groningen-Drenthe, Groningen, NL
C.V. Prowse	– Scottish National Blood Transfusion Service, Edinburgh, UK
R.A. Sacher	– Georgetown University Medical Center, Washington, DC, USA
C.Th. Smit Sibinga	– Red Cross Blood Bank Groningen-Drenthe, Groningen, NL
S.L. Thein	– Medical Research Council, John Radcliffe Hospital, Oxford, UK
E. Vellenga	– Academic Hospital Groningen, Groningen, NL

Speakers

D.J. Anstee	– International Blood Group Reference Laboratory, Bristol, UK
J.F. Apperley	– Hammersmith Hospital, London, UK
V. Boulyjenkov	– World Health Organization, Geneva, CH
S. Davies	– John Radcliffe Hospital, Oxford, UK
S. Freeman	– Tulane University Medical Center, New Orleans, LA, USA
R.S. Goodenow	– Baxter Healthcare Corporation, Biotech Group, Gene Therapy Unit, Santa Ana, CA, USA
T.H.J. Huisman	– Medical College of Georgia, Augusta, GA, USA

D.D. Koeberl – Fred Hutchinson Cancer Research Center, Seattle, WA, USA

C. Mazurier – Regional Blood Transfusion Centre, Lille, F

D.E. Onions – University of Glasgow Veterinary School, Glasgow, UK

I. Peake – The University of Sheffield, Royal Hallamshire Hospital, Sheffield, UK

M. Reid – New York Blood Center, New York, NY, USA

P.H. Reitsma – Academic Hospital Leiden, Leiden, NL

Prepared Discussants

C. Férec – Centre of Biogenetics, Blood Bank, Brest, F

FOREWORD

380 years ago, in the year 1614, Ubbo Emmius transplanted the gene of science from Ostfriesland into the education genome of the city of Groningen as developed by Regnerus Praedinius. He thereby founded the University of Groningen.

It is with great pleasure that the Faculty of Medicine as one of the founding faculties of our University, welcomes you to this 19th International Symposium of Blood Transfusion, which will cover the theme of Hereditary Diseases and their relation to Transfusion Medicine, where cell expansion, gene transfer and gene therapy are the read thread.

Since the early days there has been a specific and sincere interest in inborn errors of metabolism and hereditary disorders. This interest has resulted in a structured research, diagnostic and counselling facilities, and therapeutic approaches where various disciplines within our faculty work closely together with groups from related faculties of the University of Groningen, as well as other national and international scientific institutions.

The field of inborn errors, genetic abnormalities and mutations, and hereditary diseases covers a broad gamma of extremely interesting and exciting scientific aspects, which range from clear physical aberrations to molecular analysis of genes and genomes, coding areas and amino acid sequences. It is intriguing to realise that the balance of life seemingly depends on the position or presence of one single molecule as a part of the total complex of genetic information in the cell.

Now that these areas are more and more deeply and intensely explored, scientific options for corrective and therapeutic approaches arise from deductive, analytical, constructive, associative and alternative thinking and observations. The role of the faculty is not limited to stimulation and facilitation, but to bring the various disciplines together and make them work as a team in order to reach the goals of science and development necessary for the advancement in patient care.

The role of the faculty is also to develop new concepts, structures and compositions in the organisation of science and education in medicine. Over the past decade and a half in this respect we have noticed the activities and developments in the field of Transfusion Medicine as a more and more distinct entity within the disciplinary ranks of medical science and practice.

Where a few years ago at the 16th International Symposium on Blood Transfusion the concept of Transfusion Medicine was critically discussed and judged for its facts and fictions, it has now become clear that there should be room for this multi-faceted and interdisciplinary entity within the universum of the Alma Mater.

Increasingly, this concept becomes reality in a number of countries. Sofar, in the Netherlands the immunohaematology part of transfusion medicine has been privileged a chair in Leiden, Utrecht and Nijmegen.

The programme of this symposium – Hereditary Diseases – demonstrates the relevance and importance of Transfusion Medicine as a common denominator connecting the various disciplines and directing the research efforts towards practical implementation and new dimensions in patient care.

Gene therapy, whether short term efficacious or long term supportive, will undoubtedly bring the future closer to reality. Safety, dignity and comfort of life will increase for a group of patients with diseases, abnormalities and handicaps that sofar could only be partly supported and relieved. While the occurrence will continue, the approaches and answers will change, as this symposium will show.

Time has come to recognize the importance of Transfusion Medicine as a common denominator for the current activities, but more importantly for the future of science and research, education and development, practice and care in this dynamic and energetic part of Medicine.

The initiative of the Red Cross Blood Bank Groningen-Drenthe as initiated in 1976 under the stimulating and innovative leadership of its dynamic director is unique. Its undisputed scientific reputation has caused a fruitful and stimulating cross-fertilizing effect within our University and the Faculty of Medicine in particular.

Prof. Dr. O. Hokwerda
Faculty of Medicine
University of Groningen

I. BLOOD COAGULATION

THE MOLECULAR BIOLOGY OF HAEMOPHILIA

I.R. Peake

Introduction

The identification and cloning of the factor VIII (FVIII) and factor IX (FIX) genes in the 1980's opened up the possibility of not only detailed studies of the molecular basis of the haemophilias, but also practical techniques for accurate carrier detection and prenatal diagnosis. The cloning of the genes has also led to the production of recombinant FVIII and FIX, the former now licensed for use in several countries, and to the exciting possibility of gene therapy.

This article will concentrate on the progress that has been made in understanding the genetic basis of the haemophilias and how this information can be used as a practical basis for precise carrier detection and prenatal diagnosis. Much of the progress has of course relied upon technical developments in DNA and RNA analysis.

Methods for gene analysis

The availability, following the cloning of the FVIII genes and FIX genes, of partial and total cDNA probes for these genes immediately led to the application of restriction enzyme digestion and Southern blotting techniques. These analysis revealed large deletions in the genes of a few severely affected patients, and mutations in about 10% of patients where the DNA change created or destroyed a restriction enzyme cleavage site. Many of these, particularly within the FVIII gene were at CpG dinucleotides. This short sequence is recognised as a mutation hot spot within the human genome since the cytosine residue, following its methylation, appears to spontaneously deaminate to give a thymine (C to T) mutation. As discussed below this transition and equivalent G to A resulting from the same substitution on the non-coding DNA strand, are the commonest causative mutations in both the FVIII genes and FIX genes.

The advent of the polymerase chain reaction (PCR) has dramatically increased the mutation detection rate in haemophilia, particularly when combined with rapid DNA mismatch screening methods such as single stranded conformational polymorphism analysis (SSCP) and chemical cleavage mismatch analysis (CCMA). DNA sequencing techniques either manual or automated can then be used to identify the precise mutation. This has led to the identification by specialist laboratories of FIX gene mutations in practically all patients with haemophilia B. Because of the much greater size and complexity of the FVIII gene methods have been devised to analyze both genomic DNA and FVIII mRNA by reverse transcription to cDNA followed by PCR amplification (RT-PCR).

As well as identifying mutations, FVIII gene and FIX gene analysis has also identified a series of polymorphic changes. Both diallelic restriction fragment length polymorphisms (RFLP) and multiallelic variable number tandem repeat (VNTR) regions of DNA have been identified and successfully used as markers to track the haemophilia genes in many families world wide. The problems inherent in polymorphism analysis (non-informativeness, sporadic cases, non-availability of essential family members etc.) have often been outweighed by the overall simplicity, applicability and cheapness of these techniques when compared to current methods of mutation detection.

Haemophilia B

Factor IX gene

The FIX gene is situated at Xq27, approximately 40 megabases centromeric to the FVIII gene. It is some 34 kb in length, has been fully sequenced [1] and its 8 exons encode an mRNA of 1.4 kb. It is shown diagrammatically in Figure 1. The functional domains of FIX correspond, in general to individual exons and thus, for example, the FIX propeptide is encoded by exon 2 and the catalytic region by exons 7 and 8.

Factor IX gene polymorphisms

Seven informative polymorphisms within the FIX genes or flanking it have been reported to be useful for haemophilia B family studies by gene tracking [2]. These polymorphic markers are all diallelic RFLPs (see Figure 2) and therefore have, theoretically, an individual maximum informativeness of 50%. These can all be detected by PCR based techniques and in practice in white European and North American populations the highest individual heterozygosity is 48% (MnlI polymorphism), and only by combined use can the overall informativeness be increased to about 90% (MseI plus TaqI plus HhaI for example). Ethnic variation in heterozygosity rates for these polymorphisms is apparent and, for example the TaqI RFLP is not found in Chinese populations, whereas the MseI polymorphism appears to have a high heterozygosity rate in many different ethnic groups [3].

Factor IX gene mutations in Haemophilia B

As discussed above the advent of rapid procedures of DNA mismatch analysis has resulted in the identification of FIX gene mutations in almost all patients studied by these techniques. A database of mutations is now published yearly [4] and a summary of the mutations reported in the 1994 report is shown in Table 1. Interestingly 476 different molecular events i.e. unique mutations, are reported excluding some 29 partial or complete gene deletions. 91 different amino acid

Table 1. Haemophilia B database (1994) [4].

Haemophilia B
– 1,142 patient entries
– 476 unique molecular events
– 97 short deletions or insertions
– 291 different amino acid substitutions
– 43 STOP codon mutations
– 32% of unique mutations involve CpG dinucleotides

substitutions have been observed, indicating that not only is there no 'hot spot' area for mutations within the gene, but also that almost any amino acid change results in qualitative or quantitative FIX deficiency. In Sweden the causative mutation has been identified in almost all registered haemophilia B patients and in the UK a similarly complete database is rapidly emerging [5].

Of particular interest are the 14 different mutations which have been reported within the 5′ FIX gene promoter sequence. 13 of these are found in patients with the haemophilia B Leiden phenotype, characterised in children by moderate or severe disease with low levels of plasma FIX but which, following puberty, resolves into mild disease and then on to normality with normal FIX levels. It is believed that these mutations prevent the binding of nuclear transcription factors

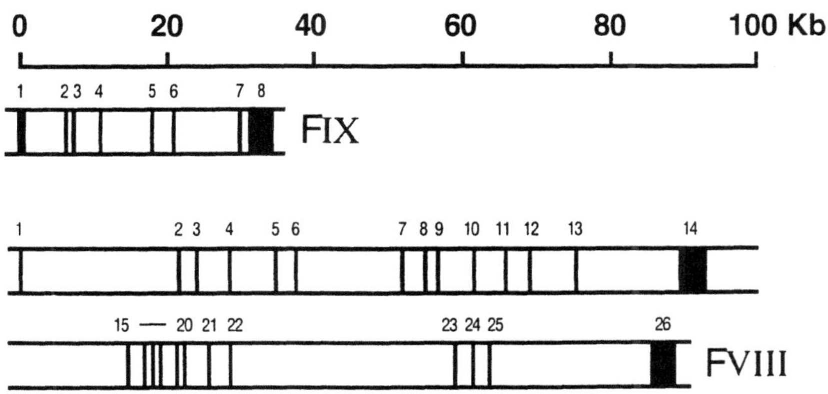

Figure 1. Diagrammatic representation of the factor IX and VIII genes.

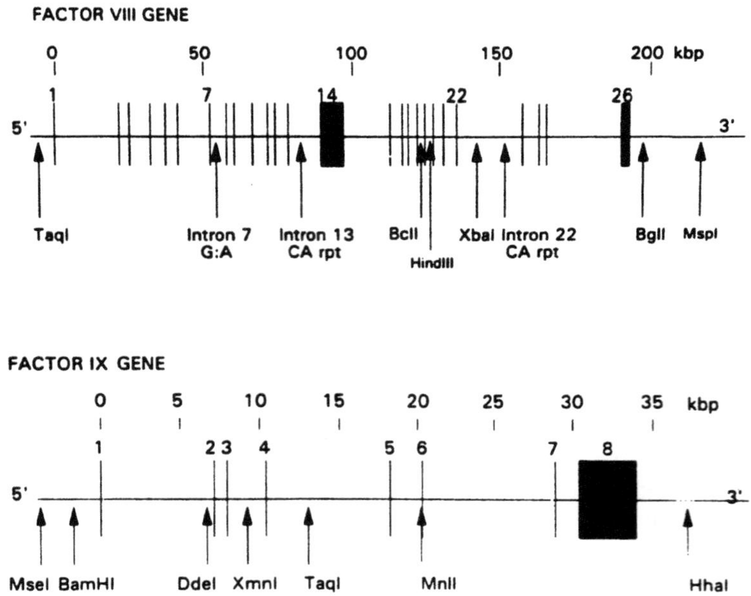

Figure 2. The localization of useful DNA polymorphisms within the factor IX and VIII genes.

to the FIX gene promoter that are essential for normal FIX production prior to puberty [6], but that the subsequent production of testosterone increases the androgenic control of transcription so cancelling out the affect of the Leiden type mutations.

Haemophilia A

Factor VIII gene

The FVIII gene is situated at the telomeric end of the long arm of the X chromosome at band Xq28. The gene encompasses 186 kb of DNA and comprises

Table 2. Haemophilia A database (1994) [9].

Haemophilia A
– 534 patient entries
– 296 unique molecular events
– 44 short deletions or insertions
78 large deletions
– 138 different amino acid substitutions
– 24 STOP codon mutations
– 25% single base pair substitutions involve CpG dinucleotides

of 26 exons varying in size from 69 bp to 3.1 kb which transcribe a mRNA of 9 kb (Figure 1). Of particular interest is intron 22 which is some 32 kb in length and contains the start sites for two further expressed genes designated F8A and F8B. The F8A gene is a 1.8 kb long intronless gene contained entirely within intron 22 and is in the opposite orientation to the FVIII gene [7]. The importance of this gene and its two copies located some 500 kb telomeric to the FVIII gene in the genetic basis of severe haemophilia A is discussed below. F8B is a chimeric gene comprising of an initial unique exon of 24 bp within intron 22 which is then spliced to exons 23 of 26 of the FVIII gene [8].

Factor VIII gene polymorphisms

Nine useful DNA polymorphisms have been described within the FVIII gene (Figure 2) [2]. Of these 6 are RFLPs, 1 in intron 7 (G/A) requires specific oligonucleotide hybridization for its detection, and the remaining 2 are multiallelic CA repeat polymorphisms (VNTR) located in introns 13 and 22. Overall the combined use of these VNTR polymorphisms results in a greater than 80% heterozygosity rate in most populations. Ethnic variations in heterozygosity rates for polymorphisms within the FVIII gene are less pronounced than seen within the FIX gene.

Factor VIII gene mutations in Haemophilia A

The size and complexity of the FVIII gene have made its analysis a daunting task. Initial studies utilising Southern blotting revealed a small number of partial or complete gene deletions in severe cases and restriction enzyme digestion particularly at CpG sites using TaqI revealed a series of missense and STOP mutations. Overall it has been estimated that about 32% of unique nucleotide-substitution based haemophilia A mutations occur at CpG dinucleotide sequences within the FVIII gene.

Recurrent mutations are also common at these sites. Table 2 summarises the data soon to be published in the latest haemophilia A database [9] obtained using the above procedures and complete gene analysis, but not including the FVIII gene inversions discussed below.

Complete analysis of the FVIII gene coding, splice and promoter regions has been attempted in two ways. Firstly by a large series of PCR amplifications of individual or groups of exons, splice sites and promoter sequences, mutations were identified in practically all mild/moderate cases, but only in about 50% of severe cases [10]. Similar results were obtained using an alternative technique or RT-PCR of FVIII mRNA, small amounts of which were isolated from leukocytes. In these studies the FVIII cDNA obtained by RT-PCR was amplified in several fragments which were then subjected to mismatch detection [11]. However, Naylor et al [12,13] subsequently noted that in those severe cases where a mutation could not be found in the coding sequence, no mRNA species crossing intron 22 could be isolated and a large DNA inversion was apparent.

These observations, combined with earlier detailed studies of this area of the X chromosome by Lakich et al [14] show that about 50% of cases of severe haemophilia A are the result of the tip of the X chromosome, one breakpoint of

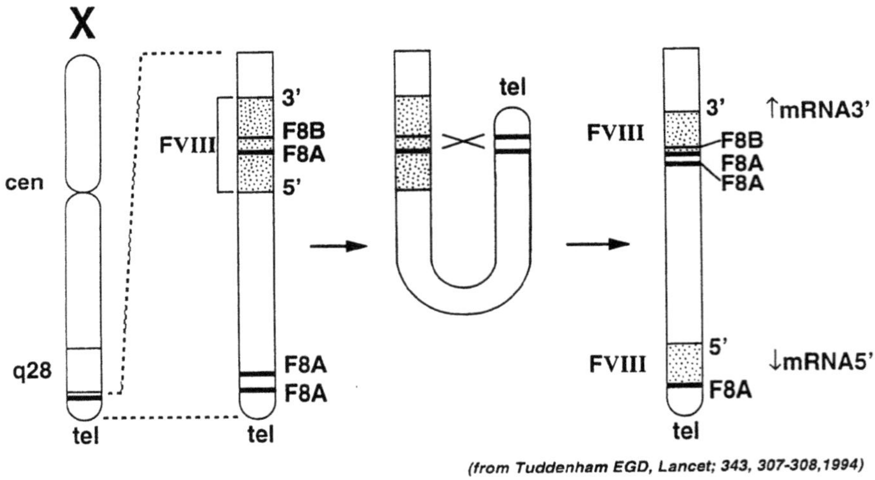

Figure 3. Diagrammatic representation of the X-chromosome inversion resulting from intrachromosomal recombination between sequences associated with the factor VIII gene intron 22 copy of the F8A gene and the distal copy of F8a. [Taken from Tuddenham EGD. Flip tip inversion and haemophilia A. Lancet 1994;343:307-08, with permission.]

which lies with intron 22 of the FVIII gene. This is shown diagrammatically in Figure 3. These inversions appear to occur by recombination between the intron 22 copy of F8A and either the distal or proximal copy. Analysis by a simple Southern blot technique [15] has shown that the former is the most common with a reported incidence of 70 to 90%. These inversions have now been reported world-wide as the cause of severe haemophilia A in about 50% of cases. Inversions detected by Southern blot should now be the first test employed in family studies in severe disease and only when it is not present are polymorphism based linkage studies or further mutation detection methods necessary.

Haemophilia mutations and disease severity

Initial studies showed, as might be expected, that patients with a total or partial gene deletion had an increased risk of inhibitor development after replacement therapy. This is also true in haemophilia A for patients with STOP mutations. The development of inhibitors in severe patients with the X-chromosome inversion was initially thought to be low [15], but this may not be the case. Mild or moderate haemophilia is generally caused by missense mutations where the substituted animo acid results in partial qualitative or quantitative deficiency.

Although an observed mutation in the FIX or FVIII gene in a haemophiliac may indicate disease severity and perhaps suggest an increased risk of inhibitor development, the studies outlined in this review have had little impact cn current treatment and until gene repair is possible, will not affect gene therapy proposals. It is however clear that gene based carrier detection and prenatal diagnosis by either polymorphism based linkage analysis or specific mutation detection has dramatically improved the reliability and accuracy of these diagnoses and helped many families with haemophilia.

References

1. Yoshitake S, Schach BG, Foster DC, Davie EW, Kurachi W. Nucleotide sequence of the gene for human factor IX (antihaemophilic factor B). Biochem J 1985;24: 3736-50.
2. Peake IR, Lillicrap DP, Boulyjenkov V, et al. Report of a joint WHO/WFH meeting on the control of haemophilia: Carrier detection and prenatal diagnosis. Blood Coagulation and Fibrinolysis 1993;4:313-44.
3. Winship PR, Nichols CE, Chuansumrit A, Peake IR. An MseI RFLP in the 5′ flanking region of the factor IX gene: Its use for haemophilia B carrier detection in Caucasian and Thai puplations. Brit J Haematol 1993;84:101-5.
4. Giannelli F, Green PM, Sommer SS, et al. Haemophilia B: Database of point mutations and short additions and deletions. Fifth edition. Nucleic Acids Res 1994;22: 3534-46.
5. Saad S, Rowley G, Tagliavacca L, Green PM, Giannelli F. First report on UK database of haemophilia mutations and pedigrees. Thromb Haemost 1994;71:571-75
6. Reitsma PH, Mandalaki T, Kasper GK, Bertina RM, Briet E. Two novel point mutations correlate with an altered developmental expression of blood coagulation factor IX (haemophila B Leiden phenotype). Blood 1989;73: 743-50.
7. Levinson B, Kenwick S, Lakich D, Hammonds G, Gitschier J. A transcribed gene in an intron of the human factor VII gene. Genomics 1990;7:1-11.
8. Levinson B, Kenwick S, Gamelp P, Fisher K, Gitschier J. Evidence for a third transcript from the human factor VIII gene. Genomics 1992;14:585-89.
9. Tuddenham EGD, Schwaab R, Seehafer J, et al. Haemophilia A database of nucleotide substitutions, deletions, insertions and rearrangements of the factor VII gene. Nucleic Acids Res 1994;22:3511-33.
10. Higuchi M, Kazazian HH Hr, Kasch L, et al. Molecular characterization of severe haemophilia A suggests that about half the mutations are not within the coding regions and splice junctions of the factor VIII gene. Proc Natl Acad Sci USA 1991; 88:7405-09
11. Naylor JA, Green GM, Montandon JA, Rizza CR, Giannelli F. Detection of three novel mutations in haemophilia A patients by rapid screening of the whole essential region of the factor VIII gene. Lancet 1991;337:635-39
12. Naylor J, Brinke A, Hassock S, Green PM, Giannelli F. Characteristic mRNA abnormality found in half the patients with severe haemophilia A is due to large DNA inversions. Human Mol Gen 1993-2:1773-75.
13. Naylor JA, Green PM, Rizza CR, Giannelli F. Factor VIII gene explains all cases of haemophillia A. Lancet 1992;340:1066-67.
14. Lakich D, Kazazian HH, Antonarakis SE, Gitschier J. Inversions disrupting the factor VIII gene are a common cause of severe haemophilia A. Nature Gen 1993; 5:236-41.
15. Goodeve AC, Preston FE, Peake IR. Factor VIII rearrangements in patients with severe haemophilia A. Lancet 1994;343:329-30.

MOLECULAR BIOLOGY OF THE VARIOUS TYPES OF VON WILLEBRAND DISEASE

C. Mazurier

Introduction

Historically discovered in 1926 by Erik von Willebrand studying bleeding patients living on an island of the Åland archipelago, von Willebrand disease (vWD) is now recognised as the most common inherited bleeding disorder. It defines a heterogeneous group of patients with quantitative or qualitative defects of the von Willebrand factor (vWF) [1] which is a large glycoprotein present in plasma, subendothelium and the alpha granules of platelets. Synthesized exclusively by both endothelial cells and megakaryocytes, vWF plays a dual role in haemostasis. It mediates platelet adhesion to the subendothelium at the site of vessel injury and its circulating form carries and stabilizes factor VIII (FVIII), [2].

In 1985, the vWF cDNA was cloned from human endothelial cell cDNA libraries by four groups [3-6]. The vWF mRNA consists of about 9000 nucleotides coding for a precursor translation product of 2813 amino acid (aa) residues named pre-pro-vWF. This pre-pro-polypeptide contains four distinct homologous domains organized in the following order: D_1-D_2-D'-D_3-A_1-A_2-A_3-D_4-B_1-B_2-B_3-C_1-C_2 [7] (Figure 1). The pre-pro-vWF undergoes an intracellular multistep biosynthetic process leading to the secretion of multimerized mature subunits of 2050 aa residues ranging from 500 to more than 10.000 kdaltons. The human genome harbours only one copy of the vWF gene that is located at the tip of the short arm of chromosome 12 in position 12p12→ter [3,6].

A partial unprocessed pseudogene for vWF is located on chromosome 22 (22q11.22-q11.23) [8]; it spans approximately 30 kbases and corresponds to exons 23-34 of the vWF gene [9]. The vWF gene consists of approximately 180 kbases and contains 52 exons (Figure 1). Exons range from 40 bp to 1.4 kbases for the largest exon (exon 28). The sequence of the entire cDNA as well as the intron/exon junctions and portions of the flanking introns have been determined five years ago [10]. In this study in which 40 kb of genomic DNA was sequenced, a number of repetitive sequences, including a multiallelic variable number of ATCT tetranucleotide repeats (VNTR) in intron 40, were identified. More than thirty biallelic polymorphisms have also been described for the vWF gene, fifteen are exonic while eight of them alter the vWF aa sequence [11]. The cloning of the vWF gene, in addition to the inreasing application of the polymerase chain

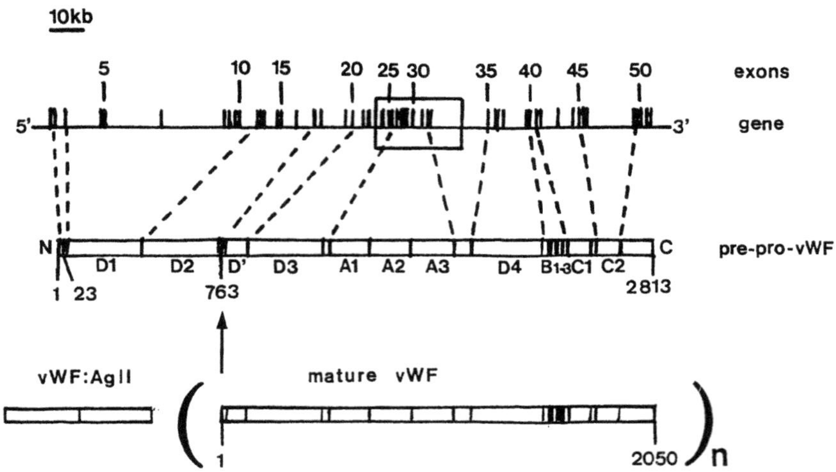

Figure 1. Structure of the vWF gene and encoded vWF protein. The structure of the gene is shown with the position of the 52 exons. The box localizes the region that is duplicated in the vWF pseudogene. The relationship between the exons and the homologous domains of the pre-pro-vWF is indicated by dashed lines. The pre-pro-vWF consists of 2813 aa residues of which 1-22 constitute the signal peptide and 23-763 correspond to the propeptide that that is named vWF:Ag II after cleavage, at the site indicated by arrow, and secretion. The mature subunit of vWF which consists of 2050 aa undergoes a complex post-translational processing and mutimerizes before storage or secretion.

reaction (PCR), led to major progress in the identification of the molecular defects responsible for the different forms of vWD. In this review of the various vWF gene defects that result in either quantitative or qualitative defects of vWF, the recently revised phenotypic classification of vWD [12] will be used. Some of the reported molecular defects have already been catalogued in a database [13] planned to be updated regularly.

Types 1 and 3 of vWD (quantitative defect of vWF)

Type 1 vWD refers to partial quantitative deficiency with normal multimeric structure of plasma vWF and is generally inherited in an autosomal dominant fashion [13]. It is the most common form of vWD accounting for approximately 75% of the diagnosed cases and presents a 1-3% prevalence in Scandinavia. Type 3 is rare, with a prevalence ranging from 0.5 to 5 per million population depending on the country [14]. Type 3 is characterized by autosomal recessive inheritance and virtually complete deficiency of vWF in both plasma and platelets

[13]. Patients with type 3 vWD have serious bleeding complications. Therefore accurate carrier detection and opportunity for prenatal diagnosis may be crucial in type 3 vWD families. In general, quantitative deficiencies in a given protein correlate with promoter mutations, nonsense mutations, frameshift mutations or deletions in the corresponding gene. The large size and number of exons of the vWF gene, as well as the presence of its partial pseudogene, have complicated the detection of molecular defects in quantitative forms of vWD. The currently identified deletions and non-deletion molecular defects in quantitative forms of vWD are summarized in Tables 1 and 2, respectively.

Type 3 vWD

The first vWF gene defects identified in type 3 vWD patients were deletions spanning the entire vWF gene [15,16]. Partial deletions were then found in other unrelated patients [17,18] (see Table 1). Gene deletions appear to correlate with a particular risk for the development of inhibitory antibodies against vWF after transfusion [18]. However, they account for only a small subset of patients as there is no evidence of gross deletions, insertions or rearrangements in most of type 3 vWD patients [19].

Once deletion has been excluded as a molecular mechanism for quantitative vWF defect, it is laborious to identify the causative gene defect by direct sequence of the entire vWF gene. A method for identifying possible defective mRNA expression in assessing DNA sequence polymorphisms located in the vWF gene exons, from both leucocyte genomic DNA and platelet mRNA, has been used in several laboratories. Defective vWF alleles associated with very low or absent platelet mRNA were thus identified in several families [20-22] (Table 2). In some cases, a single point mutations in exon 45, resulting in a premature translation termination (Arg1772ter), is possibly responsible for the associated loss of mRNA expression [21] though a direct role of the created stop codon yet has not been demonstrated. This nonsense mutation appeared to be recessive and has been shown to have a frequence of 0.23% in the Dutch population [22]. Other TGA

Table 1. vWF gene deletions identified in type 3 vWD patients.

Molecular defect	Number of independent families	Reference
Gross deletion spanning the entire vWF gene	2	[15]
	2	[16]
2.3 kbases deletion spanning the exon 42 and insertion of a novel 182 bp sequence between breakpoints	1	[17]
30 kbases deletion spanning exons 33-38	1	[18]
≃ 56 kbases deletion spanning exons 22-43	1	[18]

Table 2. Nondeletion vWF gene defects identified in types 3 and 1 vWD patients.

Molecular defect*	**Number of independent families****	**Reference**
Defective mRNA expression (no gene defect identified)	1 (3) 2 (1)	[20] [22]
Defect in exon 9: Arg(c)365ter C→T nt 1093 substitution (stop codon at position 365, in vWF prosequence)	1 (3)	[23]
Defect in exon 18: C deletion in a stretch of 6 cytosines (nt 2679-2684) leading to a stop codon in mature vWF	15 (3) 1 (3) 3 (1)	[25] [26]
Defect in exon 28: Arg896ter C→T nt 4975 substitution (stop codon at position 1659, in mature vWF)	3 (3)	[24]
Defect in exon 28: Pro503Leu and Val516Ile Three consecutive pseudogene-like substitutions: G→A: nt 3789, C→T: nt 3797, G→A: nt 3835 (2 missense codons at position 1266 and 1279, in mature vWF)	1 (1) 1 (1)	[22] [26]
Defect in exon 32: Arg1089ter C→T nt 5554 substitution (stop codon at position 1852, in mature vWF)	3 (3)	[24]
Defect in exon 45: Arg1772ter C→T nt 7603 substitution (stop codon at position 2535, in mature vWF, associated with defective mRNA expression)	3 (3) 1 (1) 1 (3)	[21] [22] [24]
Defect in exon 45: Arg1783Tyr A→T nt substitution (missense codon at position 2546, in mature vWF, associated with, but likely not causing, defective mRNA expression)	3 (3)	[21]

* The nomenclature used is described in the database [13]. Nucleotides are numbered 1 to 8439 according to the published cDNA sequence [7]. Codons are numbered 1 to 2813 with initiator ATG for Met as + 1. Amino acid residues are numbered either 1 to 2050 with Ser as + 1, when located in mature vWF, or (c)1 to (c)763, from the initiator Met as (c)1, when located in the prosequence.

** The type, 1 or 3, of vWD is in parenthesis.

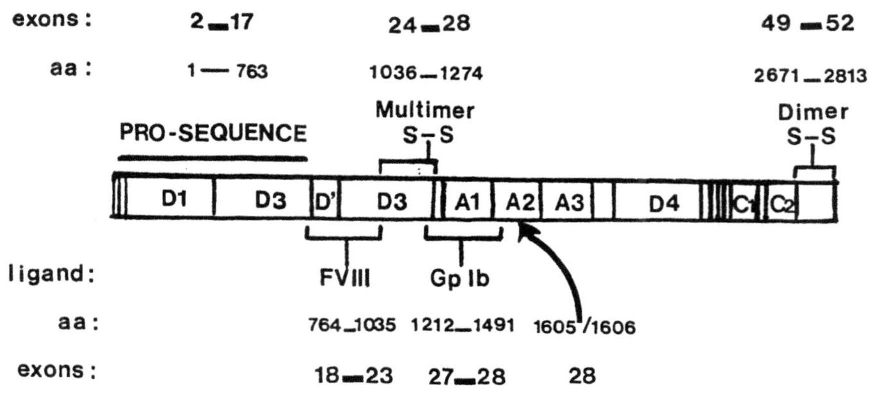

Figure 2. Schematic localization of the amino acid (aa numbered 1 to 2813) segments, within the pre-pro-vWF sequence, which are either possibly responsible for the loss of HMW multimers or involved in binding to FVIII and GPIb. The prosequence is depicted as horizontal line, interchain disulphide bonds and proteolytic site in mature vWF are depicted as S-S and curved arrow, respectively. The exons encoding these structural and functional domains are indicated on top and bottom.

stop codons resulting from C→T transition, at CpG 'hot spots', in CGA Arginine codons have also been identified in the exons 9, 28 and 32 [23, 24]. Recently, was characterized a Cytosine deletion in a stretch of 6 consecutive Cytosines in exon 18 that interrupts the reading frame and results in a stop codon [25, 26]. This Cytosine deletion has been shown to be present in half of the alleles of Swedish type 3 vWD patients [25] and likely accounts for the bleeding diathesis in the family studied, almost seventy years ago, by E. von Willebrand [26].

Type 1 vWD

Despite considerable progress in characterizing vWF gene defects in type 3 vWD, the molecular origin for the most frequent quantitative form of vWD (type 1) remains obscure. Some of the mutations identified in type 3 vWD have also been found in one of the alleles of type 1 vWD patients [22,26]. Why these mutations and defective mRNA expression [22] are apparently dominant in type 1 families whereas they are transmitted recessively in type 3 families is still an enigma. Associated subtle molecular defects might be a plausible mechanism for dominant quantitative defect of vWF because three consecutive pseudogene-like substitutions in exon 28 have been recently characterized, by two groups, in two unrelated families with type 1 vWD [22,26].

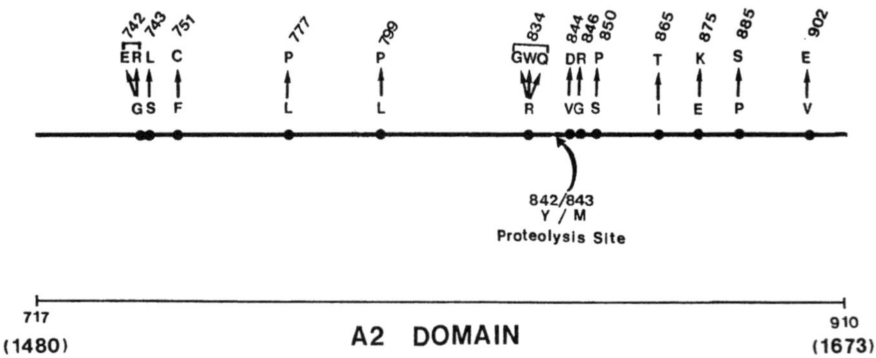

Figure 3. Mutations (arrows) within the 3′ part of vWF exon 28 that cause the phenotype IIA of type 2A vWD [13,47-50]. The aa residues are indicated by one-letter code and are numbered from the N-terminal Serine residue of mature vWF (Fig. 1). The curved arrow indicates the position of the proteolytic site within mature vWF. Numbers underneath the bottom line indicate the position of the A_2 domain corresponding to aa 1480-1673, in parenthesis, of pre-pro-vWF (Fig. 1).

Type 2 vWD (qualitative defect in vWF)

Type 2 vWD refers to qualitative deficiency of vWF and may be dominant or recessive [12]. The critical test to differentiate type 2 from type 1 is whether vWF can be distinguished from normal vWF. Abnormalities of vWF may be either structural (loss of high molecular weight multimers) or functional (loss of platelet-dependentfunction or incapacityto bind FVIII). These qualitative defects of vWF likely may result from point mutations but identifying single point mutation within the entire gene is a challenge. Therefore, an approach for detecting molecular defects in the various forms of type 2 vWD is to seek them in the exons coding either for aa sequences of pre-pro-vWF involved in the multimerization process [27, 28] and/or the proteolytic cleavage which may result in the loss of high molecular weight (HMW) vWF multimers [29] or for the specific domains of mature vWF involved in platelet or FVIII interactions [2]. These exons potentially responsible for the qualitative defects of vWF characterized in the various categories of type 2 vWD are illustrated in Figure 2.

Type 2A vWD

Type 2A vWD refers to variants with decreased platelet-dependent function that is associated with the absence of HMW vWF multimers. It corresponds closely to the previous dominant subtype IIA which accounts for approximately

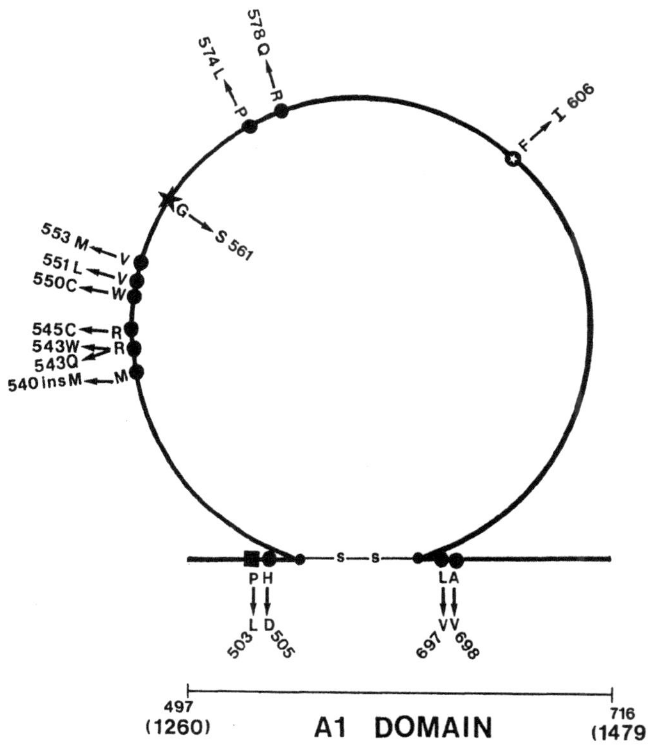

Figure 4. Mutations (arrows) within the 5′ part of vWF exon 28 that cause types 2B and 2M of vWD. The 2B mutations of subtypes IIB (full circles) [13,35,36, 51-53] and New-York or Malmö (full square) [37] are indicated. The mutations reported to cause phenotype B (full star) [39] and of a variant form of type I, likely also belonging to type 2M, (empty star) [54] are indicated. The loop is shaped by the intrachain disulphide bond (S-S) between Cysteine 509 and 695. The aa residues are indicated by one-letter code and are numbered from the N-terminal Serine residue of mature vWF. Numbers underneath the bottom line indicate the position of the A_1 domain corresponding to aa 1260-1479, in parenthesis, of the pre-pro-vWF (Fig. 1).

10-15% of vWD cases, but also includes the unfrequent previous subtypes IIC to II-I [1].

Subtype IIA: The approach used to narrow the search to a given exon was based on the previous observation of markedly increased proteolytic fragments of vWF in the plasma of type IIA vWD patients [30]. As the proteolytic site of vWF had been localized at aa 842/843 [31] encoded by exon 28 which is repeated in the pseudogen, the first strategy was to analyze the region of mRNA corresponding to this exon. By using this strategy, five years ago, two mutations (Arg834Trp and Val844Asp) were first identified in several unrelated type IIA families [32]. This strategy, as well as another one, based on specific PCR allowing to amplify

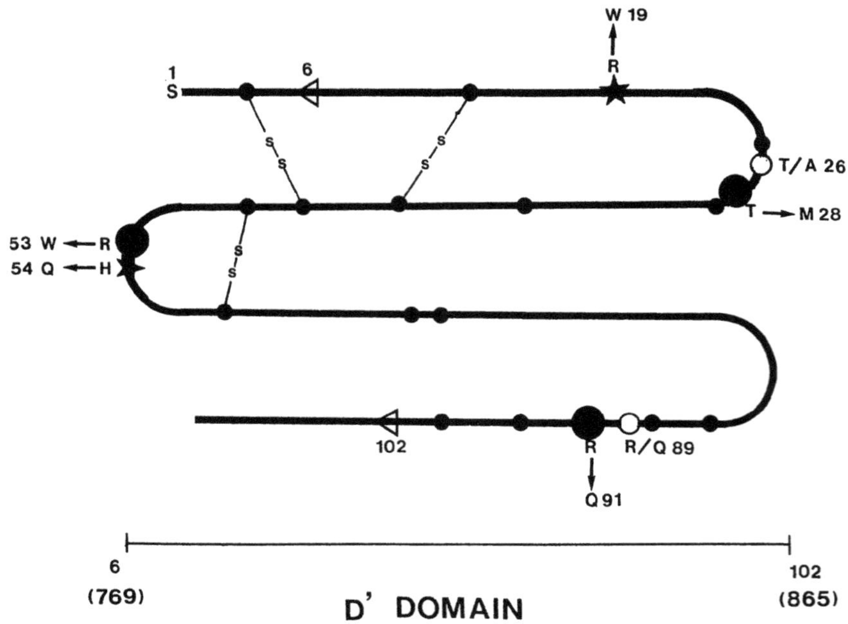

Figure 5. Mutations (arrows) within the vWF exons 18-20 that cause type 2N vWD [13]. The N-terminal sequence of mature vWF with Serine as first aa residue is rich in Cysteine (small solid circles) organized in intrachain bonds, some of them have already been paired and are localized by S-S. Changes in aa residue are either silent, as the polymorphisms in position 26 and 89 indicated by empty circles, or constitute the real mutations indicated by large solid circles in position 28, 53 and 91. The aa substitutions in 19 and 54, indicated by stars, must be associated for inducing a loss of FVIII binding of vWF. Numbers underneath the bottom line indicate the position of the D′ domain corresponding to aa 769 to 865, in parenthesis, of the pre-pro-vWF (Fig. 1).

only the authentic gene but not the pseudogene, have led to the identification of a number of missense mutations present at the heterozygous state in type IIA vWD patients [13]. With few possible exceptions, these point mutations are localized in the 3′ part of exon 28 and induce changes in 11 residues clustered within a 167aa segment of the A2 domain of vWF (Figure 3). The expression of recombinant vWF (rvWF) by mammalian cells transfected with mutant cDNA harbouring these IIA mutations has allowed to distinguish two groups of mutations. For one category of mutations, referred to as group 1, the corresponding secreted rvWF exhibits an abnormal multimeric structure with lack of HMW multimers, whereas for the other one, group 2, the multimeric pattern is normal [33]. These data suggest that phenotype IIA may result from two distinct mechanisms. Defect in intracellular transport, highly multimerized forms of vWF being retained within endoplasmic reticulum, has been shown in group 1, while increased proteolysis after secretion is assumed in group 2 [33].

Subtype IIc: The subcategory of 2A vWD patients previously named IIC defines a group of patients characterized by both a peculiar multimeric pattern with a marked predominance of the protomeric form of vWF and recessive inheritance. The approach used to seek vWF gene defect in one of these IIC vWD patients was first to sequence the exons encoding aa sequences involved in the formation of disulphide bonds involved in the multimerization (exons 24-28) and dimerization (exons 49-52) process of vWF subunits (Figure 2). As no abnormality has been found in these exons and in surrounding ones encoding the mature subunit, the sequencing analysis was enlarged to the exons 2-17 coding for the propeptide of vWF which had been previously shown to be required for multimerization. That was how a 3bp insertion and a 2bp deletion in the exons 15 and 16, respectively were detected. The IIC vWD patient was shown to be a compound heterozygous for the 2bp deletion inducing frameshift (Cys(c)709Leu, Tyr(c)710Leu) and the stop codon (Tyr(c) 711ter) on one allele and for the 3bp insertion the (c)625insGly insertion, on the other allele [34]. The direct analysis of the exon 15 in another IIC patient, whose bleeding diathesis was likely resulting from consanguineous parents, led to the identification of Cys(c)623Trp mutation on the two vWF alleles [34].

Other subtypes of 2A vWD: In the very rare patients with the phenotype IID to II-I, yet no vWF gene defect has been characterized.

Type 2B vWD

This type refers to variants with vWF increased affinity for platelet glycoprotein (GP) Ib [12]. It includes the previous phenotype IIB, with plasma vWF displaying a loss in HMW multimers, and the phenotypes "New York" or "Malmö" with normal multimeric pattern of plasma vWF. All these subtypes are inherited in an autosomal dominant fashion. Since the GPIb binding domain had been localized on a peptide fragment of vWF around a disulphide loop (Cys 509-Cys695), encoded by the 5′ part of exon 28, several groups have concentrated on this region of vWF gene (Figure 2). All the mutations identified so far, at the heterozygous state, in 2B vWD patients induce changes in aa located in, or close to, the 509-695 loop (Figure 4). Introduced in full length cDNA and transfected in eukaryotic cells, they induced rvWFs with increased affinity for platelet GPIb, confirming they are authentic mutations [13,35,37].

Type 2M vWD

Type 2M vWD refers to qualitative variants with de creased-dependentfunction that is not caused by the absence of HMW vWF multimers [12]. This subtype includes the previously characterized phenotype B described in an Australian patient [38]. An heterozygous nucleotide substitution leading to the change of Gly561 in Ser in mature vWF has been shown to be responsible for this very rare variant [39] (Figure 4).

Type 2N vWD

Type 2N vWD, previously tentatively named "Normandy", after the birth province of one proband [40], refers to qualitative variants with defective FVIII binding [12]. It is inherited recessively and about 80% of the patients diagnosed so far are either homozygous or heterozygous for a frequent nucleotide substitution in exon 20, characterized in 0.94% of the normal Dutch population [22], which induces the substitution of Gln for Arg in position 91 of mature vWF [41]. When this mutation is present on only one allele, the other one either is silent or harbours another mutation such as Arg53Trp in exon 19, or Thr28Met in exon 18, the patients being compound heterozygote [13, 41-43]. The expression of the different type 2N mutations (Figure 5) has shown that Arg91Gln mutation, as well as the association of Arg19Trp and His54Gln aa substitutions, induce dramatically decrease in vWF capacity to bind FVIII while Thr28Met and Arg53Trp mutations completely abolish this function.

Conclusion

Over the past ten years, considerable progress has been made in characterizing polymorphisms and molecular defects in the vWF gene. The analysis of the vWF gene in patients with severe quantitative defect of vWF (type 3) has first given evidence of complete or partial deletions. Then, nonsense mutations scattered all over the gene and sometimes mimicking the pseudogene sequence [44] were characterized.The identification of molecular defects and/or vWF polymorphisms in some type 3 vWD families has allowed carrier detection and prenatal diagnosis [45, 46]. However, the molecular basis for the classic dominant form of vWD (type 1) remains obscure and is a challenge for several research groups. The precise characterization of the different subtypes is required for optimal therapy of vWD patients but the progress in mutation-specific diagnosis is likely to be slow in the majority of patients who belong to type 1. However, it can be anticipated that, in time, the present phenotypic classification of type 2 vWD will be superseded by an easier and more accurate genotypic classification of the different categories of patients identified by the specific gene defects. Indeed, the selective screening of the regions of the gene potentially responsible for structural or functional vWF defects, previously identified in types 2A, 2B and 2N patients, has led to the identification of distinct clusters of mutations (missense mutations and small in-frame deletions or insertions) associated with these specific variants. Furthermore, the availability of eukaryotic expression systems has unabled corresponding mutant cDNA to be investigated and has provided considerable insights into relationship between vWF structure and function. Owing to the dual function of vWF in both primary haemostasis and coagulation, continued advance in this area may also be important for applied research in the development of new classes of antithrombotic and anticoagulant drugs.

Acknowledgements

Our gratitude goes to Prof. M. Goudemand for his continuous interest in our research work on von Willebrand disease. We thank V. Rigot for her secretarial assistance.

References

1. Ruggeri ZM, Zimmerman TS. Classification of von Willebrand disease. J Clin Lab Anal 1987;1:353-62.
2. Ruggeri ZM, War J. Von Willebrand factor. FASEB Journal 1993;7:308-16.
3. Ginsburg D, Handin RI, Bonthron, et al. Human von Willebrand factor (vWF): Isolation of complementary DNA (cDNA) clones and chromosomal localization. Science 1985;228:1401-06.
4. Lynch DC, Zimmerman TS, Collins CJ, Brown M, Morin MJ, Ling EH. Molecular cloning of cDNA for human von Willebrand factor: Authentification by a new method. Cell 1985;41:49-56.
5. Sadler JE, Shelton-Inloes BB, Sorace JM, Harlan JM, Titani K, Davie EW. Cloning and characterization of two cDNAs coding for human von Willebrand factor. Proc Nat Acad Sci USA 1985;82:6394-98.
6. Verweij CL, de Vries CJM, Distel B, et al. Construction of cDNA coding for human von Willebrand factor using antibody probes for colony-screening and mapping of the chromosomal gene. Nucleic Acids Res 1985;13:4699-717.
7. Verweij CL, Diergaarde PJ, Hart M, Pannekoek H. Full-length von Willebrand factor (vWF) cDNA encodes a highly repetitive protein larger than the mature vWF subunit. EMBO J 1986;5:1839-47.
8. Patracchini P, Calzolari E, Aiello V, et al. Sublocalization of von Willebrand factor pseudogene to 22q11.22-q11.23 by in situ hybridization in a 46, X, t (X;22) (pter;q11.21) translocation. Hum Genet 1989;83:264-66.
9. Mancuso DJ, Tuley EA, Westfield LA, et al. Human von Willebrand factor gene and pseudogene. Structural analysis and differentiation by polymerase chain reaction. Biochemistry 1991;30:253-69.
10. Mancuso DJ, Tuley EA, Westfield LA, Worrall NK, Shelton-Inloes BB. Structure of the gene for human von Willebrand factor. J Biol Chem 1989;264: 19514-27.
11. Sadler JE, Ginsburg D. A data base of polymorphisms in the von Willebrand factor gene and pseudogene. Thromb Haemost 1993;69:185-91.
12. Sadler JE. A revised classification of von Willebrand disease. Thromb Haemost 1994; 71:520-25.
13. Ginsburg D, Sadler JE. Von Willebrand disease: A database of point mutations, insertions and deletions. Thromb Haemost 1993;69:177-84.
14. Mannucci PM, Bloom AL, Larrieu MJ, Nilsson IM, West RR. Atherosclerosis and von Willebrand factor. Prevalence of severe von Willebrand's disease in western Europe and Israel. Br J Haematol 1984;57:163-69.
15. Shelton-Inloes BB, Chehab FF, Mannucci PM, Federici AB, Sadler JE. Gene deletions correlate with the development of alloantibodies in von Willebrand disease. J Clin Invest 1987;79:1459-65.
16. Ngo KV, Glotz VT, Koziol JA, et al. Homozygous and heterozygous deletions of the von Willebrand factor gene in patients and carriers of severe von Willebrand disease.

Proc Nat Acad Sci USA 1988;85:2753-57.
17. Peake IR, Liddell MB, Moodie P, et al. Severe type III von Willebrand's disease caused by deletion of exon 42 of the von Willebrand factor gene: Family studies that identify carriers of the condition and a compound heterozygous individual. Blood 1990;75:654-61.
18. Mancuso DJ, Tuley EA, Castillo R, de Bosch N, Mannucci PM, Sadler JE. Characterization of partial gene deletions in type III von Willebrand disease with alloantibody inhibitors. Thromb Haemost 1994;72:180-85.
19. Anvret M, Blombäck M, Lindstedt M, Söderlind E, Tapperpersson M, Thelander AC. Genetic and blood coagulation characterization of Swedish families with von Willebrand's disease type I and type III. New aspect of heredity. Hum Genet 1992;89: 147-54.
20. Nichols WC, Lyons SE, Harrison JS, Cody RL, Ginsburg D. Severe von Willebrand disease due to a defect at the level of von Willebrand factor messenger RNA expression. Detection by exonic PCR restriction fragment length polymorphism analysis. Proc Natl Acad Sci USA 1991;88:3857-61.
21. Eikenboom JCJ, Ploos van Amstel HK, Reitsma PH, Briët E. Mutations in severe, type III von Willebrand's disease in the Dutch population: Candidate missense and nonsense mutations associated with reduced levels of von Willebrand factor messenger RNA. Thromb Haemost 1992;68:448-54.
22. Eikenboom JCJ, Reitsma PH, Peerlinck KMJ, Briët E. Recessive inheritance of von Willebrand's disease type I. Lancet 1993;341:982-86
23. Bahnak BR, Lavergne JM, Rothschild C, Meyer D. A stop codon in a patient with severe type III von Willebrand disease. Blood 1991;78:1148-49.
24. Zhang ZP, Lindstedt M, Falk G, Blombäck M, Egberg N, Anvret M. Nonsens mutations of the von Willebrand factor gene in patients with von Willebrand disease type III and type I. Am J Hum Genet 1992;51:850-58.
25. Zhang ZP, Falk G, Blombäck M, Egberg N, Anvret M. A single cytosine deletion in exon 18 of the von Willebrand factor gene is the most common mutation in Swedish vWD type III patients. Hum Mol Genet 1992;1:767-68
26. Zhang ZP, Blombäck M, Nyman D, Anvret M. Mutations of von Willebrand factor gene in families with von Willebrand disease in the Åland Islands. Proc Natl Acad Sci USA 1993;90:7937-40.
27. Wagner DD. Cell Biology of von Willebrand factor. Ann Rev Cell Biol 1990;6: 217-46.
28. Mayadas TN, Wagner DD. Vicinal cysteines in the prosequence play a role in von Willebrand factor multimer assembly. Proc Natl Acad Sci USA 1992;89:3531-35.
29. Dent JA, Galbusera M, Ruggeri ZM. Heterogeneity of plasma von Willebrand factor multimers resulting from proteolysis of the constituent subunit. J Clin Invest 1991; 88:774-82.
30. Berkowitz SD, Dent JA, Roberts JR, et al. Epitope mapping of the von Willebrand factor subunit distinguishes fragmets present in normal and type IIA von Willebrand disease from those generated by plasmin. J Clin Invest 1987; 79:524-31.
31. Dent JA, Ware J, Kasper CK, Ruggeri ZM, Berkowitz SD. Identification of a cleavage site directing the immunochemical detection of molecular abnormalities in type IIA von Willebrand factor. Proc. Natl Acad Sci USA 1990;87:6306-10.
32. Ginsburg D, Konkle BA, Gill JC, et al. Molecular basis of human von Willebrand disease: Analysis of platelet von Willebrand factor mRNA. Proc Natl Acad Sci USA 1989;86:3723-27.

33. Lyons SE, Bruck ME, Bowie EJW, Ginsburg D. Impaired intracellular transport produced by a subset of type IIA von Willebrand disease mutations. J Biol Chem 1992;267:4424-30.
34. Gaucher C, Diéval J, Mazurier Cl. Characterization of von Willebrand factor gene defects in two urelated patients with type IIC von Willebrand disease. Blood 1994; 84:1024-30.
35. Rabinowitz I, Randi AM, Shindler KS, Tuley EA, Rustagi PK, Sadler JE. Type IIB mutation His-505→Asp implicates a new segment in the control of von Willebrand factor binding to platelet glycoprotein-Ib. J Biol Chem 1993; 268:20497-501.
36. Hilbert L, Gaucher C, de Romeuf C, Horellou MH, Vink T, Mazurier C. Leu 697→Val mutation in mature von Willebrand factor is responsible for type IIB von Willebrand disease. Blood 1994;83:1542-50.
37. Hölmberg L, Dent JA, Schneppenheim R, Budde U, Ware J, Ruggeri ZM. Von Willebrand factor mutation enhancing interaction with platelets in patients with normal multimeric structure. J Clin Invest 1993;91:2169-77.
38. Howard MA, Salem HH, Thomas KB, et al. Variant von Willebrand's disease type B. Revisited. Blood 1982;60:1420-28.
39. Rabinowitz I, Tuley EA, Mancuso DJ, et al. Von Willebrand disease type B: A missense mutation selectively abolishes ristocetin-induced von Willebrand factor binding to platelet glycoprotein Ib. Proc Natl Acad Sci USA 1992;89: 9846-49.
40. Mazurier C, Diéval J, Jorieux S, Delobel J, Goudemand M. A new von Willebrand factor defect in a patient with factor VIII deficiency but with normal levels and multimeric patterns of both plasma and platelet vWF. Characterization of abnormal vWF/FVIII interaction. Blood 1990;75:20-26.
41. Mazurier C. Von Willebrand disease masquerading as haemophilia A. Thromb Haemost 1992;67:391-96.
42. Wise RJ, Ewenstein BM, Gorlin J, Narins SC, Jesson M, Handin RI. Autosomal recessive transmission of haemophilia A due to a von Willebrand factor mutation. Hum Genet 1993;91:367-72.
43. Siguret V, Lavergne J, Cherel G, et al. A novel case of compound heterozygosity with Normandy/type I von Willebrand disease (vWD). Direct demonstration of the segregation of one allele with a defective expression at the mRNA level causing type I vWD. Hum Genet 1994;93:95-102.
44. Eikenboom JC, Vink T, Briët E, Sixma JJ, Reitsma PH. Multiple substitutions in the von Willebrand factor gene that mimic the pseudogene sequence. Proc Natl Acad Sci USA 1994;91:2221-24.
45. Peake IR, Bowen D, Bignell P, et al. Family studies and prenatal diagnosis in severe von Willebrand disease by polymerase chain reaction amplification of a variable number tandem repeat region of the von Willebrand factor gene. Blood 1990;76: 555-61.
46. Bignell P, Standen GR, Bowen DJ, Peake IR, Bloom AL. Rapid neonatal diagnosis of von Willebrand's disease by use of the polymerase chain reaction. Lancet 1990; 336:638-39.
47. Ribba AS, Voorberg J, Meyer D, Pannekoek H, Pietu G. Characterization of recombinant von Willebrand factor corresponding to mutations in type IIA and type IIB von Willebrand disease. J Biol Chem 1992;267:23209-15.
48. Pietu G, Ribba AS, de Paillette L, et al. Molecular study of von Willebrand disease: Identification of potential mutations in patients with type IIA and type IIB. Blood Coag Fibrin 1992;3:415-21.

49. Donner M, Kristoffersson AC, Berntorp E, et al. Two new candidate mutations in type IIA von Willebrand's disease (Arg834→Gly, Gly846→Arg) and one polymorphism (Tyr821→Cys) in the A2 region of the von Willebrand factor. Eur J Haemat 1993; 51:38-44.
50. Inbal A, Englender T, Kornbrot N, et al. Identification of 3 candidate mutations causing type IIA von Willebrand disease using a rapid, non radioactive, allele-specific hybridization method. Blood 1993;82:830-36.
51. Mancuso DJ, Montgomery RR, Adam P. The identification of a candidate mutation in the von Willebrand factor gene of patients with a variant form of type I von Willebrand disease. Blood 1991;78(suppl.1):67a(Abstract).
52. Donner M, Kristoffersson AC, Lenk H, et al. Type IIB von Willebrand's disease: Gene mutations and clinical presentation in nine families from Denmark, Germany and Sweden. Br J Haemat 1992;82:58-65.
53. Randi AM, Jorieux S, Tuley EA, Mazurier C, Sadler JE. Recombinant von Willebrand factor Arg578→Gln. A type IIB von Willebrand disease mutation affects binding to glycoprotein Ib but not to collagen or heparin. J Biol Chem 1992;267: 21187-92.
54. Gaucher C, Parquet-Gernez A, Hanss M, Horellou MH, Goudemand M, Mazurier C. Potential new mutations in French Families with type IIA and IIB von Willebrand's disease. Proc XX International Congress, World Federation of Hemophilia, Athens, 1992:176 (Abstract).

MOLECULAR BASIS OF THROMBOPHILIA

P.H. Reitsma

Introduction

The coagulation cascade is controlled by several anticoagulant safeguards that avoid excessive clot formation. Disorders of these anticoagulant mechanisms are an important health problem as they lead to increased risks for thromboembolic disease. Until very recently genetic defects in the antithrombin-, protein C-, and protein S genes were the best characterized hereditary risk factors for venous thrombosis. This chapter will focus on recent developments in understanding abnormalities in the protein C anticoagulant pathway [for reviews see refs 1-3].

Thrombomodulin

The protein C anticoagulant pathway consists of three key proteins. The first is thrombomodulin, which represents the endothelial receptor for the thrombin that is generated in the coagulation cascade [4,5]. Once complexed by thrombomodulin, thrombin loses its procoagulant function and turns into an anticoagulant protein. Given its function in the protein C pathway, a hereditary deficiency of thrombomodulin is a strong candidate for pathophysiological involvement in venous thrombosis. An attempt from our laboratory (Reitsma et al, unpublished) to link mutations in the thrombomodulin gene with venous thrombosis was unsuccessful in that no mutations were found in probands from 30 families with unexplained thrombophilia. The only variation discovered in this panel of individuals was a dimorphism of codon 455 such that either alanine or valine is present at this position [6]. No association could be found between this dimorphism and thrombophilia [6]. Despite these results it is not excluded that hereditary defects of thrombomodulin are to some extent involved in venous thrombosis, but it seems that they are infrequent.

Protein C

The second component of the protein C anticoagulant system is Protein C. This vitamin K-dependent glycoprotein is synthesized in the liver as a single-chain polypeptide and undergoes post-translational modification (β-hydroxylation, γ-

carboxylation, proteolytic processing, and glycosylation) to give rise to its mature two-chain form; the 41 kDa heavy chain and 21 kDa light chains are held together by a disulphide bond. Protein C is an inactive zymogen that is activated by the thrombin/thrombomodulin complex on the endothelial cell surface. Activated protein C exerts its anticoagulant effect by inactivating factors Va and VIIIa and is thought to promote fibrinolysis by neutralizing a plasminogen activator inhibitor. The structure and function of protein C have been recently reviewed [1-3].

There is little doubt about the importance of hereditary protein C deficiency in venous thrombosis. Phenotypically, two distinct types of the deficiency state can be recognised: Type I deficiency, the most common, is characterized by the parallel reduction or protein C activity and antigen levels due to the reduced synthesis or stability of normally functioning molecules. In type II deficiency, protein C activity is reduced to a greater extent than the antigen due to the synthesis of an abnormal protein C molecule exhibiting a reduced specific activity.

Heterozygous, clinically 'overt', protein C deficiency is thought to have a prevalence of between 1/16,000 and 1/36,000 in the general population [7, 8]. However, a much more frequent 'covert' form may also occur in the asymptomatic general population of whom as many as 1/200 may exhibit protein C activity levels consistent with a heritable heterozygous deficiency state [9]. The absence of thrombosis in many putative heterozygotes appears to argue against plasma protein C concentration being a prime determinant of disease. However, in many individuals/families, heterozygous protein C deficiency is clearly an important independent risk factor for thrombotic disease [10, 11] and so other factors must contribute to the likelihood of thrombosis. One important determinant of whether or not a protein C deficient individual is clinically symptomatic appears to be the coinheritance of the recently described factor V Leiden variant (see below) that is associated with APC-resistance [12]. This variant occurs at a significantly higher frequency (19%) in individuals with clinically symptomatic protein C deficiency as compared with healthy controls (3%) [12, 13].

A large variety of mutations has been shown to underlie hereditary protein C deficiency. To keep track of these mutations a mutation database has been maintained for protein C deficiency, which by August 1994 contained 307 entries (148 different) for 295 apparently unrelated probands from 16 different European and American countries (the database is an update of ref 14). The majority of these entries (256/307, 105 different) are single base-pair substitutions that either cause an amino acid replacement (missense) or create a premature termination codon (nonsense). The remaining entries are almost all insertions or deletions of one or a few nucleotides that either lead to a frameshift or to amino acid deletions or insertions.

Protein S

The third component of the protein C pathway is protein S. It circulates in plasma in two forms: free and bound to C4b binding protein, a protein of the complement system [15]. Only free protein S has anticoagulant properties [15]. Protein S acts as a cofactor of activated protein C (APC) in the inactivation of the procoagulant factors FVa and FVIIIa by potentiating the binding of APC to the phospholipid surface via a calcium ion bridge [16-18]. In addition to this, it has also been suggested that protein S may have a direct anticoagulant effect through its interaction with the prothrombinase complex [19].

Just like protein C deficiency, hereditary protein S deficiency is a risk factor for developing recurrent thromboembolic disease relativily early in life [20-27]. The genetic basis of protein S deficiency is, unlike that of protein C deficiency, still poorly studied. Several reasons account for this. First, the relatively recent characterization, in 1990 [28-30], of the protein S genes. Second, the existence of two genes per haploid genome, both located in chromosome 3 [31]. These genes, named PROS1 and PROS2, share a high degree of homology, but only the PROS1 gene is transcriptionally active [32]. Third, the large size of the PROS1 gene, greater than 80 Kb, which is composed of 15 exons separated by 14 introns [28-30].

Only 12 variant protein S alleles have been described to date; not all of these are the cause of protein S deficiency [33-41]. Included are a mutation in the PROS2 gene characterized by loss of a Msp I restriction site [33]. This mutation, although linked to the protein S deficiency in the pedigree described, probably is not causative as it is located in the pseudogene. The second variant protein S allele that has been reported is the Heerlen polymorphism, a T→C transition in exon XIII, which predicts the substitution of 460Ser by Pro [34]. This polymorphism is present in about 1% of the general population and is not associated with an increased risk of thrombosis [34]. The remaining mutations are located in the PROS1 gene: two large deletions in the middle portion of the gene [35. 36], and eight different point mutations [37-41]. All these mutations appear to be directly responsible for the protein S deficiency.

Factor V Leiden

Until very recently genetic defects in protein C-, and protein S genes were among the best characterized hereditary risk factors for venous thrombosis. When taken together these deficiencies account for maybe about 10% of the cases of familial thrombophilia. This poor understanding of thrombophilia changed dramatically in 1993 by a publication of Dahlbäck et al in which the so-called APC-resistance was described [42]. APC-resistance is a plasma abnormality characterized by a reduced prolongation of the APTT by activated protein C (APC). The LETS study by Koster et al provided further evidence that this abnormality represents a potent risk factor for venous thrombosis (relative risk of 7 in consecutive patients with a first DVT) [43].

At first the genetic basis for APC-resistance was thought to reside in a novel cofactor for APC [42]. Data published in 1994 by our research center negated the cofactor hypothesis by firmly establishing that APC-resistance is due to the loss of an APC inactivation site in activated coagulation factor V (factor V Leiden) [13]. Since then a number of other groups have corroborated these results [44-46].

In comparison with the other defects in the protein C pathway there are two unique features to the genetic basis of APC-resistance. Firstly, until now only a single defect (a G→A transition at nt 1691 leading to the replacement of ^{506}Arg by Gln) has been found to underlie APC-resistance [13, 44-46]. This contrasts with the hundreds of different genetic defects that have been shown to underlie protein C-, and protein S deficiency (see above). Secondly, in the general population the factor V Leiden mutation has an exceptionally high prevalence and is carried by as many as 1 out of every 30 individuals [13]. Heterozygosity for protein C and protein S deficiency is much less common with a prevalence of at most 1 out of 300-500 individuals.

The finding that in the overwhelming majority of cases the factor V Leiden mutation is responsible for APC-resistance has made it possible to devise a simple and specific genetic test to supplant a plasma APC-resistance test that is compromized by treatment and additional factors [13]. Given the large heterogeneity of defects in antithrombin-, protein C-, and protein S deficiency, genetic testing for these disorders will not become routine in the near future.

References

1. Esmon CT. Molecular events that control the protein C anticoagulant pathway. Thromb Haemost 1994;70:29-35.
2. Dahlbäck B, Stenflo J. A natural anticoagulant pathway: Proteins C, S, C4b-binding protein and thrombomodulin. In: Bloom AL, Forbes CD, Thomas DP, Tuddenham EGD (eds). Haemostasis and thrombosis. Edinburgh, Churchill Livingstone 1994:671-98.
3. Tuddenham EGD, Cooper DN. The molecular genetics of haemostasis and its inherited disorders. Oxford, Oxford University Press 1994.
4. Dittman WA, Majerus PW, Structure and function of thrombomodulin: A natural anticoagulant. Blood 1990;75:329-36.
5. Dittman WA, Thrombomodulin: Biology and potential cardiovascular applications. Trends Cardiovasc Med 1991;1:331-36.
6. Van der Velden PA, Krommenhoek-van Es T, Allaart CF, Bertina RM, Reitsma PH. A frequent thrombomodulin amino acid dimorphism is not associated with thrombophilia. Thromb Haemost 1991;65:511-13.
7. Broekmans AW, Conard J. Hereditary protein C deficiency. In: Bertina RM (ed). Protein C and related proteins. Edinburgh, Churchill Livingstone 1988:160-81.
8. Gladson CL, Scharrer I, Hach V, Beck KH, Griffin JH. The frequency of type I heterozygous protein S and protein C deficiency in 141 unrelated young patients with venous thrombosis. Thromb Haemost 1988;59:18-22.
9. Miletich J, Sherman L, Broze G Jr. Absence of thrombosis in subjects with heterozygous protein C deficiency. N Engl J Med 1987;317:991-96.

10. Bovill EG, Bauer KA, Dickerman JD, Callas P, West B. The clinical spectrum of heterozygous protein C deficiency in a large New England kindred. Blood 1989; 73:712-17.
11. Allaart CF, Poort SR, Rosendaal FR, Reitsma PH, Bertina RM, Briët E. Increased risk of venous thrombosis in carriers of hereditary protein C deficiency defect. Lancet 1993;341:134-38.
12. Koeleman BPC, Reitsma PH, Allaart CF, Bertina RM. APC-resistance as an additional risk factor for thrombosis in protein C deficient families. Blood 1994; 84:1031-35.
13. Bertina RM, Koeleman BPC, Koster T, et al. Mutation in blood coagulation factor V associated with resistance to activated protein C. Nature 1994;369:64-67.
14. Reitsma PH, Poort SR, Bernardi F, et al. Protein C deficiency: A database of mutations. Thromb Haemost 1993;69:77-84.
15. Comp PC, Nixon RR, Cooper MR, Esmon CT. Familial protein S deficiency is associated with recurrent thrombosis. J Clin Invest 1984;74:2082-88.
16. Walker FJ. Regulation of activated protein C by protein S. The role of phospholipid in factor Va inactivation. J Biol Chem 1981;256:11128-31.
17. Suzuki K, Nishioka J, Hashimoto S. Regulation of activated protein C by thrombin-modified protein S. J Biochem (Tokyo) 1983;94:699-705.
18. Koedam JA, Meijers JC, Sixma JJ, Bouma BN. Inactivation of human factor VIII by activated protein C. Cofactor activity of protein S and protective effect of von Willebrand factor. J Clin Invest 1988;82:1236-43.
19. Heeb MJ, Mesters RM, Tans G, Rosing J, Griffin JH. Binding of protein S to factor Va associated with inhibition of prothrombinase that is independent of activated protein C. J Biol Chem 1993;268:2872-77.
20. Schwarz HP, Fischer M, Hopmeier P. Plasma protein S deficiency in familial thrombotic disease. Blood 1984:64:1297-300.
21. Broekmans AW, Bertina RM, Reinalda Poot J, et al. Hereditary protein S deficiency and venous thrombo-embolism. A study in three Dutch families. Thromb Haemost 1985;53:273-77.
22. Bertina RM. Hereditary protein S deficiency. Haemostasis 1985;15:241-46.
23. Engesser L, Broekmans AW, Briët E, Brommer EJ, Bertina RM. Hereditary protein S deficiency: Clinical manifestations. Ann Intern Med 1987;106:677-82.
24. Tabernero MD, Tomas JF, Alberca I, Orfao A, Borrasca AL, Vicente V. Incidence and clinical characteristics of hereditary disorders associated with venous thrombosis. Am J Hematol 1991;36:249-54.
25. Allaart CF, Aronson DC, Ruys T, et al. Hereditary protein S deficiency in young adults with arterial occlusive disease. Thromb Haemost 1990;65:206-10.
26. Girolami A, Simioni P, Lazzaro AR. Heterozygous protein S deficiency: A study of a large kindred. Acta Haematol 1990;84:162-68.
27. Walker FJ. Protein S and thrombotic disease. Proc Soc Exp Biol Med 1992; 200:285-95.
28. Ploos van Amstel HK, Reitsma PH, van der Logt CP, Bertina RM. Intron-exon organization of the active human protein S gene PS alpha and its pseudogene PS beta: Duplication and silencing during primate evolution. Biochemistry 1990;29: 7853-61.
29. Schmidel DK, Tatso AV, Phelps LG, Tomczak JA, Long GL. Organization of the human protein S genes. Biochemistry 1990;29:7845-52.
30. Edenbrandt CM, Lindwall A, Wydro R, Stenflo J. Molecular analysis of the gene for vitamin K-dependent protein S and its pseudogene. Cloning and partial gene organization. Biochemistry 1990;29:7861-68.

31. Ploos van Amstel HK, van der Zanden AL, Bakker E, Reitsma PH, Bertina RM. Two genes homologous with human protein S cDNA are located on chromosome 3. Thromb Haemost 1987;58:982-87.
32. Ploos van Amstel HK, Reitsma PH, Bertina RM. The human protein S locus: Identification of the PS alpha gene as a site of liver protein S messenger RNA synthesis. Biochem Biophys Res Common 1988;157:1033-38.
33. Ploos van Amstel HK, Reitsma PH, Hamulyak K, de Die Smulders CE, Mannucci PM, Bertina RM. A mutation in the protein S pseudogene is linked to protein S deficiency in a thrombophilic family. Thromb Haemost 1989;62: 897-901.
34. Bertina RM, Ploos van Amstel HK, van Wijngaarden A, et al. Heerlen polymorphism of protein S, an immunologic polymorphism due to dimorphism of residue 460. Blood 1990;76:538-48.
35. Ploos van Amstel HK, Huisman MV, Reitsma PH, ten Cate JW, Bertina RM. Partial protein S gene deletion in a family with hereditary thrombophilia. Blood 1989;73: 479-83.
36. Schmidel DK, Nelson RM, Broxson EH Jr, Comp PC, Marlar RA, Long GL. A 5.3-kb deletion including exon XIII of the protein S α gene occurs in two protein S-deficient families. Blood 1991;77:551-59.
37. Reitsma PH, Ploos van Amstel HK, Bertina RM. Three novel mutations in five unrelated subjects with hereditary protein S deficiency type I. J Clin Invest 1994;93: 486-92.
38. Gandrille S, Borgel D, Gouault-Heilman M, Dreyfus M, Aiach M. Identification of two point mutations in the protein S alpha gene of subjects with quantitative deficiency. Circulation 1992;86:3240 (Abstract).
39. Gómez E, Ledford MR, Pegelow CH, Reitsma PH, Bertina RM. Homozygous protein S deficiency caused by one base pair deletion that leads to a stop codon in exon III of the protein S gene. Thromb Haemost 1994;71:723-26.
40. Yamazaki T, Katsumi A, Kagami K, Koyima T, Takamatsu J, Saito H. Genetic characterization of hereditary free protein S deficiency. Blood 1993; 82:1606 (Abstract).
41. Hayashi T, Nishioka J, Shigekiyo T, Saito S, Suzuki K. Protein S tokushima: Abnormal molecule with a substitution of Glu for Lys-155 in the second epidermal growth factor-like domain of protein S. Blood 1994;83:683-90.
42. Dahlbäck B, Carlsson M, Svensson PJ. Familial thrombophilia due to a previously unrecognized mechanism characterized by poor anticoagulant response to activated protein C: prediction of a cofactor to activated protein C. Proc Natl Acad Sci USA 1993;90:1004-08.
43. Koster T, Rosendaal FR, de Ronde H, Briët E, Vandenbroucke JP, Bertina RM. Venous thrombosis due to poor anticoagulant response to activated protein C: Leiden thrombophilia study. Lancet 1993;342:1503-06.
44. Sun X, Evatt B, Griffin JH. Blood coagulation factor Va abnormality associated with resistance to activated protein C in venous thrombophilia. Blood 1994;43:3120-25.
45. Greengard JS, Sun X, Xu X, Fernandez JA, Griffin JH, Evatt B. Activated protein C resistance caused by Arg506Gln mutation in factor Va. Lancet 1994;343:1361-62.
46. Zöller B, Dahlbäck B. Linkage between inherited resistance to activated protein C and factor V gene mutation in venous thrombosis. Lancet 1994;343:1536-38.

INHIBITORY SEQUENCES WITHIN THE CLOTTING FACTOR VIII cDNA BLOCK TRANSCRIPTIONAL ELONGATION AND COMPLICATE EFFORTS TOWARD GENE THERAPY FOR HAEMOPHILIA A

D.D. Koeberl, A. Krumm, A.D. Miller

Introduction

The limitations of transfusion therapy for haemophilia have prompted efforts to develop gene therapy for these disorders. The coagulation factors have rather short half-lives, and cannot be adequately replaced to prevent all episodes of bleeding in haemophiliacs [1]. Multiple transfusions are required at times of major trauma or surgery. The benefit of gene therapy would be continuous production of the deficient coagulation factor, preferably after a single treatment which would allow permanent factor replacement.

The most accepted approach to gene therapy involves the introduction of a vector into target cells, either *in vitro* or *in vivo*, which will allow those cells to synthesize a deficient protein [2]. The vector is commonly a replication-deficient virus that contains the spliced coding sequences (cDNA) for a human gene. The vector enters target cells through a process called transduction, which differs from infection with a wild-type virus in that no further spread of the retroviral vector occurs. Vectors often contain a selectable marker to allow enrichment for transduced cells in culture. Subsequently the target cells, which now synthesize a presumably therapeutic protein, can be transplanted into the appropriate host to allow analysis of protein production or therapeutic effect. Target cells have included diverse cell types, such as fibroblasts, keratinocytes, hepatocytes, and muscle cells (Table 1). Efforts toward gene therapy have been restricted to somatic cells, to avoid transmission of introduced genes through the germ line.

Retroviral vectors have several advantages, and have been widely utilized in models for gene therapy [2]. The use of packaging cell lines, which contain the viral genes necessary for vector assembly in *trans*, allows the production of large quantities of high titre vector stock. Retroviral vectors integrate into the transduced cell's genome, and are reliably transmitted to progeny cells thereafter. A number of proteins have been expressed from retroviral vectors *in vitro* and *in vivo*, and their efficacy for gene therapy has been demonstrated in the initial human gene therapy protocols [2].

Clotting factor IX (FIX), adenosine deaminase (ADA), and other cDNAs are expressed at high levels from retroviral vectors [2-4], while the FVIII cDNA is expressed at very low levels from these vectors [5-7]. For example, human

Table 1. Factor IX and factor VIII production from transduced cells.

	***In vitro* (ng/10^6 cells/24 hr)**	***In vivo* (ng/ml)**
FIX		
NIH 3T3 [4]	250	450
rat fibroblasts [4]	4.580	23
human fibroblasts [4]	1.680	190
dog hepatocytes [16]	225	10
FVIII		
NIH 3T3 [5]	1	N.D.
human fibroblasts [7]	39	N.D.
rat fibroblasts [8]	2	0

fibroblasts transduced with a retroviral vector containing the FIX cDNA produced up to 2 micrograms of FIX protein per million fibroblasts each day [4], and human fibroblasts transduced with a FVIII retroviral vector produced only about 40 nanograms of FVIII protein per million each day [7] (Table 1). In an attempt to develop an animal model for gene therapy, fibroblasts were transduced with a FVIII retroviral vector *in vitro* and transplanted into immune-deficient mice, but no human FVIII could be detected *in vivo* [8] (Table 1). FVIII RNA steady-state levels are reduced 100-fold from a FVIII retroviral vector compared to the same vector expressing other cDNAs, and consequently FVIII vector titres are reduced 100-fold compared to other vectors [7]. The consequence of low FVIII synthesis from retroviral vectors is a requirement for at least 500 million transduced cells achieve therapeutic levels *in vivo*, without allowing for any problems with release or stability of the FVIII protein [7].

The inhibitory effect of the FVIII cDNA on expression from a retroviral vector has been localized to a 1.2 kb fragment, derived from the A2 and A3 domains, which decreased steady-state RNA levels 100 to 200-fold and decreased vector titres 10-fold [7]. We have analyzed the control of expression for the FVIII inhibitory sequence (FVIII INS) in the context of retroviral expression vectors by utilizing RNA stability and nuclear run-on assays. The FVIII INS vector was found to generate vector RNA which persisted without any decrease for six hours in an assay for RNA degradation. Nuclear run-on analysis revealed that FVIII INS vectors generate a higher prevalence of upstream transcripts compared to the FVIII INS sequence, indicating the presence of a block to transcriptional elongation. The FVIII INS inhibitory sequence was localized to several smaller elements which have an additive inhibitory effect on expression.

Materials and Methods

Cell culture

PA317 amphotropic retrovirus packaging cells [9] and NIH 3T3 thymidine kinase-negative(TK-) cells [10] were cultured in Dulbecco-Vogt modified Eagle's medium (DMEM) with high glucose (4.5 grams/litre) supplemented with 10% foetal bovine serum and the antibiotics penicillin, streptomycin, and amphotericin B.

Construction of FVIII retroviral vector

The FVIII vectors pLBHSN, pLPSSN, pLBMSN, pLXHSN, pLD2SN, pLXPSN and pLSHSN were constructed as described [7, 11]. The FIX vector pLIXSN has been described [4]. The LXSN retroviral vector has been described [9].

Virus production

Transient virus production was assayed as described [7, 9]. Virus stock was prepared from vector-producing PA317 cell line by incubating medium for 16 hours with confluent layers of the cells. The PA317/LBHSN, c5, and PA317/LIXSN, c7, packaging cell lines have been described [4, 7]. Transduction with retroviral vectors at a multiplicity of infection of less than one, followed by selection with G418 to allow visualization of individual colonies, introduces a single copy of the vector to each transduced cell. Transduced NIH 3T3 and PA317 cells are pooled populations, in which the retroviral vector is chromosomally integrated in a random manner.

Nuclear run-ons

Nuclear run-ons were performed as described previously; all experiments used a 150 mM KCl buffer [12]. After the DNase I treatment and phenol-chloroform extraction of run-on transcripts, the nucleic acids were precipitated with ethanol and unincorporated nucleotides were removed by use of a Sephadex G50 spin column. Labelled transcripts were hybridized to slot blotted GeneScreen filters containing double-stranded DNA probes noted below. Double-stranded DNA probes were generated by restriction digest or PCR amplification with appropriate primers and purified from an agarose gel.

After hybridization, the filters were treated for 30 minutes at 37°C with RNAase A (10 micrograms/millilitre), and washed twice in 1×SSC, 1% SDS at 55°C for 15 minutes each. Signals from blots were quantitated with a Molecular Dynamics phosphorimager [13]. Signals were normalized to the histone H2B and beta-actin probe signals, and corrected for relative TTP content of each probe. Probes utilized have been described (Koeberl et al, submitted). The number of TTPs in relevant probes is as follows: Psi-LTR (88), Psi (171), SV40 (48), neo (177), INS (343), FIX (477). Graphs represent the signals as measured by a phosphorimager and normalized to an H2B signal for the corresponding blot, as corrected for the relative UTP content of RNA hybridizing to each probe. Signals were divided by the FIX signal from LIXSN-transduced cells for each experiment, to allow the comparison of results from different experiments.

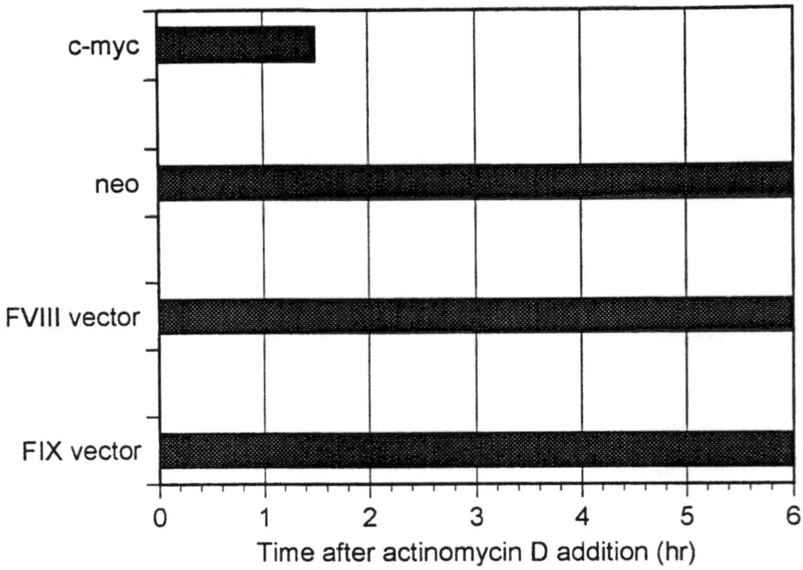

Figure 1. RNA stability assays. The persistence of vector RNAs containing FIX or FVIII INS after transcriptional arrest with actinomycin D is represented by a bar graph. Total RNA was extracted at various time points after addition of actinomycin D, from 30 minutes to 6 hours. Persistence of FVIII INS and FIX vector RNAs, as well as the neo RNA generated by each vector, was demonstrated for 6 hours after transcriptional arrest. The c-myc RNA disappeared in less than two hours, demonstrating the effect of transcriptional arrest on unstable RNAs.

Transcriptional arrest

Transcriptional arrest of subconfluent transduced NIH 3T3 cells was initiated by the addition of actinomycin D (10 micrograms/ml) to the medium. Cells were scraped and total RNA was harvested at time points from 30 minutes to 6 hours later.

Results

Steady-state RNA levels for a FVIII INS vector are not reduced due to RNA instability

A FVIII INS retroviral vector (LBHSN) consistently demonstrated steady-state RNA at 20 to 100-fold reduced levels compared to other vectors [7]. The steady-state levels of vector RNA from NIH 3T3 cells transduced with a FIX vector (LIXSN) were at least 20-fold higher than for cells transduced with a FVIII INS vector (LBHSN) [11]. The rate of degradation of FVIII INS vector RNA relative to the FIX vector RNA was analyzed to assess the role of RNA degradation in down-regulating FVIII INS expression. Medium containing actinomycin D (10

RNA polymerase distribution in FIX and FVIII vectors.

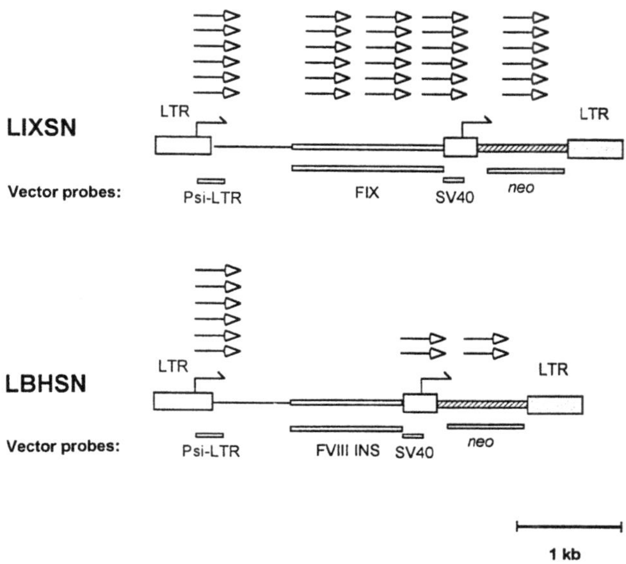

Figure 2. Nuclear run-on analyses. The signal from a nuclear run-on analysis represents the distribution of RNA polymerase II complexes in a particular sequence, as detected by DNA probes corresponding to that sequence (see text). Nuclear run-on signals for the LIXSN (FIX) and LBHSN (FVIII INS) vectors are represented by the arrows over each vector; the number of arrows corresponds to the relative signal for the section of the vector below it. LIXSN has a strong signal for transcriptional initiation (Psi-LTR probe) and for transcriptional elongation through the FIX cDNA: LBHSN has a strong signal for transcriptional initiation and no detectable signal for the FVIII INS probe, indicating the presence of a block to transcriptional elongation of FVIII INS.

micrograms/millilitre) was added to NIH 3T3 cells transduced by the viral vectors LBHSN or LIXSN, which express FVIII INS or FIX respectively. The FVIII INS vector RNA persisted for six hours without diminution, similar to the full-length LIXSN vector RNA (Figure 1). In contrast, the signal for *c-myc* RNA disappeared after one hour, when the same blot was hybridized to a mouse *c-myc* exon 1 probe (Figure 1). Disappearance of the *c-myc* signal indicates that transcriptional arrest occurred, and that labile RNAs would be expected to persist only during early time points. A smaller *neo* RNA, transcribed from the SV40 promoter, persisted for the duration of the experiment, indicating the relative stability of this transcript. The vector RNA containing FVIII inhibitory sequences is markedly more stable than the *c-myc* RNA, indicating that RNA instability is not responsible for low FVIII INS vector RNA levels.

A block to transcriptional elongation within the FVIII INS decreases transcription compared to the FIX cDNA

The relative levels of transcriptional initiation and elongation of FVIII INS compared to other vector sequences and FIX was determined by nuclear run-on analysis, which quantitates the distribution of RNA polymerase II complexes along a particular sequence [11]. Previously initiated nascent RNA molecules are elongated in the presence of radiolabelled UTP, and labelled RNA is isolated. Labelled transcripts from each preparation of nuclei are hybridized to unlabelled DNA probes slot blotted to a nylon membrane, and the signal for each probe is quantitated with a phosphorimager, normalized to a histone H2B or beta-actin signal for that blot, and corrected for relative UTP content. Nuclear run-on analyses were performed with NIH 3T3 cells transduced with the LIXSN and LBHSN vectors. The signal for a FIX cDNA probe from the LIXSN nuclear run-on was elevated 17 to 20-fold over the same probe in the LBHSN nuclear run-on [11], demonstrating a high FIX-specific signal (Figure 2). The signal for FVIII INS transcription was not above background, indicating that a block to transcriptional elongation or low transcriptional initiation was responsible (Figure 2). The signal from the upstream probe Psi-LTR was high for the LIXSN and LBHSN vectors (Figure 2). An equivalent signal for an upstream probe indicates that transcriptional initiation was not affected by the inhibitory sequences, FVIII INS compared to FIX. The LIXSN signal was as high as that from the upstream Psi-LTR signal, indicating that no significant block to elongation is present in the FIX cDNA (Figure 2). Although LBHSN revealed a high level of transcriptional initiation, very little transcription of FVIII INS was detected, and this finding is consistent with a block to transcriptional elongation within FVIII INS.

Deletion analyses of the FVIII INS fragment reveals the presence of inhibitory sequence elements which decrease expression in an additive manner

Vectors containing smaller fragments derived from FVIII INS were found to have relatively high titers. To allow the detection of possible interaction between multiple inhibitory sequence elements within FVIII INS, vectors which contained progressive deletions of the 5′ and 3′ termini of the FVIII INS fragment were constructed. After the deletion of 5′ and 3′ sequences from the FVIII INS vector (LBHSN) insert, a gradual increase in the expression of these vectors was observed; vector RNA levels increased as the size of the residual FVIII insert was decreased (Koeberl et al, submitted). No element was isolated which could account for the majority of the inhibitory effect. The D2 fragment, corresponding to the downstream 600 bp of FVIII INS, reduced vector RNA levels for LD2SN 25-fold compared to LXSN (Table 2). The smaller fragment in the vector LXPSN, 392 bp in length, had a residual six fold reduction in RNA steady-state levels (Table 2). By contrast, the smaller fragments in LSHSN, and LBMSN had no significant inhibitory effect on vector expression (Table 2). In summary, an inhibitory sequence element in the fragment XP interacts with the downstream sequence within FVIII INS to down-regulate steady-state RNA levels.

Table 2. RNA levels for FVIII INS vectors, compared to LXSN.

Vector	Insert size (kb)	Decrease, relative to LXSN (x-fold)
LBHSN	1.2	30-100
LXHSN	0.8	30
LD2SN	0.6	25
LXPSN	0.4	6
LBMSN	0.2	0
LSHSN	0.2	0
LXSN	0	0

The relative RNA level for each vector is shown, compared to LXSN. Each vector RNA level represents the signal for vector RNA from a Northern blot hybridized to a *neo* probe, normalized to the beta-actin signal for each lane. Signals were quantified with a phosphorimager.

Discussion

A block to transcriptional elongation decreases expression of the FVIII cDNA

The finding of decreased expression of the FVIII coding regions on the basis of blocks to transcriptional elongation *in vitro* suggests that the control of transcriptional elongation might be important in determining the extremely low expression of these sequences *in vivo* [8, 14]. The FVIII INS RNA is as stable as the FIX vector RNA and *neo* RNA in an assay of RNA degradation, which corroborates the relevance of the control of transcriptional elongation in the down-regulation of FVIII INS expression. The correlation of decreased steady-state RNA levels with blocks to transcriptional elongation within the FVIII INS DNA indicates that transcriptional elongation is important to the control of expression in both cases.

Earlier nuclear run-on analysis of a plasmid FVIII expression vector failed to detect the block to transcriptional elongation in the FVIII cDNA [6]. This could possibly have been due to the lack of upstream probes, which would have quantified a higher signal for transcriptional initiation compared to the signal for the FVIII cDNA [6, 15]. Thus, our finding of a block to transcriptional elongation within the FVIII cDNA does not contradict these earlier results.

Multiple sequence elements inhibit FVIII INS expression and complicate efforts to develop gene therapy for haemophilia A

We demonstrated that a single inhibitory element could not be identified within FVIII INS, because the inhibitory effect of this sequence gradually dissipated as progressive deletions were made. Two sequence elements within FVIII INS had a synergistic inhibitory effect on expression from a retroviral vector. FVIII sequences upstream of FVIII INS also appear to have an inhibitory effect on the expression of larger fragments of the cDNA [7].

Low expression of FVIII complicates efforts toward human gene therapy

The use of retroviral vectors for delivery of the FVIII cDNA is complicated by the inherent low levels of transcription of these sequences. Retroviral vectors are dependent upon transcription to produce vector RNA, and the low titers of FVIII vectors reflect inefficient transcription. Another disadvantage of the FVIII vector is the need to transduce an extremely large number of cells to have a therapeutic effect, due to the low production of FVIII protein from transduced cells [6, 7]. An advantage of integrating vectors, such as retroviral vectors, for gene therapy is that descendants of transduced cells are more likely to retain the vector. Therefore, a retroviral FVIII expression vector with a high titre and high FVIII expression would be useful for the gene therapy in haemophilia A. In order to achieve this goal, the block to transcriptional elongation in the FVIII cDNA would have to be inactivated. Although *in vitro* mutagenesis should allow this, the diffuse nature of the FVIII inhibitory sequence will complicate the task. If the 100-fold inhibition of the FVIII cDNA on vector RNA expression could be reduced to a 10-fold inhibition, the number of transduced cells needed to ameliorate severe haemophilia to a mild course would be reduced to a more feasible 50 million [7]. The transduction of hepatocytes *in vivo* might ultimately prove to be the preferred approach for gene therapy in haemophilia A, if a high titre retroviral vector could be designed, as has been possible for the FIX in haemophilia B [16] (Table 1).

Acknowledgements

We thank Mark Groudine for advice and suggestions during the course of these experiments and for providing nuclear run-on facilities.

References

1. Thompson AR. Status of gene transfer for hemophilia A and B. Thromb Haemost 1991;66:119-22.
2. Miller AD. Human gene therapy comes of age. Nature (London) 1992;357:455-60.
3. Palmer TD, Rosman GJ, Osborne WRA, Miller AD. Genetically modified skin fibroblasts persist long after transplantation but gradually inactivate introduced genes. Proc Natl Acad Sci USA 1991;88:1330-34.
4. Palmer TD, Thompson AR, Miller AD. Production of human factor IX in animals by genetically modified skin fibroblasts: Potential therapy for hemophilia B. Blood 1989;73:438-45.
5. Hoeben RC, van der Jagt RCM, Schoute F, et al. Expression of functional factor VIII in primary human skin fibroblasts after retrovirus-mediated gene transfer. J Biol Chem 1990;265:7318-23.
6. Kaufman RJ, Wasley LC, Davies MV, Wise RJ, Israel DI, Dorner AJ. Effect of von Willebrand factor coexpression on the synthesis and secretion of factor VIII in Chinese hamster ovary cells. Mol Cell Biol 1989;9:1233-42.
7. Lynch CM, Israel DI, Kaufman RJ, Miller AD. Sequences in the coding region of clotting factor VIII act as dominant inhibitors of RNA accumulation and protein production. Hum Gene Ther 1993;4:259-72.

8. Hoeben RC, Fallaux FJ, van Tilburg NH, et al. Toward gene therapy for hemophilia A: Long-term persistence of factor VIII-secreting fibroblasts after transplantation into immunodeficient mice. Hum Gene Ther 1993;4:179-86.
9. Miller AD, Rosman GJ. Improved retroviral vectors for gene transfer and expression. Bio Techniques 1989;7:980-90.
10. Wei CM, Gibson M, Spear PG, Scolnick EM. Construction and isolation of a transmissible retrovirus containing the *src* gene of Harvey murine sarcoma virus and the thymidine kinase gene of herpes simplex virus type 1. J Virol 1981;39: 935-44.
11. Koeberl DD, Halbert CL, Krumm A, Miller D. Sequences within the coding regions of clotting factor VIII and CFTR cDNAs block transcriptional elongation. Submitted.
12. Groudine M, Peretz M, Weintraub HJ. Transcriptional regulation of hemoglobin switching in chicken embryos. Mol Cell Biol 1981;1:281-88.
13. Johnston RE, Pickett SC, Burke DL. Autopadiography using storage transfer technology. Electophoresis 1990;11:355-60.
14. Wion KL, Kelly D, Summerfield JA, Tuddenham EGD, Lawn RM. Distribution of factor VIII mRNA and antigen in human liver and other tissues. Nature (London) 1985;317:726-29.
15. Kaufman RJ, Wasley LC, Dorner AJ. Synthesis, processing, and secretion of recombinant human factor VIII expressed in mammalian cells. J Biol Chem 1988;263:6352-62.
16. Kay MA, Rothenberg S, Landen CN, et al. *In vivo* gene therapy of hemophilia B: Sustained partial correction in factor IX-deficient dogs. Science 1993;262:117-19.

DISCUSSION

E. Briët, C.V. Prowse – moderators

A. Al-Hilali (Doha, Qatar): Dr. Koeberl, is the inhibitory sequence in the cDNA of factor VIII not present or is it not functioning normally?

D.D. Koeberl (Seattle, WA, USA): The question is whether this inhibitory sequence is active *in vivo* in the factor VIII gene. There is an interesting correlation in that the factor VIII RNA is expressed at very low levels where it is synthesised endogenously. The liver for instance has factor VIII RNA at about one thousand fold lower than the level seen for albumin RNA. So, there is good possibility that this is a uniform, universal effect *in vivo* and *in vitro*.

J.A. Zwiebel (Washington, DC, USA): Dr. Reitsma, with analogy to factor VIII therapy how about the factor V abnormality? Would you recommend any type of transfusion therapy for these patients in the setting of active thrombosis?

P.H. Reitsma (Leiden, NL): I like to pass on this question to our clinician dr. Briët.

E. Briët (Leiden, NL): What you suggest, as I understand, is to replace FV in patients with the FV Leiden mutation. Well, I guess that the easier way of doing this would be to treat the patients with oral anticoagulation, which would decrease the concentration of the vitamin K dependent factors in a very constant manner. This I suppose is easier than having factor V replacement on a long term basis. Of course, the idea is completely valid and I guess it is likely to work, but I think that anticoagulation is the easier way out.

C.V. Prowse (Edinburgh, UK): The kind of data that were being shown, indicate that there were effects on the APC ratio that differed between homozygotes and heterozygotes. If you do mixing experiments with factor V, is the effect of factor V progressive or is there a cut-off on how much FV you need to correct that deficiency? Is 2% enough, is 10% enough or is it just progressive?

P.H. Reitsma: First of all, the plasmas with APC-resistance do not display factor V deficiency. The procoagulantproperties of all these plasmas is perfectly normal. It is just that the response to APC in an APTT is different when you do the mixing experiment. We argued before we did these mixing experiments, that those people in which very low ratios were found were homozygous for the mutation. We did not know this for sure at that time. When you do a 50:50 mixing experiment of normal plasma with this 'homozygous' plasma, you obtain the level found in plasma from a heterozygousindividual. Therefore, in principle you can make a curve of 'cofactor activity' by different dilutions of normal plasma in homozygous plasma and obtain levels of 10% 'cofactor activity' or 20% 'cofactor activity' activities so to say, because it is not real cofactor activity, by titrating it back in a homozygousplasma to a level of 10% APC cofactor activity or 20% or whatever.

C.V. Prowse: So it is progressive. If you have double normal levels is it even more corrective than normal?

P.H. Reitsma: One way of looking at the factor V Leiden is as a defect, a loss of function. Maybe a better way of looking at factor V Leiden is as a gain of function. What you have got through the mutation is 'better' factor V. Once activated it remains longer active in plasma because it is more poorly inactivated by protein C. There is therefore no sense in trying to correct it by transfusion because the longer living factor V remains present. You will only obtain more factor V which may make the problem worse.

I. Peake (Sheffield, UK): If we consider that the presence of this resistant factor V, the amount of it, is related to the tendency towards thrombosis, then it would be true that a homozygote with 50% overall level of this material will be exactly the same as a heterozygote who has a 100% factor V of which 50% is resistant. In other words are some heterozygotes going to be as at risk of thrombosis as homozygotes, purely because they have greater overall production of factor V?

E. Briët: So you are saying that both the homozygote and the heterozygote have 100% factor V clotting activity.

I. Peake: If we consider it in terms of absolute amounts of factor V protein it is possible to have a person homozygous for this deficiency, where his total amount of factor V protein is, let us say, 50% or 60% of normal. It is possible to have a heterozygote, who has an overall factor V level at the higher level of the normal range of which half is defective. So it is possible to have a homozygote, who has exactly the same amount of resistant factor V as a heterozygote. Would you then expect them to have the same thrombotic potential?

E. Briët: I think from clinical studies it will be very difficult to answer your question, but maybe by mixing experiments you could.

I. Peake: It may be that there are heterozygotes as much at risk of thrombosis as homozygotes.

E. Briët: I suppose that there are people running around with 150% factor V or with 60% factor V and at stable levels. We would have to look whether that is true.

P.H. Reitsma: When you estimate the thrombotic risk for a homozygous individual you find an odds ratio of about 50, which is the square of the odds ratio of heterozygosity for factor V Leiden (for such an individual the odds ratio is about 7). In other words, homozygotes are at least 50 times more likely to develop thrombosis than a normal individual. The question that still remains is what happens when a factor V Leiden allele combines with a null allele of the factor V gene (i.e. a factor V allele that is completely defective). Such an individual will have factor V plasma levels of about 50% of normal, but all of this is a factor V Leiden. Is in this homozygous situation the thrombotic risk comparable to that of a heterozygote or to that of a homozygote? I think nobody knows at this moment.

R.A. Sacher (Washington, DC, USA): Dr. Reitsma or dr. Briët, have you ever detected any acquired APC resistance? Perhaps in thrombotic DIC we might have some abnormal factor V, which might be resistant to your natural anticoagulants. My question relates to whether in fact you have ever looked at any patients who have acquired thrombophilia and found APC resistant.

E. Briët: The answer is no. I have not seen patients with acquired APC resistance. The mechanism that I could envisage is that patients have circulating immune complexes, where the antibody has hidden the protein C cleavage site. But I do not know whether patients like that have ever been seen. With respect to DIC it is more difficult to envisage that you have resistant factor V since there I might see cleaved factor V circulating but not so much resistant factor V. But I guess theoretically it is possible. Like the acquired protein S deficiency cases that have been described it is always good to be on the lookout for patients like that.

C.V. Prowse: There is one group in which nobody has looked at that particular question: the patients that have repeatedly received either topical bovine thrombin or fibrin glue that contains a bovine thrombin component, where 50 cases in the literature have been described developing factor V antibodies.

E. Briët: Those patients were usually more bleeding than clotting.

C.V. Prowse: Yes, but as a patient group they are potentially immunised with factor V. Somebody pointed out that there is a fair homology between factor V and VIII. Are the sequences you are talking about located in the non-homologous regions between factor V and factor VIII?

D.D. Koeberl: I believe that they are in the homologous regions and actually one approach that Carmel Lynch tried was to develop a factor V vector and it had low expression too.

C.Th. Smit Sibinga (Groningen, NL): Could I turn to the first two presentations, where a marvellous, clear and fairly extensive overview was given of all the possibilities of abnormalities in the various structures. Could I challenge both dr. Mazurier and prof. Peake to speculate on what they think are the triggering mechanisms to get to the deletions, to get to the insertions, to get to all the abnormalities which we call mutations. How does it happen?

I. Peake: That is a very fundamental question. We know that DNA is not stable material. We know for example there are polymorphisms every 300 bases on average throughout the genome. Therefore changes are always happening and in fact there are more changes happening than we can see, because there are efficient repair mechanisms within the system to check and repair the changes. The reasons why a gene like the factor IX gene has so many different mutations in it is simply because it is a protein whose function is related very much to its overall conformation, its overall shape and any change within that seems to throw that. Therefore, that is why we have almost 500 different mutations. I think the most interesting question in terms of haemophilia is the flip-tip, the change of the tip of the X-chromosome and how that occurs and why that should occur. We now know for example that a new mutation occurs much more commonly and perhaps almost exclusively in the male gene line and not in the female. If one considers that when you have two X-chromosomes you can have cross-over recombination between those chromosomes not necessitating if you like that sort of recombination event. When you only have one X-chromosome then it can loop back on itself and cause a recombination at that level. I think that goes someway to explain that mechanism, but the overall mechanisms and mutations and why some survive and some do not is clearly related to the effect they would have on the individual and on the areas of DNA where it takes place.

E. Briët: Dr. Mazurier, a few years ago, Rodighiero[1] has done a study in school children in Italy and concluded that clinical von Willebrand's disease occurred in no less than 1% of the population. Knowing what we know about the

1. Rodighiero F, Castaman G, Dini E. Epidemiological investigation of the prevalence of von Willebrand's disease. Blood 1987;69:454-9.

recessive von Willebrand's disease and dominant von Willebrand's disease, how would you comment on that finding? Do you still agree that there is something like 1% prevalence of clinically relevant von Willebrand's disease in the population?

C. Mazurier (Lille, F): In fact, the epidemiological study of Rodighiero et al. was based mainly on the ristocetin co-factor activity (vWF:RCo) of the plasma samples of 11-14 year old children from Northern Italian schools. About 1% of them had vWF:RCo values lower than the normal range and familial or personal history of bleeding. However, I am not sure that in all these families the bleeding tendency is related to the detected vWF abnormality. Indeed I think that the link between biological abnormality and clinically relevant bleeding is difficult to establish. Lastly, I am not sure that a 1% prevalence of low vWF:RCo level means that 1% of the population is affected with symptomatic vWD.

E. Briët: So could it be then that this 1% are heterozygotes, for instance nil alleles or something like that?

C. Mazurier: Yes, it may be because the vWF gene is very large and it codes for a multidomain protein. However, most of the frequent (1% prevalence) vWF gene defects are recessive, consequently the prevalence of symptomatic forms of vWD is happily much less than 1%.

E. Briët: That is also my feeling.

C.Th. Smit Sibinga: Do you think then that there might be a likelihood, that in trying to establish gene therapy both in haemophilia as well as in von Willebrand's disease, these frequencies of mutation might stand in the way of an appropriate success of this kind of approach.

D.D. Koeberl: Well, if the approach to gene therapy were gene replacement, in other words homologous recombination, then the introduced DNA sequence would have to be targeted to the specific mutation where it is localised in the coagulation factor gene. But that is not the case. So, since the mutant coagulation factor does not interfere with coagulation factor replacement as you know, the variety of mutations should not affect gene therapy.

C.Th. Smit Sibinga: I then have another question. Both prof. Peake and I were last year in China, a fascinating country in many respects, where we were confronted with human experiments done in Shanghai about a factor IX gene therapy using fibroblasts. In two brothers the fibroblasts after having been manoeuvred were transplanted back. There was about a five years age difference between the two brothers and there was approximately the same severity of the factor IX deficiency. The younger one responded reasonably well as we could read it from the Chinese publication[1]. The older one had a little bit more difficulty in responding to the fibroblast production of the factor IX. Could it be that in the introduction of the gene in the fibroblast for the production of factor IX some inhibitory sequence could have slipped in, which blocked actually the effect on even a short term, or do you think that that is not very likely?

D.D. Koeberl: So you are asking whether the mixed success or the failure of gene therapy in that case might have been related to a complication, which altered the factor sequences. I think the more likely explanation – I saw the paper and it seemed that there was a response in one of the patients at least – for a lack of response in gene therapy utilising fibroblasts is probably due to inactivation of vector sequences, which Theo Palmer[2] saw in human fibroblasts (mouse model). They were using retroviral vectors, which probably would encounter that phenomenon. Other possibilities, other complications which might cause failure of gene therapy with fibroblasts would be if sequestration of fibroblasts occurs so that the protein would not be released depending on the location in the body. The paper was interesting but we could not interpret the results.

I. Peake: I agree entirely with what you are saying. But the other perhaps more basic problem that one must bear in mind is that the measurement of clotting factors in many laboratories wherever they are in the world is not as accurate as some of us would like to think. To measure between 4 and 6% accurately and reproducibly is something that can be very difficult. The other factor of course in that paper is that the boy whose factor IX level increased had fewer bleeding episodes, but for those of you who are involved in haemophilia care you will know that the closer you look at the patient the more times that patient comes to clinic the fewer bleeding episodes that patient has. They tend to look after themselves better, because they are doing their best for the doctor who is looking after them. So, I think these two other concerns should be built in into that particular study.

E. Briët: I fully agree, I think that the results of those experiments are well doubtful at best.

---

1. Lu D-R, Zhou J-M, Zheng B, et al. Stage I clinical trial of gene therapy for haemophilia B. Science in China (Series B) 1993;36:1342-51.
2. Palmer TD, Thompson AR, Miller AD. Production of human factor IX in animals by genetically modified skin fibroblasts: potential therapy for haemophilia B. Blood 1989;73:438-45.

Could I turn to prof. Peake once more and ask about the past time of fifteen years ago and all of us trying to measure factor VIII antigen. Now with all the mutations in factor VIII that we have found, of course, we are interested in whether we see truncated molecules in some of these mutations. Have you ever found a group of haemophilia A patients CRM positive in the inversion type of mutations?

I. Peake: No, we have not. If you remember from the inversion, although the factor VIII gene is separated by this large stretch of DNA, both separated pieces of the FVIII gene can be translated. We argued initially that perhaps when we first did our study we showed a lower instance of inhibitors in these patients with the inversion and that perhaps they were producing low amounts of FVIII. However, it is quite clear now that this is not the case and in those inversion patients we have been unable to detect any FVIII protein. There are of course FVIII mutations, the CRM positives when protein is there, particularly those mutations that for example effect the thrombin activation site of FVIII. But in the inversion patient we have never seen FVIII protein in the circulation.

C.V. Prowse: When you solve the problems and you can express FVIII with a vector, and von Willebrand factor with a vector, which target tissues should we be aiming for: the liver, or endothelium?

I. Peake: I can define what the tissues should be like. I can say the cells should live a long time, I suppose the hepatocyte might be the best one to go for, but I do not think the question has been adequately answered yet.

D.D. Koeberl: The results for FIX in hepatocytes are encouraging. The liver is an ideal candidate organ, of course, because it is a synthesis organ and is very vascular and that is where FVIII is usually synthesised.

C.V. Prowse: Has anybody tried to express von Willebrand factor in hepatocytes?

E. Briët: I suspect that there would not be very much place for gene therapy in von Willebrand's disease today. I think it is reasonable that priority has been given to the haemophiliacs. Once that tremendous problem has been solved, maybe in the very few patients with severe von Willebrand's disease we might develop gene therapy. Will you agree with that?

Dr. Mazurier, I have one other question. How often have you been approached for prenatal diagnosis in severe von Willebrand's disease?

C. Mazurier: My laboratory was involved in four prenatal diagnoses but it was not for French people. It was in collaboration with the King's College hospital of London but not necessarily for British families. In all cases it was for severe type 3 vWD.

I. Peake: I think we only have done one case of prenatal diagnosis in a severe case, when we used the VNTR to show that an unborn foetus had severe type 3 von Willebrand's disease, but that family already had one child with severe von Willebrand's disease and therefore they did not want another one.

E. Briët: Our own experience is also one case and this illustrates that the need for genetic diagnosis in von Willebrand's disease is much less; the number of requests that we get is much less than in haemophilia. Would that then mean that it is all useless, all the work we are doing on von Willebrand's disease?

C. Mazurier: I have in memory one reported case of type 2B vWD's prenatal diagnosis. Indeed severe bleeding may occur not only in type 3, but also in some variants (type 2) of vWD. I, therefore, fully understand that some people ask for prenatal diagnosis when someone in their family is affected with severe variant form of vWD.

I. Peake : Could I say that dr. Mazurier is too modest. I think all her work with the type 2N, the Normandy von Willebrand's disease, is very important. It is now clear that a lot of these patients are misclassified as mild haemophilia A. Their phenotype is very similar to mild haemophilia A or even carriers of haemophilia A. It is our experience certainly that if you look through your mild haemophilia A patients you are very likely to come up with one who is actually homozygous for type 2N von Willebrand's disease and of course that changes the diagnosis completely. So, I think the work on type 2N von Willebrand's disease is extremely important and has a bearing in haemophilia as well.

C. Mazurier: Thank you dr. Peake. I would like to say that it is not only important for genetic counselling but also for therapy. For example, if a patient with 2N vWD is infused with an immunopurified FVIII concentrate which does not contain vWF, the FVIII half-life will be very short: 2 hours instead of 8-10 hours. The second point is that 2N vWD is not very rare. Recently, a German team has found 50% of 2N vWD among 16 patients thought to have mild haemophilia A. The blood samples of these patients were sent by clinicians to this research team because they had some problems with the substitutiontherapy of these patients. Therefore, it is important not only for genetic counselling but also for therapy to differentiate real mild haemophiliacs from 2N vWD patients.

R.A. Sacher: We always see biological variation in von Willebrand's disease in particular in pregnancy. Actually we have heard reported a case of 2B, who developed spontaneousthrombocytopeniain pregnancy. But I would like to ask dr. Mazurier, do you have any understandingas to potential molecular mechanisms of biologic variability. Why would a woman who has presumably some molecular defect suddenly manifest with an elevated level of von Willebrand factor in pregnancy.

C. Mazurier: As far as 2B vWD is concerned, I cannot answer your question about the relationship between pregnancy and thrombopenia. In 2B vWD thrombopenia will develop either with age in some families or during pregnancy or periods without exercise, but we do not know why it occurs during such periods. Another point is that there is apparently a relationship between the nature of mutation of a given 2B vWD patient and the propensity to develop thrombo penia. For example, recombinant vWF mutated in position 553 shows a very large increase in affinity for platelet GP1B and the patients harbouring this mutation seem to be more often thrombopenic than the patients with some other mutations.

D.D. Koeberl: Probably a naïve question, but has anyone explored the possible role of anabolic steroids in treating haemophilia B Leiden?

E. Briët: The question is whether we tried anabolic steroids in haemophilia B Leiden. The answer is yes, and it works.

II. HAEMOGLOBIN AND RED CELLS

GLOBIN GENE REGULATION

T.H.J. Huisman

Introduction

Haematopoiesis is the process of progenitor cell proliferation, differentiation, and maturation. Its control is mediated by growth factors (glycoproteins) and membrane receptors which, when activated, modify gene expression and patterns of differentiation. The erythroid pathway results in mature red blood cells; its haemoglobin (Hb) synthesis is possible because of a selective expression of the globin genes and a stability of the appropriate mRNAs. During the first few weeks of gestation, erythroblasts in the yolk sac produce the embryonic Gower Hbs (I = $\zeta_2\varepsilon_2$; II = $\alpha_2\varepsilon_2$) and Portland Hbs (I = $\zeta_2\gamma_2$; II = $\zeta_2\beta_2$; III = $\zeta_2\delta_2$). At 10 weeks these Hb types are replaced by fetal Hbs ($\alpha_2{}^G\gamma_2$; $\alpha_2{}^A\gamma_2$) which are synthesized in definitive erythroblasts in the liver. Before birth a switch to Hb synthesis in the bone marrow occurs; these erythroblasts are committed to the synthesis of Hb A ($\alpha_2\beta_2$) and Hb A_2 ($\alpha_2\delta_2$). Thus, this complex process concerns **a)** mechanisms of cell differentiation, i.e. from the pluripotent stem cell to the erythroid cell line; **b)** activation of specific globin genes which, moreover, are expressed in different cell types; **c)** the mechanism(s) responsible for the formation of the extremely high levels of these proteins. Differential globin gene activation and regulation will be the major topic to be reviewed here. It should also be known that in non-erythroid cells the α and β clusters exist in chromatin structures which prevent digestion with DNase I, while the more open configuration in erythroid cells makes digestion possible.

The β-globin genes

The β-globin gene cluster is ~70 kb long and is located on the short arm of chromosome #11, while the α-globin gene cluster of ~30 kb can be found on the short arm of chromosome #16. The genes are arranged on the chromosomes in the same order in which they are expressed during development (Figure 1). The expression of the genes of the β-globin gene cluster undergoes three switches, namely $\varepsilon \rightarrow \gamma$ during the first month after conception, $\gamma \rightarrow \beta + \delta$ before and after birth, and in the ${}^G\gamma$ to ${}^A\gamma$ ratio after birth (from 7:3 to 4:6). Regulation of the transcription of these genes occurs, to a major extent, through the interaction of *trans*-acting factors (proteins) with *cis* regulatory sequences such as promoters, enhancers, silences, and the locus control regions (LCRs).

The sequences with the promoter which combine with the *trans*-acting proteins are an ATA box, a CCAAT box, and a CACCC box. For the β promoter these sequences are located at nucleotides (nts) –31 to –26 (ATA box), –76 to –72 (CCAAT box), and between –105 and –86 (CACCC box) relative to the Cap site. Mutations within these sequences result in decreased binding and a decreased expression of the β-globin gene resulting in (mild) thalassaemic conditions.

Although the expression of the different globin genes is partially determined by the above mentioned controlling sequences, the globin transcription in erythroid cells is largely regulated by the LCR. The LCR was first described in a cluster of five DNase I hypersensitive (HS) sites; four sites (HS-1 through 4) are located 6 to 18 kb upstream of the ε-globin gene, and the fifth (HS-5) is located 20 kb downstream of the β-globin gene. These HS sites confer both temporal and tissue specificity of gene expression by organizing the entire β-globin locus into an open domain. They also act as enhancers of globin gene transcription. Studies in transgenic mice and transfected erythroid cells have shown that the LCR allows for a high level of position-independent, copy-number-dependent, erythroid-specific expression. One segment (HS-2) of the LCR alone can confer a high level of expression in the range of about 40% of the level obtained with the complete LCR. This HS-2 appears to contain several conserved sequences that bind erythroid as well as ubiquitous nuclear transcriptional factors, while alterations in some of these sequences have dramatically changed the transcriptional enhancing activity of HS-2 in both transgenic mice and cultured erythroid cells. The locations of the sequence variations and regulatory elements are depicted in Figure 2.

Regulation of the increased γ-globin synthesis in genetic diseases, such as sickle cell anaemia (SS) and β-thalassaemia (thal) that result in variable levels of fetal Hb (Hb F), appears to depend on the presence or absence of specific mutations within these regulatory sequences as well as on non-linked factors. For instance, the Hb F levels are greatly increased in SS patients from India as compared to

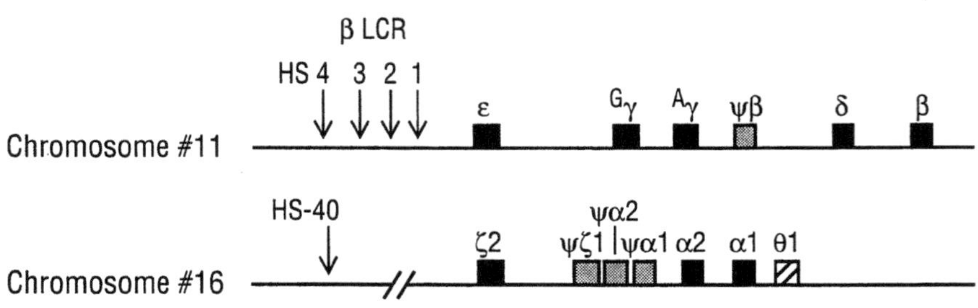

Figure 1. The β-globin gene cluster arranged on chromosome #11 and the α-globin gene cluster arranged on chromosome #6.

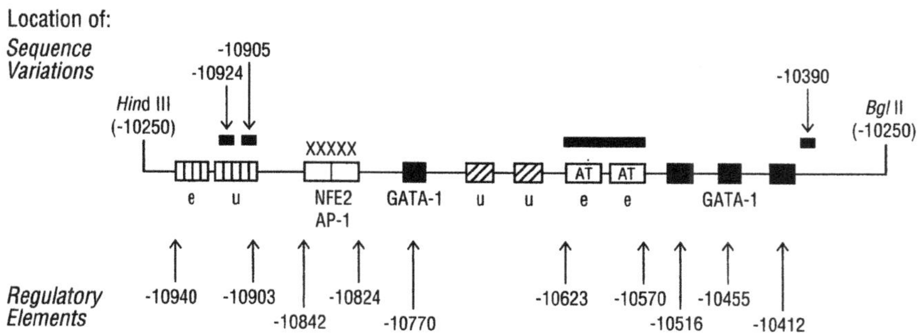

Figure 2. The locations of the sequence variations and regulatory elements of the HS-2 segment of the LCR of the β-globin gene.

those from Nigeria, SE-USA, or Kenya (Table 1). The differences are in the haplotypes of the β^S-bearing chromosomes. The patients with β^S haplotype #31 (Asian type) have much higher Hb F and $^G\gamma$ values than those with haplotypes #19 (Benin) or #20 (Kenya). The differences between these types is mainly in position −158 of the $^G\gamma$ promoter which is a C in chromosomes with haplotypes #19 or #20, and a T in those with haplotype #31. This small difference apparently promotes the expression of the $^G\gamma$-globin gene, particularly in conditions of (severe) anaemic stress.

The effect of mutations in one sequence of the LCR (LCR-2) from β^S chromosomes from patients homozygous for a haplotype with low Hb F and for that with high Hb F has also been evaluated. Several nt mutations have been found in the LCR-2 of an SS individual homozygous for haplotype #19, one being located at a site where an Sp I binding site is created. These mutations are absent in the LCR-2 of other haplotypes. These data suggest that certain mutation in the LCR-2 play a significant role in modulating $^G\gamma$ and Hb F expression. The unaltered sequence of the LCR-2 of the chromosome with haplotype #31 as compared to

Table 1. Haematological data for SS patients with different β^S haplotypes [from Adekile and Hausman, 1993].

Haplo- type	n	Age years	Hb g/dl	RBC 10^{12}/l	MCH pg	Hb A_2 %	Hb F %	$^G\gamma$
19/19	342	9.9	7.7	2.65	29.2	3.0	8.9	41.6
20/20	63	10.6	7.6	2.30	32.9	3.3	8.0	41.2
31/31	40	12.0	9.7	3.16	31.9	1.8	23.3	68.5

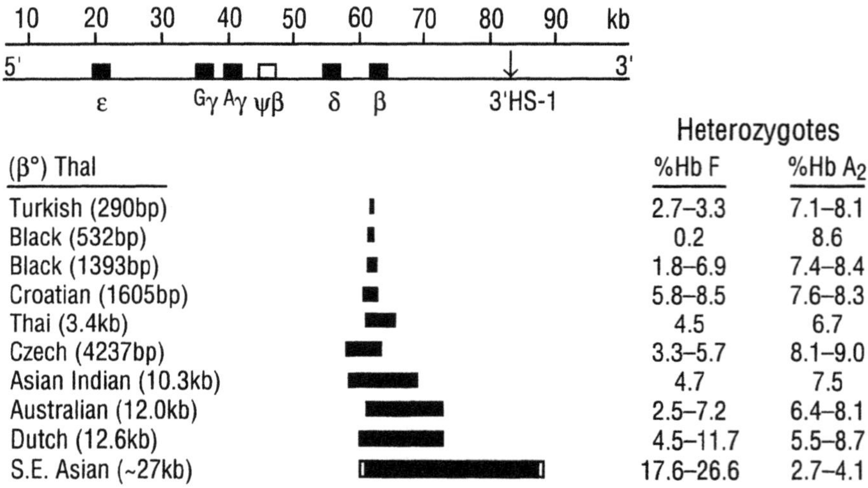

Figure 3. Heterozygosities for deletional β-thallassaemias (embryonic, foetal and adult).

the reference sequence in the Gen-Bank, may represent a chromosomal structure that allows for optimal interaction of *trans*-acting factors produced under the influence of haematopoietic stress. Conversely, the sequence variations of the LCR-2 associated with haplotypes #19 and #20 may result in chromosomal structures that are not optimal for γ-globin gene expression. The effect of the presence/absence of the 3′LCR (3′HS-1) was recently evaluated by comparing the Hb F and Hb A_2 values in patients with heterozygosities for deletional β-thalas saemias (Figure 3). These deletions concern (part of) the β-globin gene and its promoter; characteristics include a greatly elevated Hb A_2 and Hb F levels varying from 0–11%. One deletion of ~27 kb includes the 3′HS-1 and as a result the Hb A_2 levels are lower but the Hb F levels are greatly increased. No insight has yet been obtained into the mechanism(s) responsible for these significant changes.

Of the non-linked factors which influence γ-globin gene expression the age and sex should be considered. Hb F levels are generally higher in SS patients below the age of 5 years and fall sequentially thereafter. Within the three major haplotypes, the mean Hb F levels are somewhat higher among female than male patients, although the difference does not often reach statistical significance. It has also been suggested that a factor linked to the X chromosome influences the level of Hb F in both normal individuals as well as in SS patients. Females, carriers of two X chromosomes, may be homozygous for this factor and hence express, in a subset, higher levels of Hb F.

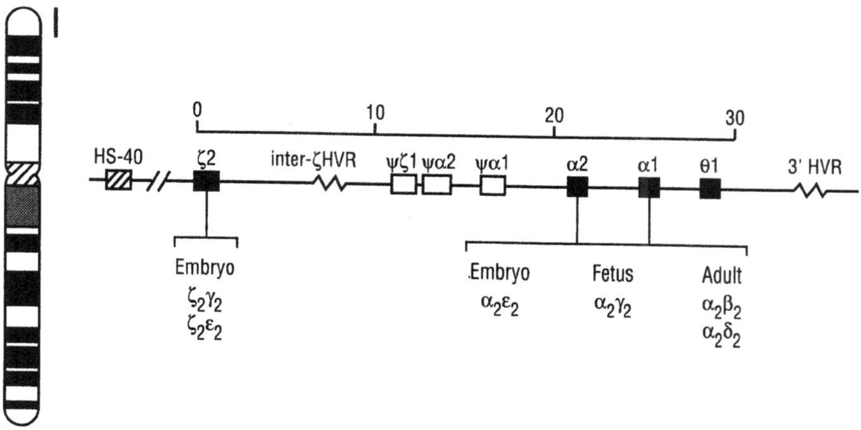

Figure 4. Hb F and Hb A_2 levels of various subjects with the same type of SS or β-thal, but with various numbers of active α-globin genes.

Several years ago we demonstrated in *in vitro* experiments that in conditions of relative α chain deficiency, the formation of Hb A ($\alpha_2\beta_2$) is preferred over that of Hb F ($\alpha_2\gamma_2$). This posttranslational mechanism has a significant effect on the Hb F levels of subjects with the same type of SS or β-thal but with various numbers of active α-globin genes (Figure 4). Indeed, several investigators have confirmed a strong inverse correlation between non-F cell levels and decreasing active α-globin number.

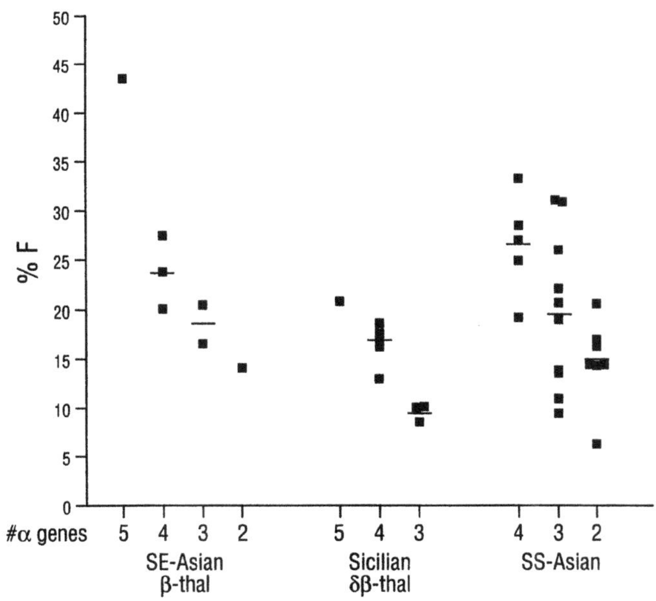

Figure 5. Variations in the structural organization of the α-globin gene cluster.

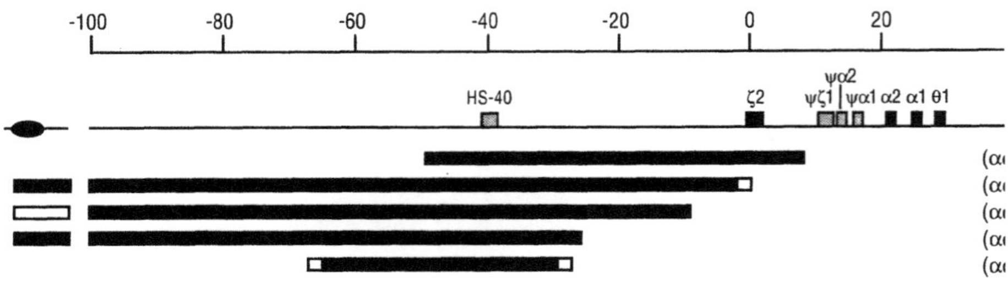

Figure 6. Five deletions outside the α-globin gene cluster, which all include the HS-40 segment.

The α-globin genes

Underproduction of α chains will result in the α-thal syndrome which is a heterogeneous group of genetic disorders characterized by variations in the structural organization of the α-globin gene cluster (Figure 5). This organization consists of an embryonic gene (ζ2), two fetal/adult genes (α2; α1), pseudogenes (ψζ1, ψα2, ψα1), and a gene with an unknown function (θ1). These genes are located at the tip of chromosome #16 as follows: Telemore-ζ-ψζ1-ψα2-ψα1-α2-α1-θ1-centromore. The two α-globin genes encode identical proteins and differ in the IVS-II and the 3′ non-coding region. In contrast, only 58% homology is observed in the 141 amino acids of the ζ and α chains; apparently a series of gene duplications and sequence mutations have resulted in these differences.

Studies of the α-globin gene cluster have shown the existence of multiple polymorphisms (point mutations, deletions, insertions), some causing α-thal. Two major groups have been identified which are known as deletional and nondeletional α-thal. Most frequent are the deletional types; one α-globin gene is absent in the α-thal-2 type (-α/) and two in the α-thal-1 type (--/). These forms are present at high frequencies in tropical and subtropical regions where *P. falciparum* malaria is (or was) endemic. At least eight different types of α-thal-2 deletions are known and 16 α-thal-1 deletions. Deletion of two α-globin genes (-α/-α or

Table 2. The quantities of Hb variants with mutations in either the α2- or α1-globin gene for heterozygotes with a normal complement of α genes (αα/αα) (average values only) [modified from Molchanova et al, 1994].

Hb variant	Mutation	n	Hb g/dl	MCV fl	MCH pg	Hb X %
A. Stable variants (α2-globin gene; genotype $\alpha^X\alpha/\alpha\alpha$)						
J-Paris_I (12 Ala→Asp)	GCC→GAC	2	16.8	114.6	33.0	24.0
I-Philadelphia (16	AAG→GAG	8	13.3	91.0	27.5	23.8
Lys→Glu)	CAC→CAA	1	11.2	104.5	29.8	28.0
Le Lamentin (20 His→Gln)	CTG→CGG	1	13.2	77.1	27.3	18.0
Montgomery (48 Leu→Arg)	AAC→AAA	2	12.7	91.8	28.7	25.1
G-Philadelphia (68	GAC→GTC	1	13.2	85.8	28.0	23.0
Asn→Lys)	AAG→AAT	2	14.1	–	–	25.0
Inkster (85 (85 Asp→Val)	AAC→AAA	1	–	–	–	21.8
J-Broussais (90 Lys-→Asn)	GCG→GAG	1	14.2	106.6	27.7	23.0
Dallas (97 Asn→Lys)	CTG→ATG	1	–	–	–	n.d.
J-Meerut (120 Ala→Glu)						
Chicago (136 Leu→Met)						
	(Average values					23.5)
B. Stable variants (α1-globin gene; gentype $\alpha\alpha^X/\alpha\alpha$)						
J-Paris-I (12 Ala→Asp)	GCC→GAC	1	13.6	96.7	29.5	20.7
J-Oxford (15 Gly→Asp)	GGT→GAT	8	14.1	101.7	30.6	22.5
Q-India (64 Asp→His)	GAC→CAC	5	13.0	93.0	29.8	16.9
Davenport (78 Asn→His)	AAC→CAC	1	13.0	77.8	26.0	19.6
J-Rajappen (90 Lys→Thr)	AAG→ACG	3	14.5	109.3	29.5	19.3
J-Broussais (90 Lys→Asn)	AAG→AAC	1	14.4	106.3	28.0	20.6
O-Indonesia (116	GAG→AAG	1	9.1	86.8	27.0	n.d.
Glu→Lys)	GCG→GAG	1	14.1	102.1	29.7	18.4
J-Meerut(120 Ala→Glu)						
	(Average values					19.7)

Standard deviation for Hb X quantitations were: I-Philadelphia 1.5; J-Oxford 1.15; Q-India 0.85; J-Rajappen 0.9.

homozygous α-thal-2, or --/αα or heterozygous α-thal-1) leads to a mild anaemia with microcytosis/hypochromia; deletion of three α-globin genes (--/-α) results
in Hb H disease (Hb H = β_4 formed from excess β chains) with moderate-to-severe anaemia and microcytosis and hypochromia; deletion of four α-globin genes (--/--) causes hydrops fetalis which is incompatible with life. The nondele tional types of α-thal are caused by mutations in the α2-globin gene (11 types) and the α1-globin gene (three types); these mutations affect RNA pro-cessing, RNA translation, or cause a posttranslational instability (unstable abnormal α chain variants).

Most important for our understanding of the α-globin genes are the observations made in patients who are heterozygous for deletions outside (5′ to) the α-globin gene cluster and have α-thalassaemic features. Five such deletions have been reported (Figure 6) and all five include a segment (HS-40) which is located ~40 kb 5′ to the ζ2-globin gene, is associated with an erythroid-specific DNase I HS site, and contains binding sites for the erythroid *trans*-acting factors GATA-1, NF-E2, and CACC box proteins. The binding of these proteins to the HS-40 fragment indeed closely resembles that observed for the LCR of the β-globin complex, that of the LCR-2 in particular.

The switch from embryonic ζ chain to the fetal/adult α chain synthesis is complete in an embryo of 10-11 weeks, although minute amounts of ζ-chain can be found in normal newborn babies and in infants with an α-thal. The mechanisms responsible for the down-regulation of the ζ gene and the up-regulation of the α genes has not been clearly defined; it appears likely that *trans*-acting factors in primitive erythroblasts promote ζ chain production or that negative regulatory factors in later erythroblasts act repressively on the ζ-globin gene.

It has been well-established that the chain products of the two α-globin genes are identical. mRNA analyses have indicated a 2- to 3-fold difference in the relative amount of α2 and α1 mRNA suggesting a major role for the α2-globin gene. Supporting evidence at the protein level has primarily been based on quantities of a few α2 and α1 variants in heterozygotes. We have recently analyzed the quantities of such variants in 20 heterozygotes with 10 different α2 mutations and in 21 heterozygotes with eight different α1 mutations and observed the values listed in Table 2. These data show only small differences in the relative amounts of these variants (α2 to α1: 1.17 to 1). These results support some older suggestions that the transcription of the α2-globin gene is considerably higher than that of the α1-globin gene, while the *in vivo* translation of the α1 gene is much more efficient than that of the α2 gene. Thus, it may be difficult, if not incorrect, to consider the α2 gene a major and the α1 gene a minor α locus, as generally assumed.

Suggested reading

1. Higgs DR. α-Thalassaemia. In: Higgs DR, Weatherall DJ (eds). The haemoglobinopathies. London: W.B. Saunders 1993:117-150 (Baillière's Clinical Haematology, Vol. 6).
2. Grosveld F, Dillon N, Higgs D. The regulation of the human globin gene expression. In: Higgs DR, Weatherall DJ (eds). The haemoglobinopathies. London: W.B. Saunders 1993:31-55. (Bailliere's Clinical Haematology, Vol. 6).
3. Molchanova TP, Pobedimskaya DD, Huisman THJ. The differences in quantities of α2- and α1-globin gene variants in heterozygotes. Br J Haematol 1994;88:300-06.
4. Öner C, Dimovski AJ, Altay Ç, et al. Sequence variations in the 5′ hypersensitive site-2 of the locus control region of β^S chromosomes are associated with different levels of fetal globin in hemoglobin S homozygotes. Blood 1992;79:813-19.
5. Stamatoyannopoulos G, Nienhuis AW, Leder P, Majerus PW, comps. The molecular basis of blood diseases. Philadelphia: W.B. Saunders 1997.
6. Adekile AD, Huisman THJ. Hb F in sickle cell anemia. Experientia 1993;49:16-27.

7. Dimovski AJ, Divoky V, Adekile AD, et al. A novel deletion of ~27 kb including the β-globin gene and the locus control region 3'HS-1 regulatory sequences: β^{o}-Thalassemia or hereditary persistence of fetal hemoglobin? Blood 1994;83:822-27.
8. Higgs DR, Vickers MA, Wilkie AOM, et al. A review of the molecular genetics of the human α-globin gene cluster. Blood 1989;73:1081-104.
9. The β- and δ-thalassemia repository (7th ed). Hemoglobin 1993;17:479-99.
10. Nathan DG. Pharmacologic manipulation of fetal hemoglobin in the hemoglobinopathies. 6th Cooley's Anemia Symposium, Ann NY Acad Sci 1990:1979-83.
11. Townes TM, Lingrel JB, Chen HY, et al. Erythroid-specific expression of the human beta-globin gene. EMBO J 1985;4:1715-23.
12. Tuan D, Soloman W, Li Q, London IM. The "β-like globin" gene domain in human erythroid cells. Proc Natl Acad Sci USA 1985;82:6384-48.
13. Fei Y-J, Liu J-C, Walker ELD III, Huisman THJ. A new gene deletion involving the α2-, α1-, and θ1-globin genes in black family with Hb H disease. Am J Hematol 1992; 39:299-303.
14. Liebhaber SA, Cash FE, Ballas SK. Human α-globin gene expression. The dominant role of the α2-locus in mRNA and protein synthesis. J Biol Chem 1986;261:15327-33.
15. Orkin SH, Goff SC. The duplicated human α-globin genes: Their relative expression as measured by RNA analysis. Cell 1981;24:345-51.
16. Proudfoot NJ. Transcriptional interference and termination between duplicated α-globin gene constructs suggest a novel mechanism for gene regulation. Nature 1986; 322:562-65.
17. Proudfoot NJ, Maniatis T. The structure of a human α-globin pseudogene and its relationship toe α-globin gene duplication. Cell 1980;21:537-44.
18. Proudfoot NJ, Gil A, Maniatis T. The structure of the human ζ-globin gene and a closely linked, nearly identical pseudogene. Cell 1982;31:553-63.

MOLECULAR PATHOLOGY OF THE THALASSAEMIA SYNDROMES

S.L. Thein

Introduction

The thalassaemias are a heterogeneous group of inherited haemoglobin disorders characterizedby a reduced output or absence of one or more of the globin chains. The common forms α- and β-thalassaemias, are among the most common genetic disorders in the world. There is increasing evidence that heterozygotes for thalassaemia are protected from the severe effects of *falciparum* malaria, this selective advantage has greatly increased the gene frequencies of many thalassaemia alleles throughout the tropical and sub-tropical regions [1]. Both α- and β-thalassaemia show a wide spectrum of clinical phenotypes ranging from severe anaemia and transfusion dependency in the homozygotes and compound heterozygotes to extremely mild forms which are clinically and haematologically silent, the so-called "silent" carrier states [2]. Furthermore, because the thalassaemias exist at a high frequency with the haemoglobin variants like Hb S, E and C in many populations, individuals may inherit more than one type giving rise to an extremely complex spectrum of clinical phenotypes. As the molecular pathology of the thalassaemias are being characterized, it has become possible to relate these heterozygous clinical phenotypes to the underlying genotypes.

Normal haemoglobin synthesis

Haemoglobin is a tetramer consisting of two identical α-like (α or ζ) and two β-like (ε, γ, δ or β) globin chains. In normal adults the major component is Hb A ($\alpha 2\beta 2$) which constitutes about 97% of the total Hb with a minor component of Hb A_2 ($\alpha 2\delta 2$) and traces of Hb F ($\alpha 2\gamma 2$). During development two major "switches" occur in the synthesis of haemoglobin; production of embryonic Hb (Hb Gower 1, $\zeta 2\varepsilon 2$; Hb Gower 2, $\alpha 2\varepsilon 2$ and Hb Portland, $\zeta 2\gamma 2$) switches after the eighth week of gestation to the production of Hb F ($\alpha 2\gamma 2$) and then just before birth to the adult Hb (Hb A and Hb A_2) [3]. At six months after birth Hb F comprises less than 5% of the total Hb and continues to fall reaching the adult level of <1% at 2 years of age. Thus while absence of α-globin chain is not compatible with life, mutations affecting the β-globin gene only become apparent clinically on completion of the switch from fetal to adult haemoglobin.

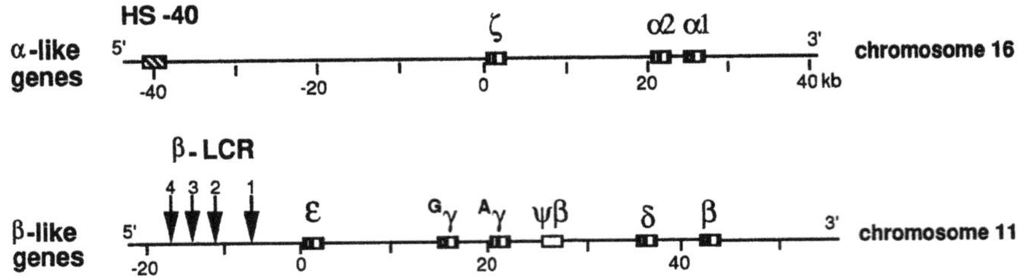

EMBRYONIC	FETAL	ADULT
ζ2ε2 (Hb Gower 1)	α2γ2 (Hb F)	α2β2 (Hb A)
α2ε2 (Hb Gower 2)		α2δ2 (Hb A2)
ζ2γ2 (Hb Portland)		

Figure 1. The α- and β-globin clusters on chromosomes 16 and 11, respectively, and the hemoglobins produced during each stage of human development. The upstream regulatory sequences of the α-cluster, HS-40, is shown as a shaded box while that for the β-cluster, β-LCR, is indicated by the four downward arrow, hypersensitive sites 1 to 4.

Each of the globin chains is encoded by a structural gene, the α-like genes located in the α-cluster which spans 30 kb on the tip of the short arm of chromosome 16 and the β-like genes, in a similar β-cluster which spans 70 kb on chromosome 11p15.5. In each cluster the genes are arranged along the chromosome in the order in which they are expressed during development (Figure 1). Immediately upstream of each gene is a promoter region which maintains local control while the entire cluster is controlled by a major regulatory element, referred to as the β-locus control region (β-LCR) in the β cluster [4], and the HS-40 [5] in the α-cluster (see Figure 1). Expression of the structural genes within each cluster is controlled by complex interactions between the local regulatory sequences and the major upstream elements of the respective LCR such that the products of the two clusters are expressed in equal amounts maintaining a balance in globin chain production throughout development. A reduced synthesis of α- or β-globin chains causes chain imbalance and a relative excess of β- or α-chains, respectively. In both instances the chain excess is harmful and leads to α- or β-thalassaemia. Interestingly, there does not appear to be an active feedback mechanism between the two clusters suggesting that they are coordinately but independently expressed.

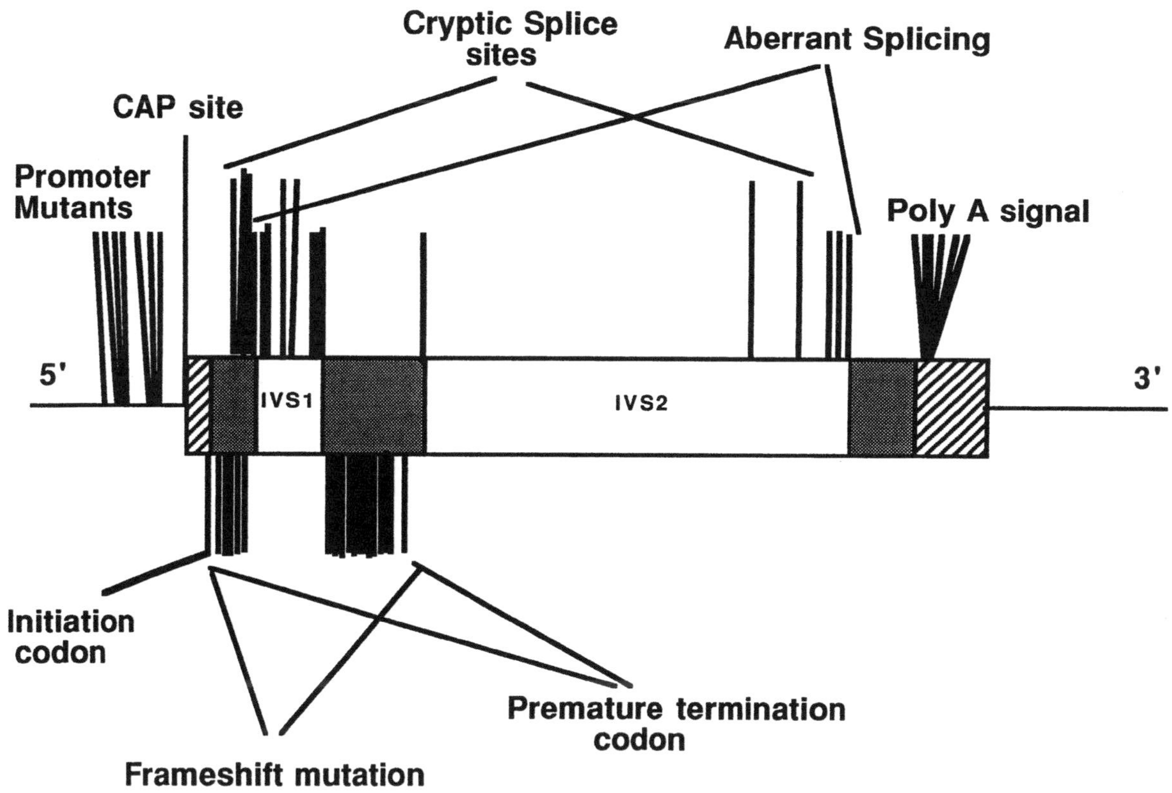

Figure 2. The β globin gene with the different classes of point mutations that cause β-thalassaemia. Point mutations can affect the promoter regions, cap site, initiation codon, splicing of the mRNA, polyadenylation site as well as cause premature termination of translation.

The interaction between the local promoter elements, enhancers and the elements of the LCR is mediated by *trans*-acting factors [6]. Much interest is focused on how those interact to produce high levels of tissue-specific and developmentally regulated expression of the globin genes. Tissue specific expression may be explained by the presence of two proteins, GATA-1 and NF-E2, that are specifically expressed in erythroid cells. Binding sites for one or more of these proteins are found in the upstream regulatory elements and some promoters of the globin genes [7]. It seems likely that these two *trans*-acting factors may form part of a network of functions involved in erythroid differentiation. The *trans*-acting factors involved in developmentally-specific expression of the globin genes, however, remain unclear.

β-thalassaemias

The β-thalassaemia syndromes result from underproduction of the β-globin chains of adult Hb A ($\alpha 2\beta 2$) giving rise to an imbalanced globin chain synthesis and excess of α-globin chains. These α chains are extremely unstable and precipitate in red cell precursors, producing an ineffective erythropoiesis and haemolytic anaemia. The severity of disease is directly related to the degree of chain imbalance.

β-thalassaemia is prevalent in regions endemic for malaria including the Mediterranean, North Africa, parts of the Middle East, India, Southeast Asia and southern China. Molecular analysis of the β-thalassaemia genes has demonstrated a striking heterogeneity; more than 160 different mutations have now been identified [8] and yet, population studies indicate that about 20 alleles account for more than 80% of the β-thalassaemia genes in the world [9]. Selective advantage of the thalassaemia phenotype in heterozygotes in these malarious regions and natural selection has greatly increased the frequencies of different mutant alleles such that in the different populations studied, the majority of the β-thalassaemias result from a small number of common mutations together with a varying number of rare ones. Each ethnic group also tends to have its own particular group of mutations. The implication of these observations is that prenatal diagnosis by direct detection is much simplified since a limited number of synthetic oligonucleotide probes may be needed.

Normal individuals have a single β-globin gene (β/β) on each chromosome 11. The mutations causing β-thalassaemia result in a deficit of β-globin production that ranges from minimal (mild β^+-thalassaemia) to a complete absence (β^o-thalassaemia). The vast majority of β-thalassaemia is caused by point mutations which affect sequences critical to the β gene function, that is, transcription, mRNA processing, translation and post-translational stability of the β-globin chain product [9,10]. Figure 2 illustrates the spectrum of point mutations that have been identified in β-thalassaemia. About 50% of the point mutations are frameshifts or nonsense codon mutations resulting in premature termination of translation of βo-thalassaemia. A substantial number of mutations affect RNA processing.

Table 1. β-thalassaemia intermedia.

Inheritance of mild forms of β-thalassaemia: - Homozygosity or compound heterozygosity for the mild β-thalassaemia alleles - Compound heterozygosity for one mild and one severe β-thalassaemia allele
Homozygosity for two severe β-thalassaemia alleles: - with co-inheritance of α-thalassaemia - with co-inheritance of genetic factors increasing Hb F expression (heterocellular HPFH, *Xmn* I-$^{G}\gamma$ site, γ promoter mutation
Compound heterozygosity for β-thalassaemia and deletion HPFH or δβ-thalassaemia
Compound heterozygosity for β-thalassaemia and Hb variants (Hb E/β-thalassaemia)
Heterozygous β-thalassaemia with triplicated α genes (ααα/ααα or ααα/αα)
Dominant forms of β-thalassaemia

Mutations that affect either of the invariant dinucleotides (GT at the 5′ donor site or AG at the 3′ acceptor site) at the splice junction, abolish normal splicing and produce β^{o}-thalassaemia. Mutations which affect the sequences flanking the splice junction reduce normal splicing to a varying degree and produce a β-thalassaemia phenotype that ranges from severe to mild β^{+}. Transcriptional mutants which affect the 5′ promoter region and mutants which affect the 3′ polyadenylation signal produce β^{+}-thalassaemia and, in general, are associated with a mild phenotype. One mutation, C→T at position −101 nt upstream of the β gene, appears to cause an extremely mild deficit of β-globin production [11]. Heterozygotes for this mutation have normal red cell indices and normal Hb A_2 levels and are the genuine "silent" carriers. Another very mild β^{+}- thalassaemia mutation involves the mRNA CAP site; homozygotes for the CAP +1 (A-C) mutation has haematologic values of a mild β-thalassaemia carrier while heterozygotes have normal red cell indices and borderline Hb A_2 levels [12]. Rarely, β-thalassaemia can be caused by deletions of the β cluster and although uncommon, these deletions provide some insight into the mechanisms responsible for the differential expression of the β-like globin genes. Three deletions are of particular interest because they remove extensive regions of the 5′ end of the β cluster but leave the β gene itself intact and yet result in β-thalassaemia [9]. We now know that these deletions silence the globin gene because they delete all or a substantial region of the major regulatory sequences in the upstream β-LCR.

Another group of deletions, ranging from 290 bp to >40 kb remove in common the 5′ promoter region of the β-globin gene. These deletions are associated with unusually high levels of Hb A_2 (3.5% to 5.5%). Individuals with two defective β-globin genes, homozygotes or compound heterozygotes, normally have severe anaemia and are transfusion-dependent (thalassaemia major). However, gradations of severity exist; some patients, despite being homozygous for β^{o}-thalassaemia (β^{o}/β^{o}) have mild disease and survive without transfusion. Similarly, some individuals have inherited only a single abnormal β-globin gene but have a thalassaemia intermedia syndrome. Table 1 lists some of the molecular interactions that have been associated with the phenotype of thalassaemia intermedia. The majority of patients are homozygotes or compound heterozygotes for β-thalassaemia and have usually co-inherited genes for α-thalassaemia or factors which may increase Hb F expression; or have one or two mild β^+-thalassaemia genes. The importance of these factors varies with the population group.

In some families β-thalassaemia intermedia is inherited as a Mendelian dominant. This group of mutations forms a distinctive sub-group referred to as dominantly inherited β-thalassaemia. A spectrum of underlying mutations have now been identified and the majority seen to involve exon 3 of the β-globin gene [13]. The rarity of these mutations, as well as their occurrence in dispersed geographical regions, suggests that they have had no selective advantage. Indeed, several of these mutations are "de novo". Genetic studies have revealed another rare form of β-thalassaemia in which the abnormality is not linked to the β complex [14] and may be due to abnormalities in the *trans*-acting factors that interact with the genes and their control regions.

α-thalassaemia

The α-thalassaemias result from under production of the α chains of fetal (Hb F $\alpha 2\gamma 2$) and adult (Hb A $\alpha 2\beta 2$) haemoglobin giving rise to an excess of γ or β chains which form the tetramers, Hb Bart's ($\gamma 4$) and Hb H ($\beta 4$).

As in β-thalassaemia, the critical factor in determining the severity of disease in α-thalassaemia is the degree of chain imbalance. The pathophysiology of α-thalassaemia, however, differs fundamentally from that of β-thalassaemia in that the anaemia is related to haemolysis due to intracellular precipitation of Hb Bart's and Hb H, rather than to ineffective erythropoiesis. Ultimately, the severity of anaemia and the amount of abnormal Hb produced is directly related to the degree of α chain deficiency.

Normal individuals have two α-globin genes ($\alpha\alpha/\alpha\alpha$) on each chromosome 16. Defects can affect one or both of the α-globin genes resulting in a reduced output (α^+-thalassaemia) or absence (α^0-thalassaemia) of α-globin from that particular chromosome [15]. In contrast to β-thalassaemia, the majority of α-thalassaemia (>95%) are caused by deletions; the phenotype of α^+-thalassaemia may result from deletions of either one or the other of the linked α-globin genes ($-\alpha/\alpha\alpha$) or from a point mutation inactivating one of the α-globin genes, usually $\alpha 2$ ($\alpha^T\alpha/\alpha\alpha$). α^0-thalassaemia results from deletions that remove both α-globin genes ($--/\alpha\alpha$). Unlike the α^+-thalassaemia deletions, α^0 thalassaemia deletions are limited in their geographical distribution. Recently several deletions which remove the upstream control region (HS-40) leaving the α-globin genes intact, have been described. These completely inactivate the α-globin gene complex. A minority of α-thalassaemia results from point mutations which affect the sequences which control the different stages of α-globin expression. Most of these affect the dominant $\alpha 2$ globin gene and in general, the non-deletion α^+-thalassaemia determinants give rise to a more severe reduction in α-chain synthesis than deletion ($-\alpha/\alpha\alpha$)α^+-thalassaemia.

Interactions between the different α-thalassaemia determinants give rise to a spectrum of clinical phenotypes which fall into three broad groups: carriers for α-thalassaemia with three or two fundamental α-globin genes ($-\alpha/\alpha\alpha$, $\alpha^T\alpha/\alpha\alpha$, $-\alpha/-\alpha$ or $--/\alpha\alpha$) who are clinically asymptomatic with mild hypochromic microcytic anaemia, Hb H disease and Hb Bart's hydrops fetalis syndrome. Hb H disease results from the interactions of α^+- and α^0-thalassaemia determinants and gives rise to a moderately severe form of haemolytic anaemia which is commonly seen in the Mediterranean, Middle East and Southeast Asia. The absence of α-globin genes ($--/--$) gives rise to lethal intrauterine haemolytic anaemia (Hb Bart's hydrops fetalis syndrome) which again occurs commonly in Southeast Asia and the Mediterranean region. Although Hb H disease is almost always inherited, it has been described as an acquired defect associated with the development of a myeloproliferative disorder predominantly in elderly males [16]. It appears to be a clonal disorder involving the neoplastic cell line. The nature of the specific defect that results in the reduction or absence of α-chain synthesis and its relationship to the haematological malignancy remains unknown.

A rare form of α-thalassaemia has also been described associated with mental retardation. It is now clear that two different forms of the α-thalassaemia mental retardation syndrome exist [17,18]. In the first group, ATR-16, the patients have relatively mild mental handicap and a variable phenotype of facial and skeletal dysmorphisms. The α-thalassaemia in these individuals are due to long deletions of at least 1 megabase which remove the α-globin gene cluster on the tip of chromosome 16. The second group is characterized by severe mental retardation and a striking homogeneous pattern of dysmorphology. These patients have a relatively mild form of Hb H disease. Studies show that the α-globin gene cluster is intact and that the syndrome segregates independently of the α cluster. The retarded patients are all males, the defect is *trans*-acting and has now been localized to chromosome Xq and is referred to as the ATR-X syndrome [19].

Elucidation of the molecular basis of this disorder should provide further insight on the regulation of globin gene expression and on the pathogenesis of some forms of mental handicap.

Conclusion

The mutations underlying the α- and β-thalassaemias are many and remarkably diverse. Interaction between these different genotypes have provided a picture of molecular mechanisms for the phenotypic diversity of monogenic diseases. Apart from providing a rationale for genetic counselling and prenatal diagnosis, analysis of these mutations have given much insight into the mechanisms regulating globin gene expression.

References

1. Flint J, Hill AVS, Bowden DK, et al. High frequencies of α thalassaemia are the result of natural selection by malaria. Nature 1986;321:744-49.
2. Weatherall DJ, Clegg JB. The thalassaemia syndromes. Oxford: Blackwell Scientific 1981.
3. Stamatoyannopoulos G, Nienhuis AW. Hemoglobin switching. In: Stamatoyannopoulos G, Nienhuis AW, Majerus PW, Varmus H (eds). The molecular basis of blood diseases (2nd ed). Philadelphia: W.B. Saunders and Co. 1994:107-55.
4. Grosveld F, Dillon N, Higgs D. The regulation of human globin gene expressio. In: Higgs DR, Weatherall DJ (eds). The haemaglobinopathies. Baillière's Clinical Haematology. London: Baillière Tindall 1993:31-55.
5. Higgs DR, Wood WG, Jarman AP, et al. A major positive regulatory region located far upstream of the human α globin gene locus. Genes Dev 1990;4:1588-601.
6. Orkin SH. Globin gene regulation and switching: Circa 1990. Cell 1990;63: 665-72.
7. Andrews NC, Orkin SH. Transcriptional control of erythropoiesis. Current Opinion in Hematology 1994;1:119-24.
8. Huisman THJ. The β- and δ-thalassemia repository. Hemoglobin 1992;16:237-58.
9. Thein SL. β-thalassaemia. In: Higgs DR, Weatherall DJ (eds). The haemoglobinopathies. Baillière's Clinical Haematology. London: Baillière Tindall 1993:151-76.
10. Kazazian HHJ, Boehm CD. Molecular basis and prenatal diagnosis of β-thalassemia. Blood 1988;72:1107-16.
11. Gonzalez-Redondo JM, Stoming TA, Kutlar A, et al. A C→T substitution at nt-101 in a conserved DNA sequence of the promoter region of the β globin gene is associated with "silent" β-thalassemia. Blood 1989;73:1705-11.
12. Wong C, Dowling CE, Saiki RK, Higuchi RG, Erlich HA, Kazazian HHJ. Characterization of β-thalassaemia mutations using direct genomic sequencing of amplified single copy DNA. Nature 1987;330:384-86.
13. Thein SL. Dominant β-thalassaemia: Molecular basis and pathophysiology. Brit J Haemat 1992;80:273-77.
14. Thein SL, Wood WG, Wickramasinghe SN, Galvin MC. β-thalassemia unlinked to the β globin gene in an English family. Blood 1993;82:961-67.
15. Higgs DR. α thalassaemia. In: Higgs DR, Weatherall DJ (eds). The haemoglobinopathies. Baillière's Clinical Haematology. London: Baillière Tindal 1993:117-50.
16. Higgs DR, Wood WG, Barton C, Weatherall DJ. Clinical features and molecular analysis of acquired HbH disease. Am J Med 1983;75:181-92.
17. Wilkie AOM, Buckle VJ, Harris PC, et al. Clinical features and molecular analysis of the α thalassemia/mental retardation syndromes. I. Cases due to deletions involving chromosome band 16p13.3. Am J Hum Genet 1990a;46:1112-26.
18. Wilkie AOM, Zeitlin HC, Lindenbaum RH, et al. Clinical features and molecular analysis of the α thalassemia/mental retardation syndromes. II. Cases without detectable abnormality of the α globin complex. Am J Hum Genet 1990b;46:1127-40.
19. Gibbons RJ, Suthers GK, Wilkie AOM, Buckle VJ, Higgs DR. X-linked α thalassemia/mental retardation (ATR-X) syndrome; localization to Xq12-q21.31 by X inactivation and linkage analysis. Am J Hum Genet 1992;51:1136-49.

THE CURRENT STATUS OF BONE MARROW TRANSPLANTATION AND GENE THERAPY IN THE MANAGEMENT OF THE HAEMOGLOBINOPATHIES

J.F. Apperley, I.A.G. Roberts

Bone marrow transplantation for the haemoglobinoplathies

Since the first successful bone marrow transplants (BMT) were reported [1-3], clinicians have been aware of their potential for the treatment of the haemoglobinopathies. To date the procedural risks of BMT have precluded its widespread use for thalassaemia and sickle cell disease. However as the risks of BMT have decreased due to a combination of increasing experience and improved techniques, it has become a viable alternative to medical treatment in selected cases. The decision to advocate transplant remains difficult, but the information now available regarding the outcome of BMT has enabled us to identify suitable patient groups.

BMT for thalassaemia

The first transplant for thalassaemia was reported in 1982 [4]. Despite the success of this procedure, the use of transplant for a non-life threatening condition was much criticised. The immediate morbidity and mortality associated with allogeneic grafts (Table 1) was thought to outweigh any benefit. However, due to the changes in the medical treatment of thalassaemia over the past three decades, it remains extremely difficult to accurately predict the clinical course in an individual patient. It is therefore even more problematic to try to balance the immediate risks of transplant against the chronic difficulties inherent in medical management.

Until the 1960s, patients were treated by blood transfusion when their anaemia became symptomatic i.e. Hb 5-6 g/dl. 12% of patients died before the age of 7

Table 1. Early morbidity and mortality of allogeneic BMT.

Side-effects of chemo-radiotherapy
Graft failure
Veno-occlusive disease
Acute GVHD
Infection

and mortality increased steadily with age. The next decade saw the initiation of transfusion programmes designed to maintain the Hb >8 g/dl. More recently, transfusion has been accompanied by chelation therapy [5], and the long term outcome of patients treated in this way is not yet known. The main causes of death are still due to the consequences of transfusional iron overload, e.g. cardiac failure, liver disease, diabetes mellitus. Compliance with chelation will undoubtedly delay the onset of these complications, but there remains a large number of patients who are either non-compliant or for whom, chelation therapy is unavailable. Even in the most compliant of individuals, the clinician must be aware of the effects of a life of transfusion-dependence and chelation therapy on the patient and their family.

The majority of data concerning the outcome of BMT for thalassaemia is derived from Pesaro groups. Their first report described a heterogeneous group of 13 patients of whom only 2 were surviving free of disease [6]. Although these results were extremely disappointing, these early transplants were highly informative with respect to the optimal conditioning regimen, and the importance of correct patient selection. In 1985 this group reported the outcome of a group of 30 patients of median age 3.5 years (range 0.5-7 years) who were conditioned with Busulphan (14-16 mg/kg) and Cyclophosphamide (200 mg/kg). This group had an overall survival of 86% and an event free survival (EFS) of 73% [7]. By 1991, Lucarelli et al were able to report on 237 children transplanted for thalassaemia. Their experience had let them to define 3 prognostic groups (Classes I-III) based on the presence or absence of portal fibrosis, liver size, and compliance with chelation therapy [8] (Table 2). Survival and EFS for the three classes were 98% and 94% (50 patients), 86% and 83% (153 patients) and 91% and 60% (35 patients) respectively. The outcome of the Class III patients had improved considerably compared to an earlier report in 1990, when the survival and EFS had been 61% and 53% respectively [9]. This had been achieved by reducing the Cyclophosphamide dose to 120 mg/kg, but at the expense of a much increased risk of graft rejection from 16% to 37%. Graft failure remains a significant problem after BMT for thalassaemia for all patients. A recent update on the survival, event free survival, rejection rate and mortality was provided at the 1994 meeting of the European Group for Blood and Marrow Transplantation (EBMT) and is given in Table 3.

Data is now available from the long term follow up of these patients. Serum ferritin levels transiently rise after BMT probably due to a combination of the

Table 2. Prognostic factors for BMT for thalassaemia.

Risk factors	**Class I**	**Class II**	**Class III**
Hepatomegaly	No	No/Yes	Yes
Portal fibrosis	No	No/Yes	Yes
Regular chelation	No	No/Yes	Yes
Total number of risk factors	0	1 or 2	3

conditioning therapy, infection, graft versus host disease (GvHD) and/or veno-occlusive disease. Thereafter they decline steadily [10]. Endocrinopathies also improve post transplant, e.g. diabetes mellitus. Growth velocity may decrease however [11]. Furthermore, gonadal dysfunction due either to pituitary of gonadal damage may be irreversible [12].

The great majority of transplants for thalassaemia have employed HLA identical siblings as bone marrows donors. However, only about one-third of patients suitable for transplant have a suitable sibling donor. The results of the transplant using alternative donors have been very disappointing. Of 17 patients transplanted in Pesaro, only 4 are alive free of disease. Seven died of transplant related mortality and six are alive with thalassaemia [13].

After more than a decade of transplantation for thalassaemia, the results have improved considerably, largely as a consequence of better patient selection. As the factors which adversely affect outcome, i.e. GvHD, CMV infection, veno-occlusive disease, interstitial pneumonitis, and organ damage due to transfusional iron overload, all become more frequent with increasing age, so it becomes important to identify patients for transplant as early as possible. The results of BMT for children with none of the three risk factors are excellent. However, this is also the group which may do extremely well on medical treatment, and some would argue should not be exposed to the risks of BMT. On the other hand patients in Class III may do poorly with transplant but by definition have failed medical therapy. The solution may be to observe patients in Class I very carefully and proceed to transplant at the first sign of liver damage of poor compliance, and to work to improving the outcome of patients transplanted for Class III disease. There is no clear answer to this dilemma. Each patient must be assessed individually with respect to disease status, availability of medical care, risk of non-compliance and the ability of the patient and their family to cope with the rigors of life-long chelation and transfusion.

Bone marrow transplantation for sickle cell disease

The first transplant describing care of sickle cell disease was reported in 1984, and was co-incidental with the use of BMT in an 8 year old girl with AML [14]. The first 5 transplants intended to cure sickle cell disease were published in 1988

Table 3. Outcome of BMT for sickle cell disease: the European experience.

	Patient numbers		
Clinical status	**Belgium**	**France**	**Total**
Alive	27	14	41
Dead	1	0	1
Cured	20	10	30
Rejection	3	2	5
Red cell independent	25	13	38

[15]. All 5 patients engrafted, although one patient later experienced graft rejection. This group recently updated their results at the 1994 EBMT meeting, when 25 patients had been transplanted. 24 patients survive and there has been only one death. Acute and chronic GvHD occurred in 45% and 17% of valuable patients respectively. The combined European experience was collated by Christine Vermylen for the 2nd International Symposium on BMT in thalassaemia in1992 and is shown in Table 4 [16, 17].

As can be seen from these results, the mortality of transplant for sickle cell disease is negligible and the morbidity surprisingly low. Graft failure is the major cause of treatment failure. The problem in sickle cell disease, is to identify patients for whom BMT is the most appropriate therapy. Despite our precise knowledge of the molecular abnormality, the clinical effects are highly variable and cannot be predicted on an individual basis. Approximately 30% of patients are severely disabled with complications such as sickle cell lung disease (SCLD), cerebrovascular disease, retinopathy, chronic renal failure and generalized osteonecrosis, 60% have less severe disease and 10% remain symptom free throughout life [18]. Patients may experience periods of recurrent severe vascular crises, interspersed with long periods of good health. This variability in the clinical course suggests that the outcome in one patient cannot be due simply to a point mutation in the DNA encoding β-globin. Some prognostic factors have now been identified, e.g. co-inheritance of α-thalassaemia, certain genetic polymorphisms of restriction enzyme sites in the β-globin gene cluster, level of expression of Hb F [19], but we are not yet able to confidently predict an individual clinical course.

At present the indications for transplant include frequent crises, cerebrovascular disease, alloimmunization, osteonecrosis and SCLD. As in thalassaemia, a number of factors must be considered prior to the recommendation of BMT, not least of which is an assurance that the patient and their family thoroughly understand the nature of their disease and the risks inherent in transplantation.

Gene therapy for the haemoglobinopathies

The haemoglobinopathies result from the absence of, or the defective production of one or more globin protein chains. Defective globin production is itself a

Table 4. Outcome of BMT for thalassaemia by patient prognostic group.

Percentage	Class I	Class II	Class III
Survival	95	88	55 (87)
Event free survival (EFS)	90	82	53 (63)
Rejection	5	6	9 (20)
Mortality	5	12	42 (13)

Figures in parentheses refers to outcome in patients in Class III conditioned with cyclophosphamide 120 mg/kg.

consequence of deletions and/or mutations in the DNA sequence encoding the globin protein. As such the haemoglobinopathies are ideal candidates for treatment by gene therapy, i.e. the replacement of the abnormal DNA by its normal counterpart. Ideally, the newly introduced globin gene would be correctly regulated and expressed for the lifetime of the patient. Recent advances in the techniques of homologous recombination make this a realistic goal for the future [20, 21]. To date, however, the majority of experimental data available concerns the expression of α-globin gene randomly inserted in the target cell genome.

The incoming globin gene must be expressed only in erythroid cells, so the obvious target cell for the gene transfer is the haemopoietic stem cell (HSC). As this is an extremely rare cell (estimated at 0.001% of nucleated cells [5, 22]), the method of transfer must be highly efficient. In practice, this is only achieved by the use of retroviral vectors, with their relatively high infection efficiency, and the ability to integrate stably into the host cell genome.

Retroviral vectors

The retrovirus itself consists of three coding regions, gag, pol and env, encoding the internal structural proteins, reverse transcriptase and the envelope glycoproteins, respectively. These RNA sequences are bound at each end by two identical 'long terminal repeats', which contain promoter and enhancer elements, and can direct integration and replication of the whole retroviral genome.

The gag, pol and env genes comprise about 8% of the retroviral genome, but can be deleted and replaced by genomic DNA encoding one or more of the globin genes, under the control of their endogenous promoter(s). This recombinant retrovirus is thus rendered incapable of producing progeny viridae, due to the lack of structural viral proteins. In order to produce large quantities of infectious virus, the recombinant, 'replication-defective' retrovirus must be introduced into a packaging cell line, itself containing the sequences encoding the necessary viral component proteins [23, 24]. In this way virus particles at concentrations up to 10^6 particles per ml can be harvested from the supernatant of the packaging cell line. These particles can then be used to infect the target haemopoietic stem cells.

Retroviral-mediated gene transfer into haemopoietic stem cells

Successful gene transfer into haemopoietic stem cells was first demonstrated in 1983 [25]. Joyner and colleagues, using a retrovirus containing a gene encoding neomycin resistance (neo^R) showed that 0.3% of CFU-GM colonies had developed resistance to the neomycin analogue, G418. In 1987, Williams et al [26] showed neoR expression in a pluripotent stem cell, i.e. the CFU-S. These early experiments were met with great excitement and enthusiasm, but by the end of the 1980s, the problems of retroviral gene transfer had also become apparent:

- Poor efficiency of infection of haemopoietic stem cells, resulting in gene expression in a small minority of cells.
- Short duration of expression in *in vivo* models. This problem is undoubtedly multi-factorial. For successful retroviral integration, the target cell must be in

division. Since the haemopoietic stem cell is likely to be a quiescent cell, its infection efficiency is predictably low. Expression seen shortly after transfer is probably a result of infection of more differentiated cells, with a finite life span. In addition, there have been reports of failure of expression despite the detection of the retroviral genome in the haemopoietic stem cells [27]. Finally it is possible that cells expressing exogenous genes secondary to retroviral gene transfer, are susceptible to antibody and complement mediated lysis due to alterations in their cell surface protein expression.
- Low levels of expression of the exogenous gene compared to its normal endogenous counterpart. This can probably be explained by the construction of the recombinant retrovirus. The exogenous genes are often expressed from promoters unrelated to the gene itself. The use of efficient and appropriate promoter and enhancer elements will be of paramount importance if we are to achieve high level, tissue specific gene expression. At present, the use of unrelated promoters is due to the size limitations of the sequence which can be inserted into the retrovirus. This size restriction also commonly necessitates the use of the cDNA rather then the genomic sequences, which may itself compound the problem.

For this reason, the short length if the genomic β-globin seemed to make the globin gene the ideal candidate for these experiments. Initial studies used the entire genomic sequence of β-globin, with its promoter, enhancer intronic and flanking sequences in a 4.4 kb fragment, which was readily accommodated within a retrovirus. Initial results were indeed encouraging. β-globin mRNA transcription

Table 5. In vitro and *in vivo* levels of transcription of human globin gene mRNA.

Globin gene	Percentage endogenous mRNA	Reference
Murine erythroleukaemia cells		
human $\gamma\beta$	5 – 40	[31]
human β	4 – 50	[30]
human β + HS 2 (1.2 kb)	100	[36]
human β + HS 2 (0.4 kb)	12	[37]
human β + HS 2 (2.7 kb)	70	[38]
Murine and human haemopoietic stem cells		
human β	0.4 – 4.0	[32]
human β	0.5 – 50	[31]
human β	5	[30]
human β	0.2 – 1.5	[33]
human β + HS 2 (2.7 kb)	10 – 40	[38]

HS 2 = Hypersensitive site 2.

could be induced in mouse erythroleukaemia (MEL) cells, but not in NIH-3T3 fibroblasts, indicating tissue specific expression [28-30]. The expression of β-globin required the presence of intronic sequences, particularly the intervening sequences 2 (IVS.2) as vectors containing only the cDNA achieved poor expression. Unfortunately the level of mRNA transcription varied widely (<1-100%) and protein expression was uniformly low [31] (Table 5).

Early attempts to transfer globin genes into murine HSCs met with even less success. mRNA transcription was seen in 18 of 104 mice surviving up to 9 months after BMT using cells infected with a β-globin containing retrovirus. Transcription was erythroid specific, but mRNA levels achieved only 0.4-4.0% of endogenous levels [32]. Similar results were obtained by other groups [31, 33]. There has been one report of successful transfer into human erythroid progenitors, BFU-E, but the frequency of infection was low at 0.04%, and mRNA transcription reached only 5% of that of endogenous β-globin [30]. These early results suggested that high levels, tissue-specific expression of β-globin using retroviral vectors may be difficult to achieve.

The identification of the locus control regions (LCR) of the α- and β-globin gene clusters may overcome the problems in obtaining high level expression [34, 35]. The LCRs are large and cannot be incorporated in full in a retroviral vector. However, three groups have recently shown increased levels of β-globin mRNA transcription in MEL cells by incorporating sequences from the LCRs [36, 38]. In addition Plavec, et al obtained much improved levels of β-globin expression in mice transplanted with cells infected with a vector containing the β-globin gene fused to the 4 major regulatory elements of the LCR [38].

In addition to the technical problems encountered in retroviral gene transfer, there are additional concerns with respect to the safety of these vectors. In particular there is a risk of recombination events in the packaging cell line resulting in the presence of wild type replication-competent viruses in the supernatant. Recently another viral vector, namely the adeno-associated virus (AAV), has been used for the transfer of the β-globin gene into MEL cells, using a construct containing part of the LCR. mRNA transcription was observed at levels comparable to that of the endogenous gene [39].

Adeno-associated virus [reviewed in 39] is a defective parvovirus which requires co-infection with adenovirus or herpes simplex virus for lytic infection. In the absence of helper virus it integrates into the host cell genome, and has been demonstrated to be stable for at least 100 passages [40]. A wide variety of cell types are permissive for AAV infection, but despite this, no disease has ever been associated with AAV in humans. The AAV genome is itself small at 4675 base pairs. This may limit its role in the gene transfer of large sequences, but at present, it holds great promise for globin gene transaction.

A number of other methods of gene transfer are currently under evaluation. The rabbit β-globin gene has been introduced into mammaham cells in a modified HSV vector [41]. Non-viral vectors, include the use of receptor-mediated endocytosis. The potential of gene therapy is only just being realised and we must anticipate rapid progress in this new and developing field.

References

1. Bach FH, Albertini RJ, Anderson JL, Joo P, Bortin MM. Bone marrow transplantation in a patient with the Wiskott-Aldrich syndrome. Lancet 1968;ii:1364-66.
2. Gatti RA, MeuwissenHJ, Allen HD, Hong R, Good RA. Immunological reconstitution of sex-linked lymphopenic immunological deficiency. Lancet 1968;ii:1366-69.
3. Koning J de, van Bekkum DW, Dicke KA, Dooren LJ, van Rood JJ, Radl J. Transplantation of bone marrow cells and fetal thymus in an infant with lymphopenic immunological deficiency. Lancet 1969;i:1223-27.
4. Thomas ED, Buckner CD, Sanders JE. Marrow transplantation for thalassemia. Lancet; ii:227-29.
5. Borgna-Pignatti C, Zurlo MG, DeStefano P, et al. Survival in thalassemia with conventional treatment. In: Buckner CD, Gale RP, Lucarelli G (eds). Advances and controversies in thalassemia therapy. New York: Alan R. Liss 1989:27-34.
6. Lucarelli G, Polchi P, Izzi T, et al. Allogeneic marrow transplantation for thalassemia. Exp Hematol 1984;12:676-81.
7. Lucarelli G, Polchi P, Galimberti M, et al. Marrow transplantation for thalassaemia following busolphan and cyclophosphamide. Lancet 1995;i;1355-57.
8. Lucarelli G, Weatherall DJ. For debate: Bone marrow transplantation for severe thalassemia. Brit J Haematol 1991;78:300-3.
9. Lucarelli G, Galimberti M, Polchi P, et al. Bone marrow transplantation in patients with thalassemia. N Engl J Med 1990;322:417-21.
10. Angelucci E, Polizzi V, Lucarelli G, Muretto P. Liver iron kinetics in thalassemic patients after bone marrow transplantation. In: Buckner CD, Gale RP, Lucarelli G (eds). Advances and controversies in thalassemia therapy. New York: Alan R. Liss 1989:291-98.
11. Galimberti M, de Sanctis V, Lucarelli G, et al. Endocrine function after bone marrow transplantation for thalassemia. Bone Marrow Transpl 1991a;7(suppl 3):74.
12. De Sanctis V, Galimberti M, Lucarelli G, et al. Gonadal function after bone marrow transplantation for thalassemia. Arch Dis Child 1991;66:517-20.
13. Galimberti M, Lucarelli G, Polchi P, et al. HLA-mismatched bone marrow transplantation for thalassemia. Bone Marrow Transpl 1991a;7(suppl 3):98-100.
14. Johnson FL, Look AT, Gockerman J, et al. Bone marrow transplantation in a patient with sickle cell anaemia. N Engl J Med 1984;311:780-83.
15. Vermylen CH, Fernandez Robles E, Ninane J, Cornu G. Bone marrow transplantation in five children with sickle cell anaemia. Lancet 1989;i:1427-28.
16. Vermylen CH, Cornu G. Bone marrow transplantation in sickle cell disease: The Belgium experience. Bone Marrow Transpl 1992;12(suppl 1):116-17.
17. Bernaudin F, Souillet G, Vannier JP, et al. Bone marrow transplantation (BMT) in 14 children with severe sickle cell disease: The French experience. Bone Marrow Transpl 1992;12(suppl 1):118-21.
18. Powards D, Chan LS, Schroeder WA. The variable expression of sickle cell disease is genetically determined. Sem Hematol 1990;27:360-76.
19. Apperley JF. Bone marrow transplant for the haemoglobinopathies: Past, present and future. In: Higgs DR, Weatherall DJ (eds). The haemoglobinopathies. Baillière's Clinical Haematology. London: Baillière Tindall 1993;6:299-325
20. Smithies O, Gregg RO, Boggs, Koralewski MA, Kuherlapati RB. Insertion of DNA sequences into the human chromosomal β-globin locus by homologous recombination. Nature. 1985; 317:230-34.

21. Thomas KR, Capecchi MR. Site directed mutagenesis by genes targeting in mouse embryo-derived stem cells. Cell 1987;51:503-12.
22. Harrison DE, Astle CM, Lerner C. Number and continuous proliferative patterns of transplanted primitive immunohematopoietic stem cells. Proc Natl Acad Sci USA 1988;85:822-26.
23. Markowitz D, Goff S, Bank A. A safe packaging line for gene transfer: Separating viral genes on two different plasmids. J Virol 1988;62:1120-24.
24. Danos O, Mulligan RC. Safe and efficient generation of recombinant retroviruses with amphotropic and ecotropic host ranges. Proc Natl Acad Sci USA 1988;85:6460-64.
25. Joyner A, Keller G, Phillips RA, Bernstein A. Retroviruse transfer of a bacterial gene into mouse hematopoietic cells. Nature 1983;305:556-58.
26. Williams DA, Lemischka IR, Nathan DG, Mulligan RC. Introduction of new genetic material into pluripotent stem cells of the mouse. Nature 1984;310:476-80.
27. Apperley JF, Luskey BD, Williams DA. Retroviral gene transfer of human adenosine deaminase in murine hemopoietic cells: Effect of selectable marker sequences on long-term expression. Blood 1991;78:310-17.
28. Cone RD, Weber-Benarous A, Baorto D, Mulligan RC. Regulated expression of a complete human β-globin gene encoded by a transmissable retrovirus vector. Mol Cell Biol 1987;7:887-97.
29. Lerner N, Brigham S, Goff S, Bank A. Human β-globin gene expression after gene transfer using retroviral vectors. DNA 1987;6:573-82.
30. Bender MA, Miller AD, Gelinas RE. Expression of the human β-globin gene after retroviral transfer into murine erythroleukemia cells and human BFU-E cells. Mol Cell Biol 1988;8:1725-35.
31. Karlsson S, Papayannopoulou T, Schweiger SC, Stamatoyannopoulos G, Nienhuis A. Retroviral-mediated transfer of genomic globin genes leads to regulated production of RNA and protein. Proc Natl Acad Sci USA 1987;84: 2411-15.
32. Dzierzak EA, Papayannopoulou T, Mulligan RC. Lineage specific expression of a human β-globin gene in murine bone marrow transplant recipients reconstituted with retrovirus-transduced stem cells. Nature 1988;331:3541-44.
33. Bender MA, Gelinas RE, Miller AD. A majority of mice show long-term expression of the β-globin gene after retroviral transfer into haematopoietic stem cells. Mol Cell Biol 1989;9:1426-36.
34. Grosveld F, Blom van Assendfeldt G, Greaves DR, Kollias G. Position-indepedent high-level expression of the human β-globin gene in transgenic mice. Cell 1987;51:975-85.
35. Higgs DR, Wood WG, Jarman AP, et al. A major positive regulatory region far up-stream of the human α-globin gene locus. Genes Devel 1990;4:1588-1601.
36. Novak U, Harris EAS, Forrester W, Groudine M, Grelin R. High-level β-globin ex-pression after retroviral transfer of locus activation region-containing human β-globin gene derivatives into murine erythroleukaemia cells. Proc Natl Acad Sci USA 1990; 87:3386-90.
37. Chang JC, Liu D, Kan YW. A 36-base-pair core sequence of locus control region enhances retrovirally transferred human β-globin gene expression. Proc Natl Acad Sci USA 1992;89:3107-10.
38. Plavec I, Papayannopoulou T, Maury C, Meyer F. A human β-globin gene fused to the human β-globin gene locus control region is expressed at high levels in erythroid cells of mice engrafted with retrovirus-transduced hematopoietic stem cells. Blood 1993;81:1384-92.

39. Walsh CE, Lieu JM, Miller JL, Nienhuis AW, Samulski RJ. Gene therapy for human haemoglobinopathies. Proc Soc Exp Biol Med 1993;204:289-300.
40. Cheung A, Hoggan MD, Hauswirth WW, Berns KI. Integration of the adeno-associated virus genome into latently infected Detroit-6 cells. J Virol 1980;33:739-48.
41. Smiley JR, Smibert C, Everett RD. Expression of a cellular gene cloned in herpes simplex virus: Rabbit β-globin is regulated as an early viral gene in infected fibroblasts. J Virol 1987;61:2368-77.

THE MOLECULAR BIOLOGY OF BLOOD GROUPS: RELEVANCE TO THE STUDY OF ERYTHROID MATURATION AND THE CLINICAL MANAGEMENT OF HAEMOLYTIC DISEASE OF THE NEWBORN

D.J. Anstee, P.A. Judson

The structure of blood group-active proteins and their antigens

In the past few years rapid advances have been made in our understanding of the molecular background of human blood group antigens. There are 23 different blood group systems found on human red cells. Two of these systems (CH/RG, LE) are not intrinsic to the red cell but acquired from plasma. Four systems (ABO, H, P, LE) are defined by carbohydrate structures and cDNAs corresponding to the glycosyl transferase responsible for ABO, H and LE antigens have been cloned and sequenced (reviewed in Lowe 1993 [1], Anstee, et al 1994a [2]). The antigens of 18 blood group systems are defined by the sequence of proteins which are intrinsic to the red cell. The primary sequence of proteins responsible for the antigens of 15 of these systems is known from sequencing cDNA (reviewed in Anstee 1994 [3]). Partial sequence information is available for the JK (urea transporter) protein [4]. The proteins giving rise to SC and DO antigens have been identified but no sequence information is yet available [5, 6].

Those proteins that have been cloned display a diverse array of structures. In some cases, the function of the proteins is known in other cases the function can be proposed by analogy with structurally homologous proteins of known function. The antigens of the DI, CO, RH, XK and JK systems are located on proteins with multiple membrane traverses. The DI antigens are on band 3, the anion transport protein and CO antigens on the water transporter (CHIP 28, Aquaporin-1 (AQP-CHIP)). The JK antigens are associated with urea transport and, by inference, it would be expected that the RH and XK polypeptide also have membrane transport functions.

Glycophorins which express antigens of the MNS (GPA, GPB) and Gerbich (GPC, GPD) systems have heavily sialylated extracellular domains with no clearly defined function. It seems likely, however, that they serve as a barrier to membrane fusion.

The FY antigens are located on a chemokine receptor whilst the IN antigens are on CD44, a well characterised hyaluronic acid binding glycoprotein. The LW glycoprotein is structurally analogous to the group of integrin binding proteins known as ICAMs (intercellular adhesion molecules). The Xg^a protein has a striking structural similarity with CD99 (syn 12E7, E2) a molecule implicated in cell adhesion, whilst the LU glycoprotein is a novel member of the immunoglobulin superfamily, a family of molecules associated with receptor/cell adhesion functions.

The YT antigens are located on the cell surface enzyme acetylcholinesterase and the Kell protein shares structural homology with zinc metalloendopeptidases. Two proteins CD55 (syn DAF) and CD35 (CR1) which carry the antigens of the Cromer and KN systems respectively, function in the regulation of complement.

The molecular basis of the antigens expressed by these proteins is known in several cases and since this has been reviewed in detail recently (Anstee 1994 [3], Anstee, et al 1994a [2]) only a brief description will be given here. In most cases the molecular basis of blood group antigens on proteins can be traced to a single nucleotide base within a codon which gives rise to a particular amino acid essential for antigen expression. The blood group polymorphisms Di^a/Di^b, Co^a/Co^b, Fy^a/Fy^b, Yt^a/Yt^b and E/e result from such point mutations. Occasionally point mutations can have additional consequences. A point mutation causing the loss of the Dr^a antigen (Cromer blood group system) also allows the use of the cryptic splice site and in so doing results in a dramatically reduced expression of CD55 in the red cell membrane of rare individuals with the Dr(a-) phenotype [7].

Most blood group-active red cell membrane proteins are glycosylated (exceptions are Rh polypeptides, the JK polypeptide and the XK polypeptide). In some cases a single nucleotide base change can alter the glycosylation pattern of a protein and this glycosylation change is also relevant to antigen expression. For example, the rare antigen Wb (Gerbich blood group system) results from a single base change which converts Asn 8 to Ser. This change causes the loss of an N-glycosylation site and the creation of a potential O-glycosylation site [2]. Genetic rearrangements which result in the duplication of exons may also create novel antigenic sites in the translated protein because a novel sequence is generated at the exon-exon boundary. The Ls^a antigen of the Gerbich blood group system is an example of this phenomenon [2]. By far the greatest antigenic complexity of the red cell blood groups is found in the MNS and RH systems. In these cases the complexity derives from the fact that the antigens are the products of at least two adjacent genes (GYPA and GYPB in the MNS system and the CE and D genes in the RH system) and this gives rise to opportunities for non-homologous crossing over and gene conversion. Finally, antigens may be dependent upon protein: protein interactions. The Wr^b antigen is defined by the amino acid sequence of band 3 but is only expressed when band 3 is associated with Glycophorin A [8].

Consideration of the relative abundance of blood group-active proteins reveals that few are expressed at more than 20,000 copies/cell. The most abundant proteins are band 3 and GPA, both of which are expressed at 106 copies/ cell and probably associate together in the membrane. GPB (250,000 copies/ cell) and Rh polypeptides (200,000 copies/cell) probably associate together. The only other major blood group active protein is CHIP-28 which is also expressed at 200,000 copies/cell (50,000 tetramers). In fact, the mature red cell has relatively few major surface proteins and the only major proteins not yet uniquely marked by blood group antigens (although they have ABH-active oligosaccharides) are the glucose transporter (500,000 copies/cell) and the Rh glycoprotein (200,000 copies/cell). The Rh glycoprotein associates in the membrane with Rh polypeptides.

Study of the expression of blood group-active proteins during erythropoiesis may provide useful information concerning the various elements that control erythroid gene expression

Most of the blood group-active red cell proteins described above have a broad tissue distribution. Only band 3, the Rh polypeptides, GPA and GPB could be described as erythroid specific (band 3 and GPA are also found in a minor cell population in the kidney). Band 3/GPA and the Rh complex (Rh polypeptides/ Rh glycoprotein/GPB) appear to be associated in the red cell membrane as functional complexes. GPA facilitates the membrane assembly of band 3 [9]. The Rh complex may be associated with band 3/GPA under certain conditions, for example in South East Asian Ovalocytes (see Anstee, et al 1994b [10] for discussion).

The high abundance and erythroid specificity of the Rh polypeptides, GPA and band 3 make them suitable markers for the study of erythroid genes is controlled by DNA binding proteins, or transcription factor, which respond to extracellular signals. Erythropoietin (EPO) is an important cytokine controlling erythroid maturation. There is an increase in cell surface expression of EPO-receptors (EPO-R) during the BFU-E to CFU-E transition followed by a decreased expression and complete loss by the reticulocyte stage (reviewed in Barber and D'Andrea 1992 [11]). The level of EPO-R transcripts increases proportionally with the level of the major erythroid transcription factor GATA-1 [12]. A useful model for the study of the maturation of human erythroid progenitors is the two-phase liquid culture system [13,14] which has the advantage over conventional cultures in semi-solid media because the cells can be harvested readily for further testing. The procedure is divided into an EPO-independent phase and an EPO-dependent phase. Peripheral blood mononuclear cells from normal individuals are cultured in the presence of a combination of growth factors provided by 5637 bladder carcinoma cell line conditioned medium, for 7 days. The culture is depleted of lymphocytes by treatment with cyclosporin A, and the non-adherent cells cultured in the second phase in the presence of EPO. EPO was shown to induce the up regulation of GATA-1, which peaked on days 7-9 of phase 2, just preceding a rise in globin gene mRNA [15]. We have recently prepared rodent monoclonal antibodies specific for the extracellular domain of human band 3 [16] and used these together with monoclonal antibodies to epitopes on the extra cellular domains of GPA, the Rh polypeptides and the Rh glycoprotein to look at the expression of band 3, GPA and Rh polypeptides in liquid culture using flow cytometry. The results (Figure 1) show a progressive increase in the expression of these proteins to a peak at 9-13 days after EPO is added to the cultures, which mirrors the appearance of haemoglobin. These results are consistent with previous

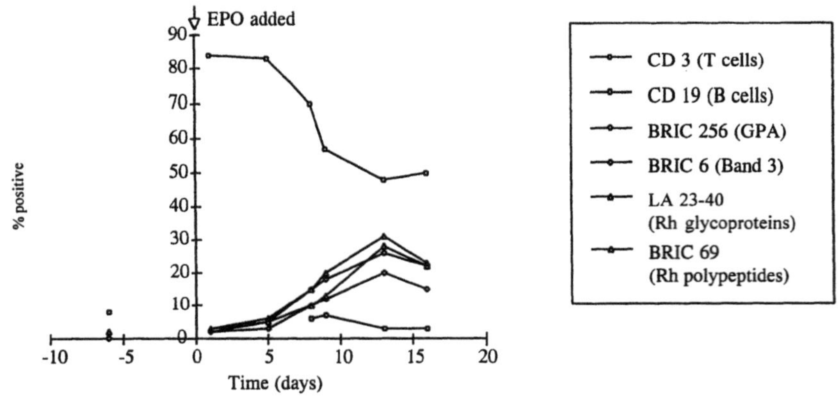

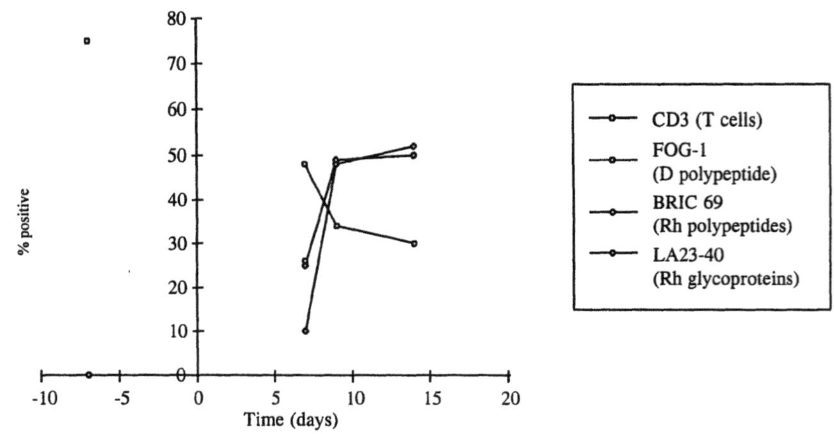

Figure 1. Expression of erythroid cell surface proteins in liquid culture. Two-stage liquid culture of peripheral blood mononuclear cells was set up on day –7. The EPO dependent second stage was started on day 0 and monoclonal antibodies used to measure the time course of the appearance of antigens by flow cytometry. Results for two separate cultures are shown.

reports that GPA and band 3 appearance correlates with appearance of mature erythroblasts (reviewed in Fukuda 1993 [17] and Tanner 1993 [18]), but we have as yet been unable to dissect the finer elements of the timing of the expression of these proteins. The two-phase liquid culture system as well as other *in vitro* models of erythroid development have been used to study the assembly of the membrane skeleton (reviewed by Hanspal and Palek 1992 [19]). These studies suggest that the initiation of band 3 synthesis is a critical step in the assembly of the membrane skeleton (band 3 interacts with the skeleton through ankyrin) and that band 3 synthesis increases dramatically from early to late erythroblasts. The liquid culture system should be of value in providing a source of erythroblasts for the study of the synthesis and assembly of normal and abnormal membrane proteins, and the role of transcription factors.

There are a number of inherited conditions in which abnormal expression of a blood group-active red cell surface protein results not from a structural gene abnormality but from erythroid-specific alterations in regulation of the gene, for example Fy(a-b-) phenotype, Lu(a-b-) phenotype, In(Lu) type. Further analysis of such abnormal cells may provide a useful approach to the elucidation of the various elements that control erythroid gene expression. Investigation of the red cells of an anaemic patient with a novel form of congenital dyserythropoietic anaemia (CDA) characterized by unusual membranous cytoplasmic inclusions in erythroblasts and circulating red cells [20] revealed the unique blood group phenotype In(a-b-) Co(a-b-) [21]. The In blood group antigens are located on the well characterized hyaluronic acid binding protein CD44 [22]. CD44 was shown to be absent from the red cells of this patient but normal levels were found in lymphocytes and granulocytes.

The recent demonstration that CO antigens are located on the water transporter CHIP-28 (AQP-CHIP) [23] allowed for the biochemical investigation of the Co(a-b-) phenotype of this patient and revealed a gross deficiency of CHIP-28 [24]. The patient did not express any obvious renal, neurological, ocular or endothelial disorder suggesting that the CHIP-28 deficiency is limited to red cells. CD44 is encoded by a gene on human chromosome 11p13 [25] whilst CHIP-28 is encoded by AQP-1, a single structural gene on human chromosome 7p14 [26]. The patient also expressed other erythroid abnormalities: persistent expression of ε and ζ embryonic globins and large amounts of $A\gamma$ and $B\gamma$ foetal haemoglobins [27]. These results suggest a fundamental defect in erythroid ontogeny. One possibility suggested by Agre et al [24] is that the patient is homozygous for a mutated form of an erythroid transcription factor which is normally needed to suppress embryonic and foetal globin genes but will induce expression of CD44 and CHIP-28. It is possible that investigation of unusual blood group phenotypes like this which result from erythroid specific abnormalities in gene regulation will further illuminate the mechanisms which regulate erythroid maturation in normal cells.

A clinical application deriving from knowledge of the molecular basis of blood group antigens

The successful elucidation of the molecular basis of several blood group antigens has opened up the possibility of using the polymerase chain reaction (PCR) to determine the blood group genotype of foetuses at risk from haemolytic disease of the newborn (HDN). The antibodies usually responsible for HDN are anti-D with anti-c and anti-K the next most important. The risk of alloimmunization due to anti-D in a subsequent pregnancy has been reduced dramatically by administration of prophylactic anti-D to D negative women after miscarriage, the birth of a D positive baby or obstetric procedures which may cause foetomaternal haemorrhage [28]. Nevertheless, foetomaternal sensitization to anti-D still occurs when prophylaxis is omitted or when foeto-maternal haemorrhage occurs before prophylaxis is given. No prophylactic treatment is available to prevent foeto-maternal sensitisation to other blood group antigens.

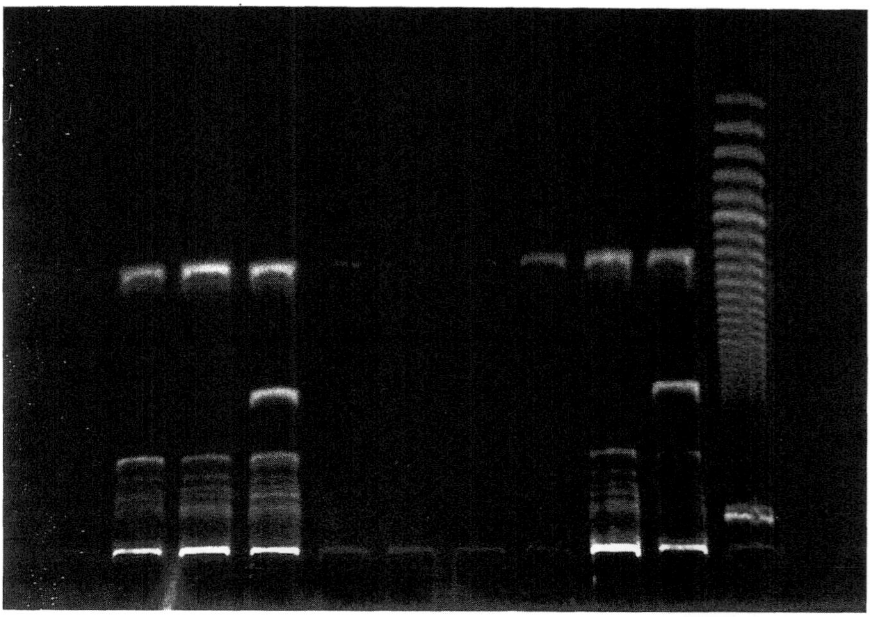

Figure 2. Determination of D type using exon 10.
PCR products were separated on a 6% (w/v) acrylamide gel. Amplicons of 244 bp (exon 10) and 120 bp (exon 5) were obtained. Results for foetal DNA obtained from amniotic fluid of four foetuses, all of which typed as D negative, are shown in tracks 4-7. Results for adults of phenotype -D-, Cde, CDe, cde, cdE are shown in tracks 2, 3, 8, 9 and 10, respectively.

Recently, considerable progress has been made elucidating the genes giving rise to Rh polypeptides (for recent reviews see Cartron and Agre 1993 [29], Anstee and Tanner 1993 [30], Colin et al 1994 [31]). It is clear that there are at least two genes, denoted respectively D gene and CE gene by Colin et al [31]. Southern analysis has suggested that there is a gross deletion of the D gene in most D negative individuals of Caucasian origin, however, this deletion has not yet been precisely defined. It is not yet clear whether a similar deletion of the D gene is responsible for the D negative phenotype in other racial groups. Indeed, there is evidence to suggest that the absence of this gene is not the basis of the D negative phenotype in some Japanese [32], and the black D negative complex cCde^{S} contains an internally deleted D gene in which exon 10 gives a normal PCR product [33]. A PCR assay based on the assumption that exon 10 of the D gene is deleted in all D negative individuals has been developed by Bennett et al. [34] (Figure 2). Simsek et al [35] reported five discrepancies when analysing 200 DNA samples from individuals of known Rh phenotype utilising the method of Bennett et al [34]. Two individuals of phenotype CcDe gave false negative reactions and three of phenotype Cce gave false positive reactions. An alternative PCR method (based on the observation of Arce et al. 1993 [36]) utilised primers targeting intron 4 of the CE gene, (since this intron in the D gene has a large deletion) did not yield discrepancies [35]. A method based on differences between the D and CE genes in their respective exon 7s has also been described [37]. Other authors have noticed the presence of D gene products in individuals of phenotype Ce [38, 39]. Discrepancies in these various assays which are based on selected regions of difference between the CE and D genes are not surprising. D is not an antigen defined by a single amino acid but a term given to a collection of antigens defined by different regions of the polypeptide. Unequal crossover or gene conversion events between the D and CE gene products, partial deletions and regulatory defects could all be anticipated to result in discrepant results when genomic and serological assays are compared. In view of this it would seem prudent to devise PCR assays which measure the presence or absence of several different regions of D gene (multiplex assays) in order to give the most complete picture of the status of the gene in foetuses at potential risk of HDN.

PCR assays for the determination of the c or E antigen status of a foetus at risk from HDN due to anti-c or anti-E respectively, have also been described [40, 41]. These methods rely on the assumption that the critical residues for c and E are defined by two positions on the CE gene at nt 307 (Pro 103) and nt 676 (Pro 226) respectively, and that the corresponding positions in the D gene remain constant. In addition to Rh antibodies, a whole array of other antibody specificities have been implicated as the cause of HDN (anti-K, Fy^a, Fy^b, Jk^a, Jk^b, Di^a, Di^b, Kp^a, k, S, s, U, M, Yt^a, Do^a, Co^a, Wr^a [42]). The molecular basis of many of these antigens is known (Table 1) and that for K will shortly be published (Redman personal communication) and so it should be possible to devise foetal DNA typing methods in most cases of maternal sensitisation should there be evidence that the foetus is at risk. One such case was recently referred to our laboratory for foetal genotyping of FY. The mother presented (22/40) with an anti-Fy^a of titre 1:2048 which gave a chemiluminescence test consistent with moderate to severe HDN. The father was Fy(a+b+). Foetal genotyping was carried out on DNA obtained from amniotic fluid using RFLP analysis since the Fy(a+) sequence has a novel Ban I restriction site [43]. The genotype was Fy(a+b+). The foetus required four intra-uterine transfusions during the course of the pregnancy, was delivered at 27/40 and did receive phototherapy.

In an analysis of three studies (from the USA, UK, Germany) on the prevalence of different immune red cell alloantibodies Mollison 1979 [42] noted that if anti-D is excluded, approximately 50% of the antibodies were anti-c or anti-E, 29% anti-K and 11% anti-Fy^a with all other antibodies comprizing the remaining 10%. It can therefore be anticipated that the major demand for foetal DNA typing at least in European populations will be for D, c, E, K and Fy^a.

Table 1. Critical amino acids defining blood group antigens.

System	Glycoprotein	Antigen	Nature and position of critical amino acid	Reference
FY	FY glycoprotein	Fy^{a}*	Gly (44)	Mallinson et al 1994 [43]
		Fy^{b}*	Asp (44)	
DI	Band 3 (AE-1)	Di^{a}*	Leu (854)	Bruce et al 1994 [44]
		Di^{b}*	Pro (854)	
		Wr^{a}*	Lys (658)	
		Wr^{b}	Glu (658)	
MNS	Glycophorin A	M*	Ser (1)/Gly (5)	Wasniowska et al 1977 [45]
		N	Leu (1)/Glu (5)	
	Glycophorin B	S*	Met (29)	
		s*	Thr (29)	Dahr et al 1982 [46]
YT	Acetylcholinesterase	Yt^{a}*	His (322)	Bartels et al 1992 [47]
		Yt^{b}	Asn (322)	
CO	CHIP-28	Co^{a}*	Ala (45)	Smith et al 1994 [23]
		Co^{b}	Val (45)	

* Antibodies to these antigens have been reported to cause HDN [42].

Acknowledgements

Figure 2 is reproduced from a project report "Molecular genetic analysis of the D gene: use in prenatal diagnosis of foetal D genotype" submitted by Michelle Ayres in partial fulfilment of the requirements for the MSc in Biotechnology, University of the West of England, Bristol. We thank Andrew Hadley, Gary Mallinson and Neil Avent for helpful discussions and Sherrie Ayles for assistance with the preparation of the manuscript.

References

1. Lowe JB. The blood group-specific human glycosyltransferases. In: Tanner MJA, Anstee DJ (eds). The red cell membrane and red cell antigens. Oxford, UK: Baillières Clinical Haematology 1993:465-92.
2. Anstee DJ, Spring FA, Parsons SF, et al. Molecular background of human blood group antigens. In: Tippett P, Hackel E (eds). Human genetics '94, a revolution in full swing. Bethesda MD: American Association of Blood Banks 1994:1-52.
3. Anstee DJ. Blood group antigens defined by the sequences of red cell surface proteins. Transf Med 1995;5:1-13
4. Gunn RB, Gargus JJ, Frohlich O. The Kidd antigens and urea transport. In: Agre P, Cartron JP (eds). Protein blood group antigens of the human red cell. Baltimore: Johns Hopkins 1992:88-100.

5. Spring FA, Herron R, Rowe G. An erythrocyte glycoprotein of apparent Mr 60,000 expresses Sc1 and Sc2 antigens. Vox Sang 1990;58:122-25.
6. Banks J, Hemming NJ, Poole J. Evidence that the Gy^a, Hy and Jo^a antigens belong to the Dombrock blood group system. Vox Sang 1995;68:177-82.
7. Lublin DM, Mallinson G, Poole J, et al. Molecular basis of reduced or absent expression of decay accelerating factor in Cromer blood group phenotypes. Blood 1994;84:1276-82.
8. Bruce LJ, Ring SM, Anstee DJ, Reid ME, Wilkinson S, Tanner MJA. Changes in the blood group Wr (Wright) antigens are associated with a mutation at amino acid 658 in human erythrocyte band 3: A site for interaction between band 3 and glycophorin A in the red cell membrane under certain conditions. Blood 1995;85:541-47.
9. Groves JD, Tanner MJA. Glycophorin A facilitates the expression of human band 3-mediated anion transport in *Xenopus* oocytes. J Biol Chem 1992;267:22163-70.
10. Anstee DJ, Hemming NJ, Tanner MJA. Functional factors in the red cell membrane: Interactions between the membrane and its underlying skeleton. Immunol Invest 1995;24:187-98.
11. Barber DL, D'Andrea AD. The erythropoietin receptor and the molecular basis of signal transduction. Semin Hematol 1992;29:293-304.
12. Zon LI, Youssoufian H, Lodish H, et al. Regulation of the erythropoietin receptor promotor by cell specific transcription factor GATA-1. Blood 1990;76(suppl 1): 174a(abstract 688).
13. Fibach E, Manor D, Oppenheim A, et al. Proliferation and maturation of human erythroid progenitors in liquid culture. Blood 1989;73:100-03.
14. Wada H, Suda T, Miura Y, et al. Expression of major blood group antigens on human erythroid cells in a two-phase liquid culture system. Blood 1990;75:505-11.
15. Daylot N, Fibach E, Ronchi A, Rachmilewitz EA, Ottolengh S, Oppenheim A. Erythropoietin triggers a burst of GATA-1 in normal human erythroid cells differentiating in tissue culture. Nucleic Acids Res 1993;21:4031-37.
16. Smythe J, Gardner B, Spring FA, Anstee DJ. Rat monoclonal antibodies to extracellular epitopes on band 3, the human erythrocyte anion exchange protein. Transf Med 1993;3(suppl 1):(abstract p95).
17. Funkuda M. Molecular genetics of the Glycophorin A gene cluster. Semin Hematol 1993;30:138-51.
18. Tanner MJA. Molecular and cellular biology of the erythrocyte anion exchanger (AE-1). Semin Hematol 1993;30:34-57.
19. Hanspal M, Palek J. Biogenesis of normal and abnormal red blood cell membrane skeleton. Semin Hematol 1992;29:305-19.
20. Wickramasinghe SN, Illum N, Wimberley PD. Congenital dyserythropoietic anaemia with novel intra-erythroblastic and intra-erytrocytic inclusions. Brit J Haematol 1991;79:322-30.
21. Parsons SF, Jones J, Anstee DJ, et al. A novel form of congenital dyserythropoietic anaemia associated with deficiency of erythroid CD44 and a unique blood group phenotype [In(a-b-), Co(a-b-)]. Blood 1994;83:860-68.
22. Spring FA, Dalchau R, Daniels GL, et al. The In^a and In^b blood group antigens are located on a glycoprotein of 80,000 MW (the CDw44 glycoprotein) whose expression is influenced by the In(Lu) gene. Immunology 1988;64:37-43.
23. Smith BL, Preston GM, Spring FA, Anstee DJ, Agre P. Human red cell Aquaporin CHIP. I. Molecular characterisation of ABH and Colton blood group antigens. J Clin Invest 1994;94:1043-49.

24. Agre P, Smith BL, Baumgarten R, et al. Human red cell Aquaporin CHIP. II. Expression during normal fetal development and in a novel form of congenital dyserythropoietic anaemia. J Clin Invest 1994;94:1050-58.
25. Goodfellow PN, Banting G, Wiles WV, et al. The gene MIC4, which controls expression of the antigen defined by monoclonal antibody F10.44.2 is on human chromosome 11. Eur J Immunol 1982;12:659-63.
26. Moon C, Preston GM, Griffin C, Jabs EW, Agre P. The human Aquaporin gene: Structure, organisation and chromosomal location. J Biol Chem 1993;268:15772-78.
27. Tang W, Cai S-P, Eng MC, et al. Expression of embryonic ζ-globin chains in a 10 year old girl with congenital anaemia. Blood 1993;81:1636-40.
28. Clarke CA, Whitfield AG, Mollison PL. Deaths from Rh haemolytic disease in England and Wales in 1984 and 1985. Brit Med J 1987;294:1001.
29. Cartron J-P, Agre P. Rh blood group antigens: Protein and gene strucutre. Semin Hematol 1993;30:193-208.
30. Anstee DJ, Tanner MJA. Biochemical aspects of blood group Rh (Rhesus) antigens in red cell membrane and red cell antigens. In: Tanner MJA, Anstee DJ (eds). Oxford, UK: Baillières Clinical Haematology 1993;6.1:401-22.
31. Colin Y, Bailly P, Cartron J-P. Molecular genetic basis of RH and LW blood groups. Vox Sang 1994;67(suppl 3):67-72.
32. Umenishi F, Kajii E, Ikemoto S. Molecular analysis of Rh polypeptides in a family with Rh D positive and Rh D negative phenotypes. Biochem J 1994; 299:207-11.
33. Blunt T, Daniels GL, Carritt B. Serotype switching in a partially deleted Rh *D* gene. Vox Sang 1994;67:397-401.
34. Bennett PR, Le van Kim C, Colin Y, et al. Prenatal determination of fetal Rh D type by DNA amplification. New Engl J Med 1993;329:607-10.
35. Simsek S, Bleeker PMM, von dem Borne AEGKr. Prenatal determination of fetal Rh D type. New Engl J Med 1994;330:795.
36. Arce MA, Thompsom ES, Wagner S, et al. Molecular cloning of Rh D cDNA derived from gene present in Rh D positive but not Rh D negative individuals. Blood 1993;82: 651-55.
37. Wolter LC, Hyland CA. Rhesus D genotyping using polymerase chain reaction. Blood 1993;82:1682-83.
38. Carritt B, Steers FJ, Avent ND. Prenatal determination of fetal Rh D type. Lancet 1994;344:205-6.
39. Hyland CA, Wolter LC, Saul A. Three unrelated Rh *D* gene polymorphisms identified among blood donors with Rhesus CCee (r′r′) phenotypes. Blood 1994;84:321-24.
40. Faas BHW, Simsek S, Bleeker PMM, et al. Rh E genotyping by polymerase chain reaction amplication with sequence specific primers (PCR-SSP). Vox Sang 1994;67(suppl 2):1(abstract 0003).
41. Le van Kim C, Mouro I, Brossard Y, Chavinie J, Cartron J-P, Colin Y. PCR-based determination of Rh c and Rh E status of fetuses at risk of Rh c and Rh E haemolytic disease. Brit J Haematol 1994;88:193-95.
42. Mollison PL. Blood transfusion in clinical medicine. 7th ed. Blackwell, Oxford, 1979:668.
43. Mallinson G, Soo K, Anstee DJ. The molecular basis of the Fy^a and Fy^b antigens. Transf Med 1994;4(suppl 1):45(abstract p69).
44. Bruce LJ, Anstee DJ, Spring FA, Tanner MJA. Band 3 Memphis Variant II: Altered stilbenedisulphonate binding and the Diego (Di^a) blood group antigen are associated with the human erythrocyte band 3 mutation Pro 854→Leu. J Biol Chem1994;269:

16155-58.

45. Wasniowska K, Drzeniek Z, Lisowska E. The amino acids of M and N blood group glycopeptides are different. Biochem Biophys Res Comm 1977;76:385-90.
46. Dahr W, Beyreuther K, Kardowicz M, Kruger J. N-terminal amino acid sequence of sialoglycoprotein D (Glycophorin C) from human erythrocyte membranes. Eur J Biochem 1982;125:57-62.
47. Bartels CF, Zelinski T, Lockridge O. Mutation of codon 322 in the human acetylcholinesterase gene (AChE) accounts for the Yt blood group polymorphism. Amer J Hum Genet 1993;52:928-36.

GENETIC ABNORMALITIES IN BLOOD GROUP SEROLOGY

M.E. Reid

Introduction

Laboratory and clinical investigation of red blood cell (RBC) incompatibility between patient and donor in the context of transfusion has led to the identification of blood groups whose expression is genetically determined. Blood group antigens are polymorphic, inherited, structural characteristics that are located on proteins, glycoproteins or glycolipids on the exofacial surface of the RBC membrane.

For decades, blood group antigens have been recognized to be clinically important in the immune destruction of RBCs in allogeneic blood transfusions, maternofoetal blood group incompatibility, autoimmune haemolytic anaemia and organ transplantation. The polymorphism of blood groups has been exploited as a tool to monitor *in vivo* survival of transfused RBCs either by differential haemagglutination or flow cytometry. By virtue of their relative ease of detection by haemagglutination and generally straightforward mode of inheritance, blood group antigens have been used in genetic, forensic and anthropological investigations. Blood group antigen profiles have been used to predict inheritance of diseases that are encoded in close proximity to the gene encoding the blood group antigen. The presence or absence of certain antigens has been implicated in susceptibility or resistance to certain diseases.

The persistence of blood group loci in evolution suggests that blood group antigens are located on biologically important structures. These antigens have been used as markers of polymorphisms and anomalies in inheritance to identify samples for study. Molecular biology and immunochemical analysis on appropriate samples have revealed knowledge about the structure and function of RBC membrane components on which the antigens are carried. These studies have also revealed genetic abnormalities as a consequence of gene rearrangements which can serve as models for other systems.

Table 1. Blood group systems.

Name	Number antigens	Gene product	Chromosomal location	Possible function
ABO	4	Glycosyltransferase	9q34	Glyclosylation
P	1	Glycosyltransferase	22q11-qter	Glyclosylation
Lewis	3	Glycosyltransferase	19p	Glyclosylation
Hh	1	Glycosyltransferase	19q	Glyclosylation
MNS	37	Glycophorin A,B	4q28-q31	SA/receptor
Gerbich	7	Glycophorin C,D	2q14-q21	SA/receptor
Duffy	6	Fy glycoprotein	1q22-q23	Receptor
Kell	21	Kell glycoprotein	7q33	Enzyme
Yt	2	Acetylcholinesterase	7q22	Enzyme
Diego	4	Band 3 (AE1)	17q12-q21	Transport
Colton	3	CHIP	7p14	Transport
Kidd	3	Jk glycoprotein	18q11-q12	Transport
Rh	45	CcEe and D polypeptides	1p36-p3	Transport
Lutheran	18	Lutheran glycoprotein	19q13.2	Adhesion
LW	3	LW glycoprotein	19p13	Adhesion
Indian	2	CD44	11p13	Adhesion
Xg	1	Xg^a glycoprotein	Xp22.3	Adhesion
Cromer	10	CD55 (DAF)	1q32	Complement regulation
Knops	5	CD35 (CRI)	1q32	Complement regulation
Chido/Rodgers	9	C′ component 4 (C4)	6p21.3	Complement regulation
Kx	1	Kx glycoprotein	Xp21.1	Unknown
Scianna	3	Sc glycoprotein	1p34-p32	Unknown
Dombrock	5	Do glycoprotein	not known	Unknown

SA = Sialic acid; CHIP = Channel-forming integral protein

Blood group antigens

Over 250 distinct antigens have been recognized by the Working Party on Terminology for RBC Surface Antigens of the International Society of Blood Transfusion([1]; committee meeting minutes; ISBT meeting, July 1994). Almost 200 of these antigens are accommodated within 23 blood group systems (Table 1) while the others are found either on RBCs of nearly all individuals (high prevalence of public antigens) or occur rarely (low prevalence or private antigens). Four of the blood group systems (MNS, Rh, Lutheran and Kell) are highly polymorphic and all the chromosomal locations have been determined.

Recently, many genes encoding the proteins that carry blood group antigens have been cloned and sequenced [reviewed in 2] and in some instances the amino acid substitutions giving rise to blood group polymorphisms have been determined. As described in the previous chapter, this knowledge is being used in the clinical laboratory for such applications as the prenatal determination of foetuses at risk for haemolytic disease of the newborn. Determination of a predicted antigen-negative status of a foetus on amniocytes at 12 weeks gestation would prevent the need to frequently monitor by amniotic fluid and blood sampling. The genes still to be cloned are those encoding the proteins carrying

Table 2. Size and orientation of integral RBC membrane components carrying blood group antigens.

Antigens	Proteins	Amino acid residues	Orientation of *N*-terminus
Single spanning proteins			
M,N	GPA	131	Exofacial
S,s	GPB	72	Exofacial
Ge3	GPC	128	Exofacial
Ge2	GPD	107	Exofacial
Kell	Kell	732	Cytoplasmic
IN	CD44	341	Exofacial
LW	LW	241	Exofacial
LU	Lutheran	597	Exofacial
KN	CD35 (CR1)	1998	Exofacial
Xg^a	XG	180	Exofacial
Glycosylphosphatidylinositol-linked proteins			
YT	AChE	557	Exofacial
CR	CD55 (DAF)	347	Exofacial

Polytopic proteins

Antigens	Proteins	Amino acid residues	Predicted no. of spans	Orientation	
				N-terminus	*C*-terminus
RH	RhD	416	12	Cytoplasmic	Cytoplasmic
	RhCcEe	416	12	Cytoplasmic	Cytoplasmic
	Rh glycoprotein	409	12	Cytoplasmic	Cytoplasmic
FY	Duffy	338	9	Exofacial	Cytoplasmic
DI	Band 3	911	14	Cytoplasmic	Cytoplasmic
CO	CHIP	269	6	Cytoplasmic	Cytoplasmic

antigens in the Kidd, Dombrock and Scianna blood group systems. A candidate gene for the McLeod phenotype has been cloned but it is not known whether it encodes Kx antigen [3]. The deduced amino acid sequence of proteins carrying blood group antigens has provided a key to their potential functions (Table 1) and structure (Table 2) [4-20]. As shown in Table 2, eight of the blood group systems are carried on single-spanning proteins, only one of which is oriented with its *C*-terminus to the exofacial (outside) surface of the RBC membrane. Two systems are carried on glycosylphosphatidylinositol (GPI) linked proteins and four are carried on polytopic proteins.

Blood Group Systems Null Phenotypes

A majority of the blood group systems have a null phenotype that is due to the absence of carbohydrate or protein from the RBC membrane. Carbohydrate antigens do not appear to be of vital importance to the integrity of the RBC membrane since their absence does not compromise the cell. Thus, RBCs of the rare Bombay (O_h) phenotype in the ABO blood group system lack the immunodominant carbohydrates that confer A, B and H antigens but have normal morphology, function and *in vivo* survival [21]. In contrast, RBCs that lack certain proteins may have altered morphology and function. For example, RBCs with the rare Rh_{null} phenotype lack proteins expressing antigens in the Rh blood group system and have stomatocytic morphology, possible abnormality of membrane potassium and sodium transport, and reduced *in vivo* survival [21-25]. RBCs with the McLeod phenotype lack the Kx protein, are acanthocytic and have a reduced *in vivo* survival [26, 27]. RBCs with the dominant type Lu(a-b-) phenotype also may be acanthocytic [28] while a proportion of RBCs with the Gerbich-negative Leach phenotype are elliptocytic [29-33]. This is now thought to be due more to a slight reduction of the RBC membrane skeletal protein 4.1, which interacts with the glycophorins, than to the absence of glycophorin C (GPC) and glycophorin D (GPD) [34, 35].

The knowledge gained by molecular analysis has broadened our understanding of the pathogenesis of RBC disorders associated with blood group null phenotypes. Some null phenotypes are notorious in that the absence of the protein(s) on which the antigens are carried has no known detrimental effect on the integrity of the RBC. RBCs with En(a-), U- or M^kM^k phenotypes lack, respectively, glycophorin A (GPA), glycophorin B (GPB) or both. The cells are normocytic and have a normal *in vivo* survival. The RBCs lacking GPA have an increased glycosylation of protein band 3 [reviewed in 36]. RBCs with the Ko phenotype lack the Kell glycoprotein and the only observed membrane change is an increased expression of the Kx antigen [reviewed in 27]. RBCs with the recessive type of Lu(a-b-) phenotype have no known alterations [37]. Other normocytic RBCs with null phenotype include Co(a-b-) which have a reduced osmotic water permeability [38], Jk(a-b-) RBCs which resist lysis in urea [39], INAB RBCs which may have an increased susceptibility to complement lysis [40, 41] and Fy(a-b-) RBCs which resist invasion by *Plasmodium vivax* and *Plasmodium knowlesi* [reviewed in 42]. Of these null phenotypes, the molecular basis of En(a-), U-, M^kM^k, Leach, Co(a-b-) and INAB phenotypes has been published and will be described below.

There are examples where, although RBCs serotype as null phenotypes, they actually possess reduced quantities of the protein on which the blood group is carried. JMH-negative RBCs have small amounts of 76-kDa JMH protein and in two families this phenotype has been associated with congenital dyserythropoietic anaemia (CDA) [43]. One individual whose RBCs type as In(a-b-), Co(a-b-) has a novel form of CDA [44] and has been described in the previous

Table 3. In vivo and *in vitro* changes associated with null phenotypes of blood groups carried on integral RBC proteins.

Phenotype	Protein	Morphology	*In vivo/in vitro* changes
En(a-)	Absent GPA	Normocytic	Hyperglycosylation of band 3
U-	Absent GPA	Normocytic	Possible resistance to malaria
M^kM^k	Absent GPA and GPB	Normocytic	Hyperglycosylation of band 3
Ko	Absent Kell glycoprotein	Normocytic	Increased Kx
Lu(a-b-)	Absent Lu protein	Normocytic	Not known
Co(a-b-)	Absent CHIP	Normocytic	Reduced osmotic water permeability
Jk(a-b-)	Not known	Normocytic	Resist lysis in urea, inability to maximally concentrate urine
Fy(a-b-)	Absent Fy glycoprotein	Normocytic	Resist invasion by some malarial parasites
INAB	Absent CD55 (DAF)	Normocytic	Increased sensitivity to C′ *in vitro*
K_{mod}	Down-regulated Kell glycoprotein	Normocytic	Increased Kx
JMH-	Down-regulated JMH protein	Normocytic	Associated with CDA in 2 families
IN(a-b-)/C0(a-b-)	Down-regulated CD55 and aquaporin-1	Normocytic	Associated with CDA in 1 person
Lu(a-b-) (dominant type)	Down-regulated Lu, CD44 CD44, AnWj, MER2	Acanthocytic	*In vitro* storage defect
Rh_{mod}	Down-regulated Rh polypeptides	Stomatocytic	Mild haemolytic anaemia
Rh_{null}	Absent Rh, Rh-related and LW polypeptides and down-regulated GPB	Stomatocytic	Mild haemolytic anaemia
McLeod	Absent Kx protein	Acanthocytic	Weakened expression of Kell antigens; reduced cell survival; late onset muscular dystrophy
Leach	Absent GPC and GPD	Elliptocytic	Slightly reduced protein 4.1; slightly reduced survival

CDA = Congenital dyserythropoietic anaemia.

chapter. RBCs with the dominant Lu(a-b-) phenotype have reduced expression of Lutheran, In^a and In^b (carried on CD44), AnWj and MER2 antigens [reviewed in 45]. These Lu(a-b-) RBCs may be acanthocytic [28]. K_{mod} RBCs, which have a weak expression of Kell antigens, are also normocytic and have no known clinical manifestation [8]. Similarly, Rh_{mod} RBCs have a weak expression of Rh antigens [reviewed in 25]. The underlying genetic events giving rise to these down-regulated proteins are not understood but are under intense investigation.

Three null phenotypes result in reduced *in vivo* RBC survival with accompanying mild haemolytic anaemia. RBCs with these phenotypes (Rh_{null}, McLeod and Leach) are, respectively, stomatocytes, acanthocytes and elliptocytes. The genetic events giving rise to the Rh_{null} phenotype are being studied but as yet have not been fully resolved. It is apparent, however, that genes encoding D, Cc and Ee antigens are deleted, inactive or poorly functioning [6]. It is thought that the McLeod phenotype arises from a deletion of a part of the X-chromosome that includes the gene encoding the Kx antigen [reviewed in 27]. A candidate gene for the McLeod phenotype has been cloned but it has not yet been established that it encodes Kx antigen [3]. Two mechanisms have been described that give rise to the Leach phenotype [35, 46-48] an will be described below. A summary of observed *in vivo* and *in vitro* changes associated with null phenotypes of blood group antigens carried on red blood cell membrane proteins is given in Table 3.

Molecular basis of some null phenotypes

En(a-)Fin, U- and M^kM^k phenotypes

Genes encoding GPA and GPB are homologous and adjacent on chromosome 4. These glycophorins carry MNS blood group system antigens and the associated null phenotypes lack GPA, GPB or both. The GPA gene has seven exons while the GPB gene has six exons, of which exon 3 is a pseudo or non-coding exon. Next to the GPB gene is the GPE gene, the product of which has not been shown conclusively to be present in the RBC membrane. The GPE gene has a genomic structure similar to the GPB gene and is also composed of six exons, of which exons 3 and 4 are pseudoexons. Exon 1 and part of exon 2 from these 3 genes encode a leader sequence that is cleaved from the mature membrane-bound protein. A deletion of exons A2-A7 and exon B1 gives rise to the rare En(a-)Fin phenotype. RBCs with this null phenotype lack GPA and, thus, all antigenic determinants carried on GPA. Similarly, deletion of exons B2-B6 and exons E1 precludes production of GPB and RBCs from such individuals have the S-s-U-phenotype. A larger deletion that includes exons A2-A7, B1-B6 and E1 results in the M^kM^k genotype which is the true null phenotype of the MNS blood group system. In all three, genomic DNA has been studied by Southern blot hybridization but the causes for the deletions have not been reported. There is a vast literature on the molecular genetics of this family of glycophorin genes and the reader is referred to recent reviews [36, 49, 50].

Leach phenotype

RBCs with the Leach phenotype lack GPC and GPD and, thus, all Gerbich blood group antigens which are carried on one or both of these glycophorins. There are two mechanisms that give rise to this phenotype: a deletion of exons 3 and 4, and a nucleotide substitution and a nucleotide deletion at positions 131 and 134, respectively [35, 36, 46, 47, 51, 52].

Southern blot analysis of genomic DNA from three unrelated individuals with the Leach phenotype (PL, JC, MWB) revealed a deletion of 7-kilobases that encompass exons 3 and 4 [35, 46, 47, 51]. In one study [51], mRNA was detected in circulating reticulocytes and a 140-bp fragment was amplified when using primers spanning exons 1 and 2. No polymerase chain reaction (PCR) products were detected in this Leach phenotype using primers flanking either exons 1 and 3 or exons 1 and 4. When the Leach cDNA fragment was cloned and sequenced, the nucleotide sequence was identical to that of normal GPC cDNA. Although the mRNA could encode an *N*-terminal fragment of GPC, this protein isoform(s) would not be expressed in the membrane because it lacks the transmembrane and cytoplasmic domains.

A fourth individual with Leach phenotype RBCs (LN) had GPC mRNA of normal size on Northern blots and a normal map of genomic DNA by Southern analysis using the restriction enzymes Pst1, Bam HI and Hind III [35]. In contrast, the restriction map using Msp1 was different from the normal control. PCR amplification of mRNA from the donors lymphocytes and subsequent sequencing revealed two significant mutations: G^{131} to T^{131} substitution changed Trp^{44} to Leu^{44}; and a C^{134} deletion changed Pro^{45} to Arg^{45}. This single nucleotide deletion caused a -1 frameshift and a premature stop codon (TAA) at codon 55. If the mRNA is translated, it would be predicted to produce a protein consisting of 55 amino acid residues which would lack the transmembrane and cytoplasmic domains of GPC. This product has not been found on the RBC surface. Interestingly, RBCs from LN have been shown to have a low molecular weight protein, possessing the epitope recognized by a monoclonal antibody to the *C*-terminus of GPC [53, 54]. This protein stably associates with the membrane. When RBC membranes from LN were extracted at low ionic strength to dissociate the membrane skeleton, approximately half of the protein 4.1 content was liberated, compared to a quarter from normal RBC membranes and nearly three quarters from RBCs with the other Leach phenotype (PL). These results suggest that GPC and GPD may contain two types of binding site for protein 4.1; one sensitive to proteases and the other resistant. It is possible that the GPC gene in LN has a novel consensus sequence such that a truncated protein with the *C*-terminal sequence of GPC is transcribed and translated. This is an example where an RBC with a null phenotype has a grossly normal gene as determined by Northern blot analysis and by Southern blot analysis using several restriction enzymes.

INAB phenotype

Studies on genomic DNA and mRNA, prepared from peripheral blood of the original INAB proband, explain the lack of the RBC membrane decay-accelerating factor (DAF, CD55) in this individual [55]. A single nucleotide substitution (G to A) at position 314 resulted in Trp^{53} (TGG) changing to a stop codon (TGA). Thus, this truncated protein lacks the carboxyl-terminal signal for GPI anchoring. RBCs that lack DAF have an *in vitro* increased susceptibility to lysis [40, 56].

Co(a-b-) phenotype

Preston et al [38] have recently shown that rare humans who lack Co^a and Co^b blood group antigens also lack RBC channel-forming integral protein (CHIP) because of mutations in aquaporin-1. These workers obtained blood samples and urine sediment from one Co(a-b-) member of three kindred and have identified three different mutations. Aquaporin-1 from proband 1 had a deletion of exon 1 and, thus, a translation failure. Aquaporin-1 from proband 2 had a nucleotide insertion (T) at position 307 resulting in a frame-shift after Gly^{104} and a major disruption in CHIP structure. Aquaporin-1 from proband 3 had a nucleotide substitution of C to T at position 113 in Leu replacing Pro^{38}. Residue 38 is located at the end of the first lipid bilayer spanning α-helix and either Pro or Gly at this position is likely to be a structural requirement of CHIP and related proteins. This mutation encodes a non-functioning CHIP molecule, a small amount of which is present in RBCs from proband 3. In transfection experiments, two days after *Xenopus* oocytes were injected with cDNA from proband 3 or a normal individual, mutant CHIP was expressed in slightly lower amounts than was the normal CHIP control. After three days, the amount of the mutant CHIP in the oocytes was substantially reduced compared to the normal controls and may explain the small amount of CHIP in RBCs from proband 3.

RBCs from all three probands had an osmotic water permeability at 37°C that was approximately 80% of normal. Since none of the Co(a-b-) individuals suffer from haematological, renal, ocular, respiratory, gastrointestinal, reproductive or neurological dysfunction, it implies that other mechanisms compensate for the absence of CHIP.

Conclusion

The molecular basis of the blood group null phenotypes described above, illustrates that, in some cases, a single nucleotide substitution can have a profound effect on the integrity of the RBC. In the clinical laboratory, the molecular understanding can have valuable applications in the prenatal diagnosis of foetuses at risk for haemolytic disease of the newborn, genotype determination in paternity or forensic cases, antigen typing when sera are poorly reactive or not generally available and antigen typing of recently transfused patients. Further, cDNA from appropriate genes transfected into carried cell systems and have potential utility in the identification of blood group antibodies in the absorption of unwanted antibodies to provide an absorbed serum sample suitable for compatibility testing.

References

1. Lewis M, Anstee DJ, Bird GWG, et al. Blood group terminology 1990. Vox Sang 1990;58:152-59.

2. Telen MJ, Rao N. Recent advances in immunohematology. Curr Opinion in Hematol 1994;1:143-50.
3. Ho M, Chelly J, Carter N, Danek A, Crocker P, Monaco AP. Isolation of the gene for McLeod syndrome that encodes a novel membrane transport protein. Cell 1994; 77:869-80.
4. Anstee DJ. Blood group-active surface molecules of the human red blood cell. Vox Sang 1990;58:1-20.
5. Anstee DJ, Mallinson G. The biochemistry of blood group antigens. Some recent advances. Vox Sang 1994;67(suppl 3):1-6.
6. Colin Y, Bailly P, Cartron J-P. Molecular genetic basis of RH and LW blood groups. Vox Sang 1994;67(suppl 3):67-72.
7. Cherif-Zahar B, Bloy C, Le van Kim C, et al. Molecular cloning and protein structure of a human blood group Rh polypeptide. Proc Natl Acad Sci USA 1990;87:6243-47.
8. Le van Kim C, Mouro I, Cherif-Zahar B, et al. Molecular cloning and primary structure of the human blood group RhD polypeptide. Proc Natl Acad Sci USA 1992;89:10925-29.
9. Avent N, Ridgwell K, Tanner MJA, Anstee DJ. cDNA cloning of a 30 kD erythrocyte membrane protein associated with Rh (rhesus)-blood-group-antigen expression. Biochem J 1990;271:821-25.
10. Chaudhuri A, Polyakova J, Zbrzezna V, Williams K, Gulati S, Pogo AO. Cloning of glycoprotein D cDNA, which encodes the major subunit of the Duffy blood group system and the receptor for the *Plasmodium vivax* malaria parasite. Proc Natl Sci Acad USA 1993;90:10793-97.
11. Bartels CF, Zelinski T, Lockridge O. Mutation at codon 322 in the human acetylcholinesterase (ACHE) gene accounts for the YT blood group polymorphism. Am J Hum Genet 1993;53:928-36.
12. Preston GM, Agre P. Isolation of the cDNA for erythrocyte integral membrane protein of 28 kilodaltons: Member of an ancient channel family. Proc Natl Acad Sci USA 1991;88:11110-14.
13. Smith BL, Preston GM, Spring FA, Anstee DJ, Agre P. Human red cell aquaporin CHIP. 1. Molecular characterization of ABH and Colton blood group antigens. J Clin Invest 1994;94:1043-49.
14. Medof ME, Lublin DM, Holers VM, et al. Cloning and characterization of cDNAs encoding the complete sequence of decay-accelerating factor of human complement. Proc Natl Acad Sci USA 1987;84:2007-11.
15. Caras IW, Davitz MA, Rhee L, Weddell G, Martin DW jr, Nussenzweig V. Cloning of decay-accelerating factor suggests novel use of splicing to generate two proteins. Nature 1987;325:545-49.
16. Lee S, Zambas E, Marsh WL, Redman CM. Molecular cloning and primary structure of Kell blood group protein. Proc Natl Acad Sci USA 1991;88:6353-57.
17. Spring FA, Bruce LJ, Anstee DJ, Tanner MJA. A red cell band 3 variant with altered stilbene disulphonate binding is associated with the Diego (Di^a) blood group antigen. Biochem J 1992;288:713-16.
18. Parsons SF, Mawby WJ, Anstee DJ. Lutheran blood group glycoprotein is a member of the immunoglobulin superfamily of proteins. Vox Sang 1994;67(suppl 2):1.
19. Ellis NA, Ye T-Z, Patton S, German J, Goodfellow PN, Weller P. Cloning of *PBDX*, an MIC2-related gene that spans the pseudoautosomal boundary on chromosome Xp. Nature Genet 1994;6:394-400.

20. Ellis NA, Tippett P, Petty A, et al. *PBDX* is the *XG* blood group gene. Nature Genet 1994;8:285-90.
21. Schmidt PJ, Vos GH. Multiple phenotype abnormalities associated with Rh_{null} (---/---). Vox Sang 1967;13:18-20.
22. Nash R, Shojania AM. Hematological aspect of Rh deficiency syndrome: A case report and a review of the literature. Am J Hematol 1987;24:267-74.
23. Lauf PK, Joiner CH. Increased potassium transport and ouabain binding in human Rh_{null} red blood cells. Blood 1976;48:457-68.
24. Ballas SK, Clark MR, Mohandas N, et al. Red cell membrane and cation deficiency in Rh_{null} syndrome. Blood 1984;63:1046-55.
25. Lauf PK. Membrane transport changes in Rh_{null} erythrocytes. In: Stean EA (ed). Cellular antigens and disease. Washington DC: American Association of Blood 1977:41.
26. Wimer BM, Marsh WL, Taswell HF, Galey WR. Haematological changes associated with the McLeod phenotype of the Kell blood group system. Brit J Haematol 1977; 36:219-24.
27. Marsh WL, Redman CM. Recent developments in the Kell blood group system. Transf Med Rev 1987;1:4-13.
28. Udden MM, Umeda M, Hirano Y, Marcus DM. New abnormalities in the morphology, cell surface receptors, and electrolyte metabolism of *In(Lu)* erythrocytes. Blood 1987;69:52-57.
29. Anstee DJ, Parsons SF, Ridgwell K, et al. Two individuals with elliptocytic red cells apparently lack three minor red cell membrane sialoglycoproteins. Biochem J 1984; 218:615-19.
30. Daniels GL, Shaw M-A, Judson PA, et al. A family demonstrating inheritance of the Leach phenotype: A Gerbich negative phenotype associated with elliptocytosis. Vox Sang 1986;50:117-22.
31. Reid ME, Martynewycz M-A, Wolford EE, Crawford MN, Miller LH. Leach type Ge-red cells and elliptocytosis. Transfusion 1987;27:213-14(letter).
32. Rountree J, Chen J, Moulds MK, Moulds JJ, Green AM, Telen MJ. A second family demonstrating inheritance of the Leach phenotype. Transfusion 1989;29(suppl): 15S(abstract).
33. McShane K, Chung A. A novel human alloantibody in the Gerbich system. Vox Sang 1989;57:205-8.
34. Discher D, Knowles D, McGee S, et al. Mechanical linkage between red cell skeleton and plasma membrane is not a demonstrated function of protein 4.1. Blood 1993;82 (suppl 1):309a.
35. Telen MJ, Le van Kim C, Chung A, Cartron J-P, Colin Y. Molecular basis for elliptocytosis associated with glycophorin C deficiency in the Leach phenotype. Blood 1991;78:1603-6.
36. Cartron J-P, Rahuel C. Human erythrocyte glycophorins: Protein and gene structure analysis. Transf Med Rev 1992;6:63-92.
37. Daniels G. The Lutheran blood group system: Monoclonal antibodies, biochemistry and the effect of In(Lu). In: Pierce SR, Macpherson CR (eds). Blood group systems: Duffy, Kidd and Lutheran. Arlington, VA: American Association of Blood Banks 1986:133.
38. Preston GM, Smith BL, Zeidel ML, Moulds JJ, Agre P. Mutations in aquaporin-1 in phenotypically normal humans without functional CHIP water channels. Science 1994; 265:1585-87.

39. Heaton DC, McLoughlin K. Jk(a-b-) red blood cells resist urea lysis. Transfusion 1982;22:70-2.
40. Telen MJ, Green AM. The Inab phenotype: Characterization of the membrane protein and complement regulatory defect. Blood 1989;47:437-42.
41. Tate CG, Uchikawa M, Tanner MJA, et al. Studies on the defect which causes absence of decay accelerating factor (DAF) from the peripheral blood cells of an individual with the Inab phenotype. Biochem J 1989;261:489-95.
42. Hadley TJ, Miller LH, Haynes JD. Recognition of red cells by malaria parasites: The role of erythrocyte-binding proteins. Transf Med Rev 1991;5:108-13.
43. Bobolis KA, Lande WM, Telen MJ. Markedly weakened expression of JMH in a kindred with congenital hemolytic anemia. Transfusion 1991;31(suppl):46S.
44. Parsons SF, Jones J, Anstee DJ, et al. A novel form of congenital dyserythropoietic anemia associated with deficiency of erythroid CD44 and unique blood group phenotype [Inab(a-b-), Co(a-b-)]. Blood 1994;83:860-68.
45. Tippett P. Regulator genes affecting red cell antigens. Transf Med Rev 1990;4:56-68.
46. Tanner MJA, High S, Martin PG, et al. Genetic variants of human red cell membrane sialoglycoprotein β. Study of the alterations occurring in the sialoglycoprotein β gene. Biochem J 1988;250:407-14.
47. High S, Tanner MJA, Macdonald EB, et al. Rearrangements of the red cell membrane glycophorin C (sialoglycoprotein β) gene. Biochem J 1989;262:47-54.
48. Chang S, Reid ME, Conboy J, Kan KW. Molecular characterization of erythrocyte glycophorin C variants. Blood 1991;77:644-48.
49. Fuduka M. Molecular genetics of the glycophorin A gene cluster. Semin Hematol 1993;30:138-51.
50. Reid ME. Some concepts relating to the molecular genetic basis of certain MNS blood group antigens. Transf med 1994;4:99-111.
51. Winardi R, Reid M, Conboy J, Mohandas N. Molecular analysis of glycophorin C deficiency in human erythrocytes. Blood 1993;81:2799-803.
52. Reid ME, Spring FA. Molecular basis of glycophorin C variants and their associated blood group antigens. Transf Med 1994;4:139-49.
53. Cartron J-P, Le van Kim C, Colin Y. Glycophorin C and related glycophorins: Structure, function and regulation. Semin Hematol 1993;30:152-68.
54. Pinder JC, Chung A, Reid ME, Gratzer WB. Membrane attachment sites for the membrane cytoskeletal protein 4.1 of the red blood cell. Blood 1993;82:3482-88.
55. Lublin DM, Mallinson G, Poole J, et al. Molecular basis of reduced or absent expression of decay-accelerating factor in Cromer blood group phenotypes. Blood 1994;84: 1276-82.
56. Merry AH, Rawlinson VI, Uchikawa M, Daha MR, Sim RB. Studies on the sensitivity to complement-mediated lysis of erythrocytes (Inab phenotype) with a deficiency of DAF (decay accelerating factor). Brit J Haematol 1989;73:248-54.

DISCUSSION

S.L. Thein, P.C. Das – moderators

C.Th. Smit Sibinga (Groningen, NL): Dr. Thein's presentation showed the development in the haemoglobin sequence from embryonic, to the foetal, to the adult. When we come to the point of thinking of where to start in gene therapy, it could mean that we should try to get to the most early stage, unravel the mechanisms where things go wrong and try to correct at the embryonic stage or could it also be possible that a correction is being made at a later stage in the development of the molecules, i.e. at the foetal stage.

S.L. Thein (Oxford, UK): If I understood rightly, you are asking whether we should intervene at the foetal stage rather than after birth?

C.Th. Smit Sibinga: There is a development, a basic mechanism for the production based on the genetic information and the engineering that then happens in the body. This starts with an embryonic type of haemoglobin, which develops during the foetal stage and then matures into the adult, eventually.

S.L. Thein: It is difficult I think to intervene at such an early stage, even shortly after birth, because of the difficulty to predict with a 100% accuracy the clinical course of the disease. So the answer to the question then is really, assuming that the parents have refused prenatal diagnosis, that one should wait till a later stage to see how the child behaves. But I also think now with the better prognosis in bone marrow transplantation we should consider this as a first line treatment. Perhaps I could ask dr. Apperley what her views are regarding gene therapy.

J.F. Apperley (London UK): Well, I think I agree. At the moment everything is in its infancy and for these individuals it is extremely difficult to predict how severely they will have to be affected and therefore how aggressive one ought to be with intervention. If you knew from other members of the family that a particular individual was going to have a bad course or if you could predict with great accuracy by the molecular biology that an individual is going to have a bad course, you might for instance consider collecting umbilical cord blood at the time of the birth, introducing genes into that and doing an autologous transplant at that stage. But I really do not think we are at that point yet. I mean we have got a long way to go to demonstrate that we can get enough expression of any of these genes by gene transfer technology to change the phenotype of the patient. So, until you can do that you cannot move backwards in the time of intervention.

C.Th. Smit Sibinga: It is, as you said, likely that you aim for the stem cell in this particular situation. Could it be thinkable that one collects at a certain point in time autologous stem cells from these patients, bring them into a stage of culture, genetically manoeuvre the information in the stem cell and then transplant them back. Would that be an option?

J.F. Apperley: That is exactly what would be the aim. At this point there are several problems in that idea. The first is that although we can collect what we think are stem cell populations as identified by surface antigen expression. On the ability to propagate long term culture, we do not really know the morphology of the phenotype of the long term repopulating cell. If you look at experimental data, there is very little evidence that we really do expand the stem cell. We can certainly expand a long term culture initiating CD34 positive cell, but we do not know as yet that we can expand the stem cell. In fact, in the experiments that have been done in the mice even though you can expand the CD34 population by one thousand fold you still need the same number of stem cells to transplant any other mice. That is the first problem. But I think that with the discovery of more growth factors that will come, and if you could add an unlimited number of stem cells to the ability to introduce your gene at exactly the right place along the lines of homologous recombination then you have the absolute perfect treatment. Because the problem we have to face in the haemoglobinopathies at the moment with gene transfer is in the great majority of patients, because there is a problem with the balance of production of the genes. You actually have to ablate the individuals own haemapoietic stem cells to introduce the manipulative ones. If we can avoid that problem that would be a great advantage.

C.Th. Smit Sibinga: So the option is realistic as such for the future?

J.F. Apperley: For the far future I think.

P.F.W. Strengers (Amsterdam, NL): Dr. Apperley, at the end of your presentation you mentioned you used a few vectors. You said to prefer to have more research on the adeno-associated virus. Is there any reason that you are afraid of the use of other virus vectors, especially the retroviruses and the wild type. Could this be a problem in the patient and therefore a reason, an indication that this is a danger in the development of the use of gene therapy?

J.F. Apperley: This is a very important issue, which I think will be covered in more detail later on in the conference. At the moment one has to obtain a source of virus which contains a gene of interest and because one introduces exogenous DNA sequences into the retrovirus obviously you get expression of the globin gene. You interfere with the retrovirus' own mechanism and render it replication defective. So, in order to get large quantities of virus we have to use various tricks, which I am sure have already been mentioned such as packaging cell lines. A problem is that the packaging cell lines are at the moment suboptimal, because they have to be processed in the laboratory. As they contain wild type sequences there is always a problem of recombination. So the danger is that you have a source of retrovirus, that contains the globin gene for instance but is mixed with wild type virus which, if introduced into the individual may cause a problem. There is already a problem in the primate system, where the monkeys developed T-cell lymphomas following retroviral gene transfer. The second problem is a problem of random integration of the retrovirus into the genome, which if it goes into the wrong place may activate oncogenes or suppress tumour suppressor genes. One can think of all sorts of things they might do. To be honest this seems a much more theoretical risk than a practical risk, because there have already been thousands of mice transplanted in this way now and none of them seem to have gone into those sort of problems. Prof. David Onions will also talk about these issues[1]. We have no idea for instance whether the recombinant retrovirus that we introduce into the patient cells has the ability to recombine with endogenous human retroviruses such that you can generate a potentially harmful organism. All these things have to be taken into account before we go into a disease which is not immediately life-threatening.

D.D. Koeberl (Seattle, WA, USA): First a comment and then a question for dr. Apperley. The point about possible risks using integrated vectors for gene therapy is well taken. However, the comment about the risk for generation of wild type retrovirus from packaging cell lines, I just say that there has been rigorous testing for helper virus from packaging cell lines. The lines that are currently used for human gene therapy trials have not yielded any helper virus, because multiple recombination events would be necessary to produce wild type virus recombination between the vectors and the retroviral genes in the packaging cell line genome. So, there is a theoretical risk for wild type virus being generated from packaging cell lines. But those that are currently used for human gene therapy have not yet generated any helper virus.

Then a question – I was interested to see in the ADA experiment that there was transient expression of ADA despite the persistence of the retroviral vector. I was curious about the promotor used in that vector because of the evidence that viral promotors can be inactivated *in vivo* or whether it was a tissue specific globin promotor or some other.

J.F. Apperley: There are two parts of that question.
The first part regards the safety of retroviruses. I am obviously a proponent of gene transfer technology, but I think one has to temper one's enthousiasm with some reality. To be fair the reason why some of the safety testing sofar has been

---

1. See pp. 209-20.

negative is perhaps because we have not got the right safety test. I would not be so presumptuous just to say that the packaging lines we have currently are going to be the best ones for clinical use. I think there is quite a lot of work to do on that.

The second part of the question referred to something that somebody who works in the field picked up on and may not be immediately apparent to the audience. I showed you some data on a protein electrophoresis strip and a Southern blot. I only talked about the electrophoresis strip. You may remember that we tried to introduce human ADA into mouse cells and then transplant mice with that construct. We lost the expression between 10 and 14 weeks. The Southern blots done on the blood taken from these mice at the same time points to see if the retrovirus was still present. The anomaly you picked up was that despite the presence of the provirus at twenty weeks, there was seemingly no protein expression. Now unfortunately due to the limitations, we have only been able to take 20 microlitres of blood from a mouse every 2 or 3 weeks. We only looked at DNA presence and protein expression. We do not know whether mRNA was present and not being translated, mRNA was not present which might indicate some defect in the DNA, or whether protein was being produced and then being mobbed up, if you like, by antibody production. I think all those three possibilities exist and to my knowledge nobody has successfully demonstrated one or other as being the cause in every single case. It is a well known fact now in gene transfer that if you use a retroviral construct that has two genes in it, one for selection and one for expression, that very often you get downregulation of one gene at the expense of another. The simpler the construct the more likely you are to see long term expression[1].

J.F. Harrison (Brentwood, UK): Prof. Huisman, I was very interested in the case you reported of the sickle cell patient who was treated with hydroxyurea and produced a high level of haemoglobin F. I wonder if you could tell us something more about that. Do other patients respond in this way and is this a long-term response?

T.H.J. Huisman (Augusta, GA, USA): In our institution we have treated sickle cell anaemia patients for about five years and the treatment is to some extent haplotype dependent. Patients with haplotype 3, which is the Senegal type, respond in general very well. So do the patients with haplotype 19, which is the Benin type. It is indeed individually rather variable. In our institution that depends also on whether the patients are very serious about their own treatment, if they are complying with the taking of the drugs, but the most sincere patients seem to respond very well. There also has been a study done in Curaçao of about 8 patients, also patients with different haplotypes. They have been treated for a

1. Apperley JF, Luskey BD, Williams DA. Retroviral gene transfer of human adenosine deaminase in murine hemopoietic cells: effect of selectable marker sequence on long-term expression. Blood 1991;78:310-17.

considerable period of time and they all responded reasonably well to this particular oral treatment. The foetal haemoglobin indeed increases considerably, not only the foetal human globin, but also the F cells. If one determines this by flowcytometry with specific monoclonal antibodies one can see that indeed the patient, who has a 30% of foetal haemoglobin obtained during this treatment, has then foetal haemoglobin distributed over the red cells rather equally. About 70-80% of all the red cells contain foetal human globin and that is indeed the reason why crises diminish in number, why the red cells survive much longer, and why the haemoglobin level increases. Compliance is usually measured by looking at the MCV values, because the cells increase by size considerably and if for some reason it does not occur, it almost invariably indicates that the patient is not taking the medication.

S.L. Thein: I do not think it is so straightforward. In terms of haemoglobin F levels they may respond very well, but this is not the only factor; it is well known that the Arab-Indian patients for instance with high haemoglobin F do not have less sickling pain. The response of hydroxyurea, I think is not just due to the increase in the haemoglobin F levels. There is an increase in the MCV and in fact we should also be looking at what it does to the platelets and the white cells, because there is a decrease in the viscosity which is an important factor in the clinical course in sickle cell disease.

E. Briët (Leiden, NL): I would like to know from dr. Apperley whether you think that the availability of L1 has had any change in the conservative management of patients with these diseases and whether that has had an influence on your assessment of the suitability of bone marrow transplantation.

J.F. Apperley: The simple answer to that question is: not yet. Obviously the various lines of treatment for the haemoglobinopathies improved medical care with respect to verticulation or collation that is more acceptable to the patient and easier to take. It is going along with the same way bone marrow transplantation is improving and gene therapy is coming on line and things like hydroxyurea are being evaluated. I think we have to pursue all these areas and assess the outcome logically and then allow the results of that to impact on our decision to go one way or the other, but at the moment the availability of L1 is certainly not influencing us.

P.C. Das (Groningen, NL): Dr. Apperley, you showed that the Lucarelli group in Italy has classified these class I, II and III and chances of success depend on that. On the other hand you also showed that if there is no family donor there is a bad chance of having success. Now Italians of course do have large families, but in other countries we do not. How do you visualise that the future would be? Would it be looking for more donor panels or do you suggest something else?

J.F. Apperley: Well, I think this is a very good point. I should emphasise that the 500 transplants referred to, that were abled to be grouped in class I and class III were HLA identical sibling transplants in individuals under the age of 17. Lucarelli of course is not only transplanting Italian thalassaemics. In fact I suspect very few of his 500 originally came from Italy and family size is a problem for him as well. There are various options available; first of all if you are talking about children there is always a potention to use the haplotypical identical parent and the chances of that succeeding obviously are better if you do it very early in the child's life, because the chance of rejection, the chance of GVH is much lower. But as I showed in the mismatch results they are not particularly good. The second option is the development of unrelated bone marrow donor panels. There are now 2.5 million individuals who have volunteered to donate bone marrow for transplant recipients. Now the difficulty here is that in general, as blood bankers will know, the persons who volunteer to donate their blood or their bone marrow tend to be relatively well educated, often Caucasian middle class individuals. The difficulty with things like thalassaemia and sickle cell anaemia is of course the ethnic groups that we need to get a good database of HLA identical donors, are very small. For instance, I can give you an example in the UK. We have 250,000 donors on the Antony Nolan panel in London and 259 of them are Afro-Caribbean. So the chance of finding a donor for an Afro-Caribbean patient is very, very small. Now obviously the one way to go for this, which again is of great interest for blood bankers, is umbilical cord blood banks, which could for instance target the ethnic population. This is obviously being addressed at the moment. There are banks in most of the European countries being developed. I think we have to see whether umbilical cord blood comes through as the great saviour of transplantation. The theoretical advantage is obviously being that you have captive audiences of mothers giving birth to children. So you have thousands of babies born every day in Europe who could potentially donate from their cord and secondly that it may cause less GVH disease because the transplant material is immunological naïve.

C.Th. Smit Sibinga: Could I raise another question out of curiosity to prof. Huisman? You showed a map with the variations in sickle cell patterns, specifically on the African and Asian continent. What struck me was the white part on the bottom of Africa, that is South Africa, supposed to be a reasonably developed country, where a lot of research must have been on. Why is it that you do not know the classification of sickle cell disease occurring in South Africa? Most of the blacks are Bantu's and Zulu's if I am well informed. Is there any information available?

The second question: a couple of years ago I came across peculiar information – there seems to be a tribe isolated right in the centre part of Asian India with sickle cell anaemia, as the only tribe present there with that type of disease. Have you any information on that and classified that type?

T.H.J. Huisman: The map identified the different haplotypes, the chromosomes carrying the β^S gene among the African population. Now indeed South Africa is a well developed country with very good research institutes. But the haemoglobin S incidence in the population of South Africa appears to be very low and therefore information about haplotype distribution is insufficient to be listed in this particular map. The cases that I have studied were primary sickle cell anaemia cases and Indians, who had immigrated and were established in South Africa. They all had that Indian type of sickle cell anaemia haplotype number 31. The tribes in the central part of India, their sickle cell anaemia generally is much milder. We studied about 50 sickle cell anaemia patients from that area and of these 49 had that haplotype 31 with the elevated foetal haemoglobin. Their haematology was not always as optimal as expected, mainly because of acquired abnormalities that interfered with that particular patient, but in general they did much better.

R.Y.J. Tamminga (Groningen, NL): Prof. Huisman, you talked about hydroxyurea treatment in sickle cell disease raising the Hb F level. We also heard something about indications for bone marrow transplantation in sickle cell disease. What do you think one should do with a child with lots of complaints? What are your indications for starting hydroxyurea and what is the place in your opinion of bone marrow transplantation in those children?

T.H.J. Huisman: I can tell you that in our centre we have done an evaluation of the interest about bone marrow transplantation. Among the population that we are serving the interest is relatively low. Moreover, the technique in the United States is expensive and that is often prohibitory in applying it to the patients that are usually not insured for medical care. Treatment with hydroxyurea is much cheaper, it is easier and is at the moment in a testing stage. It is a national programme in the United States, it is applied in 10 to 20 different centres. In ours we have about 80 patients that we are treating with that drug and in general the results are encouraging. I showed one of the better patients that was treated with this particular drug. I do not think that bone marrow transplantation will have a great future in patients with sickle cell anaemia for multiple reasons. There are other patients with haemoglobinopathies where this might be applicable. For instance we studied recently two patients with a very severely unstable haemoglobin. A young girl and a young boy both 3 to 4 years old with a severe haemolytic anaemia due to this unstable haemoglobin. Some of these unstable haemoglobins precipitate even already in early erythroblasts where you can see the Heinz bodies appearing. These patients do not have a future, they are more severe than any thalassaemia patient that I have ever seen. They are the prime candidates for bone marrow transplantation.

J.F. Apperley: I think that I have tried to emphasise throughout my talk and in answering the questions, that in trying to decide whether transplantations are the right treatment for any individual patient one assesses that patient without regard to the other patients. So if you have a situation where a child is very badly affected, is having recurrent crises or already had a stroke and is on a life-long transfusion programme, you may try hydroxyurea and it may not produce the benefits you want. If that child has a suitable donor, that might be on that individual case the choice for that child. It might not be the choice for the child in the next bed. I think that is the situation we are at for the moment.

C.Th. Smit Sibinga: Dr. Anstee, I was intrigued by your statement that in the situation of D absence there is an entire absence of the polypeptide. That puzzled me, because I remember a couple of years ago that Fred Plapp told us here in this particular meeting that that is not really the case[1]. If you invert red cell membranes you could come along a number of D antigens, polypeptides, which have just sinken through the membrane and are not in the extraphacial but in the intraphacial side. How is the state of the art then today?

D.J. Anstee (Bristol, UK): Well, I think it is very clear that the polypeptide is not in a membrane in that sense. As far as I am aware, several groups have tried to repeat the work that Fred Plapp published some years ago without success. There are many different genetic mechanisms that could create D negative, which would mean that a fragment, a part of the polypeptide was translated. So, you might find part of the polypeptide inside the cell, but it could not get incorporated into the membrane. I think it is very clear that there is no D polypeptide in red cell membranes from D negative individuals.

R.Y.J. Tamminga: Dr. Anstee, you showed us an overview of all the blood groups on the erythrocytes. I assume that they are mature erythrocytes.

What about the precursor cells, the erythroblasts, do they have the same pattern of blood groups or do they have other blood groups on their surface?

D.J. Anstee: Yes, what I showed was blood group proteins on mature erythrocytes. Several of these proteins appear very late in the maturation process, for instance the major transport protein band 3 appears very late, as do RH and glycophorin A. The other molecules that I showed, the ones of minor abundance in the mature cell, are likely to be expressed in the earlier lineages, because they are molecules which are found on other haematopietic cells as well. CD44 is expressed at higher levels on earlier erythroid cells than on the mature red cell. So, in those cases the molecules are being downregulated with maturation rather than upregulated as is the case with band 3.

---

1. Plapp FV, Rachel JM, Beck ML, Sinor LT. Solid phase red cell adherence tests in blood banking. In: Smit Sibinga CTh, Das PC, Greenwalt TJ (eds). Future developments in blood banking. Martinus Nijhoff Publ. Boston, Dordrecht, Lancaster, 1986: 177-206.

R.L. Mcshine (Groningen, NL): Dr. Anstee or dr. Reid, as you know one of the mysteries in haematology is the poor correlation between the concentration of IgG molecules on the red cell and the rate of red cell destruction *in vivo*. Have the molecular biologists an answer to this mystery?

M.E. Reid (New York, NY, USA): The strength and type of an *in vitro* alloantibody/antigen reaction can, to some extent, be correlated to the number of copies of the antigen per RBC and the distance of the antigen from the lipid bilayer. The target antigen for many autoantibodies often goes undetermined. Even when the antibody recognises a determinant on Rh glycoproteins or on glycophorin A, the rate of *in vivo* destruction is not predictable. Thus, to my knowledge, in situations involving either alloantibodies or autoantibodies, molecular biologists have not provided an answer to the question of what can be used to predict the rate of *in vivo* destruction of RBCs.

P.C. Das: Dr. Reid, you showed that in certain diseases like Hodgkin's lymphoma the antigeneic expression is changed or weakened. That is an intriguing phenomenon. Would you like to elaborate how it is done?

M.E. Reid: In certain diseases, the antigenic expression of a blood group antigen is changed or weakened as a result of translocation or stress haemopoiesis. If a translocation of part of a chromosome that induces a disease occurs in the area that includes a gene encoding a blood group antigen, the antigen will be changed or weakened as a result of the translocation. Any disease that increases the rate of transit of RBC precursors through the glycosylation organelles can result in a general reduction of glycosylation of RBC membrane components. Any blood group antigen that is dependent on CHO for its expression may be effected; however, most commonly there is a weakened expression of A, B and I antigens and a concomitant increase in expression of i antigen.

III. WHITE CELLS AND MALIGNANCIES

THE ROLE OF THE BLOOD BANK IN HUMAN GENE THERAPY TRIALS

S.M. Freeman[1], A.J. Marrogi[1], K.A. Whartenby[2], C. Abboud[3]

Introduction

Molecular biology has developed over the last two decades as the structure and function of many genes and their regulation have begun to be elucidated. This basic understanding of gene expression in cells led to studies to genetically transfer genes into cells. Initial studies in gene transfer for gene therapy purposes focused on diseases in which the gene of interest is mutated and thus led to treatment of a genetic disease resulting from the dysfunction of a single gene (e.g., Lesch-Nyhan Syndrome) [1, 2]. The mutated gene leads to a dysfunctional protein or unexpressed gene. The early studies for gene therapy focused on these genetic diseases since it was hypothesized that replacing a single gene defect would be the easiest and most ethical approach to the first clinical gene therapy trial [3]. In order to genetically modify a renewable population of cells so that the gene would be expressed for the lifetime of an individual, gene transfer into haematopoietic stem cells to correct a lymphocyte defect, adenosine deaminase deficiency (ADA), seemed the most likely approach. Currently, there are six main groups of target diseases for stem cell gene transfer. Disease affecting red blood cells, such as sickle cell anaemia and thalassaemia, could be cured by insertion of a normal globin gene into stem cells. Neutrophil deficiencies that are caused by an enzyme defect (e.g., chronic granulomatous disease) lead to chronic infections, and can be corrected by insertion of the normal gene that corrects the oxidative pathway [4]. Storage disease can be corrected through stem cell gene transfer, which would correct the genetic defect within the monocyte cell population. Gene transfer into haematopoietic stem cells can correct genetic deficiencies affecting lymphocytes, as with ADA. Although AIDS is an acquired infectious disease rather than a genetic one, experimental protocols using bone marrow gene therapy are ongoing with the hypothesis that genetic material, such as ribozymes, inserted into the host genome are able to inhibit the AIDS virus by binding to and cleaving the viral RNA [5]. Drug resistance genes are being inserted into stem cells in the

1. Department of Pathology, Tulane University Medical School.
2. Center for Biologics, Food and Drug Administration.
3. Department of Medicine, University of Rochester Medical Center.

Table 1. Comparison of retroviral vectors and AAV vectors.

	Retrovirus	**AAV**
Transduction	High	High
Integration	Random	Specific
Cell division	Required	Not required
In vivo expression	Moderate	Unknown

treatment of cancer. In addition, bone marrow marking studies in leukaemic patients will provide relevant information in regard to cancer therapy and treatment of genetic diseases.

To provide materials for the early clinical gene therapy trials, an appropriate delivery system for the modification of bone marrow stem cells was developed over the decade beginning in 1980 [6]. A system for human gene transfer studies needed to satisfy a number of conditions. First, the gene needed to be expressed efficiently. Second, the gene needed to be transferred to a relatively high (>1%) proportion of the bone marrow cells. Third, the vector needed to be safe. A retroviral vector developed from the Moloney Murine Leukemia Virus met these criteria. Retroviral vectors insert into transcriptional active sites and thus lead to high levels of gene expression. The receptor for the retrovirus is ubiquitous and thus expressed on virtually all cells, which allows high level transduction of cells. Finally, the retroviral vector could be genetically modified to eliminate all the viral genes to produce a safe gene transfer system [7, 8].

This review will focus on: biology of stem cell gene expression, cell culture and expansion, gene marking studies, bone marrow gene therapy, and lymphocyte gene therapy. We hope this review will serve to detail the rapid growth of gene therapy clinical trials using haematopoietic cells, the problems to date, and the challenge of the future.

Biology of gene transfer and expression

Transduction

Gene transfer into stem cells has been studied for the past decade. The two main modes to genetically alter the stem cell has been physical and biologic. Physical methods include electroporation and calcium-phosphate transfection, while biological methods have focused on using RNA and DNA viral vectors. Physical methods to transfect bone marrow stem cells yielded poor results because of the inefficiency of the gene transfer and the toxicity of the procedure to the cells. Thus, initial studies focused on using retroviral vectors, which have the advantage of transducing cells efficiently and generating high levels of expression [9, 10]. Through the insertion of appropriate promotors and their regulatory units along with a gene of interest, gene expression in bone marrow has been achieved. Currently, methods to improve expression by designing a vector which can lead to long term gene expression in the stem cell are being studied. An area of recent study is the use of the adeno-associated viral vector (AAV) for gene transfer (Table 1).

The main viral vector used to transduce stem cells is derived from the Molony Murine Leukemia virus (M-MLV) [11]. This retrovirus contains the standard RNA viral genes: gag, pol, and env genes, which code for the viral core protein, reverse transcriptase, and envelope protein, respectively. In addition, the retrovirus contains a 5' and 3' long terminal repeat (LTR) and a psi sequence. The LTR has promotor, enhancer, and integration functions and the psi sequence is important for packaging the viral RNA into the virion. By deleting the trans viral genes (gag, pol and env) and inserting a therapeutic gene for interest, a retroviral vector was produced. This retroviral vector was packaged into a one time infectious viral particle by using a packaging cell that provides the viral proteins in trans.

Although retroviral vectors can lead to high levels of expression in cultured cells, the ability to obtain gene expression *in vivo* is often unsuccessful. This was demonstrated by Verma and colleagues using fibroblasts expressing the factor IX gene [12]. They observed that gene-modified fibroblasts implanted into mice lost their ability to secrete the factor IX protein due to *in vivo* inactivation of the promotor-gene unit. Using a fibroblast specific promotor, they were able to extend gene expression for months. However, not all fibroblast specific promotors performed in this capacity. This situation has also been demonstrated in bone marrow cells. Vectors that generate high levels of expression in immortalized haematopoietic cell lines do not necessarily generate high levels of gene expression in haematopoietic stem cells. Recent studies by Karlsson and colleagues evaluated expression of a gene in haematopoietic stem cells under control of different promotors to determine which promotor-gene unit led to the highest levels of gene expression in the haematopoietic stem cells [13]. Using the glucocerebrosidase gene (GC), they evaluated protein expression in long term reconstituted mice that had received bone marrow transduced with a number of retroviral vectors. They compared gene expression: 1) from the LTR with or without a selectable marker gene and 2) from a promotor (PGK, SV40, HSV-TK) in the forward or reverse orientation without a selectable marker gene. The best expression and copy number was found in the haematopoietic cells which contained the retroviral vector with the GC gene promoted by the LTR without a selectable marker. However, they and others have found that retroviral copy number does not necessarily correlate with expression [14]. The next best GC expression was obtained when the PGK promotor was in the forward orientation without a selectable marker, which was also reported by others [10].

These results show that retroviruses containing two genes do not function efficiency *in vivo*, possibly due to inactivation of the promotor gene unit by the LTR [15, 16]. However, other investigators have shown that the LTR may not be the most effective promotor in haematopoietic stem cells and itself may become inactivated. Keating and colleagues found that the CMV promotor was the strongest in generating expression of the CAT gene in long term bone marrow cultures. These discrepancies in identifying the best promotor for haematopoietic stem cells may relate to the gene being expressed rather than the promotor being tested. That is, each gene may need to be tested with a variety of promotors to determine which promotor will generate high levels of expression in bone marrow with that gene.

To further increase gene expression within bone marrow cells, strategies to increase the transduction efficiency of these cells must be analyzed. Retroviral vectors have advantages as a method to transduce stem cells since they insert into transcriptionally active sites and thus can lead to high levels of gene expression. In addition, since the receptor for the retroviral vector is ubiquitous, the retrovirus binds to almost all cells. Retroviral vectors have the significant disadvantage that in order for the vector to insert into the host genome, the cell must divide [17]. Since haematopoietic stem cells are relatively quiescent in terms of cell division, only 1-10% of the stem cells can be transduced [18]. Strategies to genetically alter non-dividing cells are currently being analyzed, and include the use of adeno-associated viral vectors and haematopoietic growth factors to stimulate stem cell division.

Adeno-associated viral (AAV) vectors have recently been shown to transduce mammalian cells [19]. AAV vectors have the advantage that they can transduce non-dividing cells and specifically integrate into the host genome at chromosome 19 [20]. Gene transfer into transformed haematopoietic cell line have been achieved using the globin gene [21]. Using the β-galactosidase gene as a marker, Nienhuis and colleagues recently showed that an AAV vector could be used to genetically modify haematopoietic progenitor cells. Further studies need to be performed to determine how effective these vectors will be in obtaining long term *in vivo* gene expression.

Growth factors

Another strategy being used to more efficiently transduce bone marrow is to increase the number of haematopoietic stem cells undergoing division. Since less than 5% of the stem cells are in the S or M phase of the cell cycle [22] and retroviral vectors only transduce dividing cells, one potential method to increase the cell cycling of stem cells and thus their transducibility, is to stimulate the stem cells to divide. Initial studies to cycle stem cells focused on pre-treatment of animals with chemotherapeutic agents before harvesting the bone marrow. 5-fluorouracil was used in this approach and found to increase the number of stem cells and the transducibility of the cells following treatment [23]. However, with the advent of haematopoietic growth factors, which have been used to expand bone marrow stem cells in culture and peripheral blood stem cells *in vivo* [24], studies began to determine whether exposure of stem cells to growth factors would increase their transduction efficiency. Nienhuis and colleagues demonstrated that the combination of IL-3 and IL-6 was more effective in increasing stem cell transduction than either of the growth factors alone, although IL-3 was required for stem cell survival, as measured by spleen colony forming units [25].

Although haematopoietic growth factors have been used to increase transduction efficiency of stem cells by increasing the cycling of these cells, the cycling rate is not the only critical factor involved in the transduction efficiency. Haematopoietic cells that are more actively dividing, such as CML cells, are only slightly more transducable [26].

Stroma

The bone marrow micro-environment plays an important role in haematopoiesis both *in vitro* and *in vivo* [27]. Impairment of this micro-environment by drugs will lead to a decrease in haematopoiesis [28] and is essential for stem cell support in culture [29]. Bone marrow stroma cells have also been shown to play a significant role in the transducibility of bone marrow. This was first demonstrated through the increased efficiency of gene transfer into bone marrow by co-cultivation of bone marrow cells with retroviral producer fibroblasts [30, 31]. The mechanism for this effect was initially thought to be due to the close proximity of the retrovirus with the stem cell during co-cultivation. However, since the extracellular matrix of the bone marrow micro-environment consists of fibroblasts, macrophages, endothelial cells, and adipocytes, the increased transduction efficiency observed with co-culture may be related to establishment of a micro-environment as opposed to closer proximity of the retrovirus to the stem cell.

Williams and colleagues explored this possibility by using a fibronectin fragment to coat plates on which bone marrow stem cells and retroviral stock were used for transduction [32, 33]. They found that when the carboxy-terminal fragment of fibronectin was used to coat the tissue culture flasks, there was an increase in the transduction efficiency of the haematopoietic stem cells. Further studies by Belmont and colleagues showed that transduction of human bone marrow in the presence of stromal support produced a higher transduction efficiency [34, 35]. The transducibility of bone marrow cells could be further enhanced by adding growth factors to the culture medium. The haematopoietic growth factors IL-3 and IL-6 have been shown to increase retroviral mediated gene transfer [33, 34], while the addition of leukaemia inhibitory factor (LIF) and mast cell growth factor (MGF) could also increase the transduction efficiency four fold over stroma alone [36]. However, growth factors are not able to replace the role of stroma.

A recent study by Kohn and colleagues has further demonstrated the role of the haematopoietic stromal micro-environment by *in vivo* xenogeneic experiments [37]. Stromal cells synthesize stem cell factor and IL-6 [33] and in combination with IL-3 , which is produced by T lymphocytes, stimulate the growth of haematopoietic stem cells. By transplanting human bone marrow along with human stroma which was genetically engineered to secrete IL-3, they showed that long term reconstitution (>4 months) was achieved in immunodeficient mice.

The future challenges of bone marrow stem cell transduction will continue to center on increasing gene expression and transduction efficiency by studying promotor gene interactions in stem cells, growth factor stimulation of stem cell division, and stromal support of stem cell growth and division.

Stem cell gene therapy

Transduction of bone marrow with retroviral vectors was initially demonstrated using murine haematopoietic cells. Reconstruction of irradiated animals with the transduced marrow was then shown using a retroviral vector containing the neomycin resistance gene (neo^R). Transduced cells containing retroviral DNA were identified within haematopoietic organs (spleen, bone marrow), Other genes were subsequently expressed within animals which include adenosine deaminase (ADA), dihydrofolate reductase (DHFR), and β-globin. Early studies showed difficulty with efficient transduction and long term *in vivo* expression [38]. Recent advances in transduction techniques and promotor utilization has led to improved results, but as discussed above, these have not achieved long term, high level *in vivo* gene expression.

The use of haematopoietic growth factors, has allowed the isolation of peripheral blood stem cells (PBSC) in large numbers. Normally, PBSC exist in the circulation in relatively small numbers (<0.05%). Using growth factors allows the expansion of the circulating PBSC approximately three logs [39-41]. The stem cells can be harvested by apheresis whereby the stem cell donor who has received five consecutive daily doses of G-CSF is apheresed on two consecutive days [42, 43]. The harvested PBSC have been used for bone marrow transplantation [44].

Studies by Gianni have demonstrated that human PBSC can be transduced at a higher efficiency than bone marrow stem cells, possibly due to an increased cycling of the growth factor-stimulated PBSC [45, 46]. Murine studies likewise have shown the increased transducibility of the PBSC. Mice treated with G-CSF and stem cell factor showed a 250 fold increase in PBSC, and these cells could be transduced at a three fold higher efficiency than chemotherapy-mobilized bone marrow stem cells [47]. Furthermore, the PBSC may engraft quicker than the bone marrow derived stem cell [42, 43]. A number of clinical gene therapy trials are currently underway that use PBSC [48]. Future studies need to determine if long term gene expression can be achieved by reconstituting mice with the transduced PBSC.

Cord blood has been shown to be a rich source of haematopoietic stem cells and can be used for bone marrow transplantation [49-51]. The cord blood cells can be transduced at higher efficiencies than PBSC [52]. There are currently a number of clinical gene therapy trials that use transduced cord blood cells to replace a genetic defect. The initial trials focused on using cord blood from neonates with adenosine deaminase deficiency (ADA). The cord blood from these neonates was transduced at birth by an ADA containing retroviral vector and then infused into the neonate [48]. Cord blood gene transfer will continue to play a significant role in future gene therapy protocols.

Expansion of transduced stem cells and provision of a selective growth advantage may aid in engraftment and increased numbers of gene modified cells in the peripheral circulation. Bone marrow stem cells can be expanded *in vivo* with growth factors as evidenced by more rapid engraftment and increased peripheral blood cells post transplantation. However, the ability to expand a gene-modified stem cell population was shown when bone marrow stem cells were transduced with a positive selectable marker gene. The multi-drug resistance gene (MDR) and the dihydrofolate reductase gene (DHFR) have been used as selectable gene markers in bone marrow cells. Using MDR modified bone marrow to reconstitute mice, Bank and colleagues have shown that by treating the reconstituted mice with chemotherapeutic regimens, the percentage of gene-modified peripheral blood cells could be increased from <1% to >7%. Thus, the use of selectable markers may partially aid in overcoming low bone marrow transduction efficiency by generating an *in vivo* selection effect [53, 54].

Clinical trials

Gene marking studies

Labelling cells with a marker gene permits the tracking of the marked cells in tissues or blood following implantation. Moreover, using the polymerase chain reaction (PCR), one marked cell in a population of 100,000 unmodified cells can be detected [55]. There are two categories of gene marking protocols currently active that are designed to address questions related to cancer therapy (Table 2). In one, there is an attempt to determine the fate of reinfused anti-tumour lymphocytes in patients undergoing treatment for advanced malignant melanoma. In the other, gene labelling is being employed to determine the contribution of residual bone marrow tumour cells to relapse in patients who have undergone autologous bone marrow transplantation. In addition, genetic marking of stem cells has been used to analyze the contribution of peripheral blood stem cells and bone marrow stem cells to haematopoietic population after transplantation.

Rosenberg and colleagues have developed a method of adoptive immunotherapy to treat cancer, in which autologous anti-cancer lymphocytes are administered to tumour-bearing patients. The lymphocytes are first isolated by culturing biopsied tumour tissue with the addition of interleukin 2 (IL2) [56]. These tumour infiltrating lymphocytes (TIL) are stimulated to divide with IL-2 and frequently exhibit cytotoxicity against the tumour cells *in vitro*. The large numbers of TIL that are subsequently reinfused have been shown to induce an anti-tumour response in some patients [57].

Since a majority of these patients have not achieved a long term response, questions were raised concerning the fate of the administered TIL. Previous attempts to track TIL migration and survival *in vivo* had been inconclusive due to the limitations imposed by conventional radionuclide labelling, including the short half-life of radioisotopes and the leeching out of the radiolabel with its

Table 2. Clinical trials using haematopoietic stem cells.

- Bone marrow marking with neo
- Bone marrow gene transfer with MDR
- Peripheral blood stem cell marking with neo
- Peripheral blood stem cell gene transfer (i.e., ADA)

subsequent incorporation into neighbouring non-TIL cells [58]. The first NIH-approved human gene transfer experiment addressing these concerns was begun at the NCI in 1988. TIL were genetically marked with the bacterial neomycin resistance gene using a retroviral vector called LNL-6 [59]. Stable integration of the retroviral vector into the host genome resulted in permanent labelling of the transduced cells and their progeny. TIL transduced *in vitro* with the LNL-6 retroviral vector were infused into patients and tracked using PCR amplification of neo^R DNA sequences in peripheral blood cells and tumour tissue. With this method, neo^R-containing TIL could be detected consistently in the circulation for three to eight weeks and in tumour biopsies for up to 64 days [60]. In addition, retrovirally marked cells from 4 of 5 evaluable patients undergoing this procedure could be recovered and grown in culture in the presence of the toxic neomycin analogue, G418, indicating that the cells were expressing the neo^R gene. There was no evidence of replication competent virus in the infused TIL, nor was there evidence of retroviral infection in patients who received transduced TIL, as measured by seroconversion on Western blots.

A second category of gene marking pertains to patients undergoing autologous bone marrow transplantation (ABMT). In this procedure, bone marrow is harvested from the patient and used for subsequent reconstitution in a "rescue" procedure that follows high dose chemotherapy. A number of malignancies are being treated in this fashion, including leukaemia, lymphoma, breast cancer, and ovarian cancer. Since tumour cells may contaminate the harvested bone marrow, techniques to purge the marrow of contaminating tumour cells are being developed. These purging methods include exposure of the marrow to cytotoxic anti-tumour monoclonal antibodies or to chemotherapeutic agents such as 4-hydroperoxycyclophosphamide. Since it is unknown whether residual tumour cells in reinfused bone marrow contribute to relapse following ABMT, a number of investigators are genetically marking purged bone marrow prior to transplant. It is hypothesized that the subsequent detection of the marker gene in recurrent tumour will indicate that tumour cells present in transplanted bone marrow contributed to relapse [61]. Deisseroth and colleagues hope that they may be able to compare different purging methods in the same patient by using two dissimilar (and distinguishable by PCR) neo^R vectors to transduce batches of bone marrow that were purged differently [62]. Thus, the presence of one or the other vector in a relapsed tumour may be attributed to the failure of a particular purging method.

Brenner and colleagues studied cancer patients (AML, neuroblastoma) undergoing ABMT. They transduced the bone marrow cells with a neo^R containing retroviral vector and detected the gene in peripheral blood cells in 5 of 5 patients eighteen months post-transplantation [63]. In addition, of two patients who relapsed, both contained the neo^R gene in the tumour cell population, thus indicating the importance of bone marrow tumour cells to relapse in cancer patients undergoing ABMT [64].

Future bone marrow marking studies will continue to focus on understanding engraftment and the role of tumour cells in the bone marrow of cancer patients undergoing autologous transplantation. Engraftment issues will focus on whether bone marrow or peripheral blood stem cells are a better source of haematopoietic progenitor cells. This can be accomplished by marking each population with a different retroviral vector that can be detected by PCR and simultaneously infusing the two marked populations. Similarly, the contribution and success of bone marrow tumour purging studies can be studied. By splitting the bone marrow harvest into aliquots for purging with different methods and then marking the purged marrow with a different retroviral vector, the success of each purging method can be determined by analyzing the relative contribution of each retroviral vector in the gene-modified tumour cell population.

Conclusions

Gene therapy for the treatment of disease using bone marrow stem cells has made significant strides in the past several years. A number of issues are currently being evaluated that relate to more efficient gene transfer and expression. Future challenges in the improvement of *in vivo* gene expression include identifying an appropriate promotor for HSC gene expression, determining the best combination of growth factors for cell cycling, and analyzing the use of stromal cells as a support system. The Blood Bank will serve a significant role in the transduction and processing of the bone marrow since it is one of the few areas that can satisfy the regulatory requirements necessary for implementation of gene therapy technology. The challenge for the Blood Bank staff is to remain abreast of the developing gene transfer technology so that the Blood Bank can assist in the ongoing and future gene therapy clinical trials.

References

1. Edwards NL, Jeryc W, Fox IH. Enzyme replacement in the Lesch-Nyhan syndrome with long-term erythrocyte transfusions. Adv Exp Med Biol 1984;165A:23-26.
2. Dick JE, Magli MC, Huszar D, Philips RA, Bernstein A. Introduction of a selectable gene into primitive stem cells capable of long-term reconstitution of the hemopoietic system of W/Wv mice. Cell 1985;42:71-79.
3. Karlsson S. Treatment of genetic defects in hematopoietic cell function by gene therapy. Blood 1991;78:2481-92.
4. Cobb CS, Malech HL, Leto TL, et al. Retrovial mediated restoration of p47phox protein to EBV-transformed B lymphocytes from a patient with chronic granulomatous disease. Blood 1992;79:1829-35.
5. Sullenger BA, Gallardo HF, Ungers GE, Gilboa E. Overexpression of TAR sequences renders cells resistant to human immunodficiency virus replication. Cell 1990;63: 601-8.
6. Freeman SM, Zwiebel JA. Gene therapy of cancer. Cancer Invest 1993;11:676-88.
7. Mann R, Mulligen RC, Baltimore D. Construction of a retrovirus packaging mutant and its use to produce helper-free defective retrovirus. Cell 1983;33:153-59.
8. Miller AD, Law MF, Verma IM. Generation of helper-free amphotropic retroviruses that transduce a dominant-acting, methotrexate-resistant dihydrofolate reductase gene. Mol Cell Biol 1985;5:431-37.

9. Cone RD, Mulligan RC. High-efficiency gene transfer into mammalian cells: Generation of helper-free recombinant retrovirus with broad mammalian host gene. Proc Natl Acad Sci USA 1984:6349-53.
10. Sorrentino BP, Brandt SJ, Bodine D, et al. Selection of drug-resistant bone marrow cells *in vivo* after retroviral transfer of human MDR-1. Science 1992;257:99-103.
11. Linial ML, Miller AD. Retroviral RNA packaging: Sequence requirements and implications. Curr Top Microbiol Immunol 1990;157:125-52.
12. Scharfmann R, Axelrod JH, Verma IM. Long term *in vivo* expression of retroviral-mediated gene transfer in mouse fibroblast implants. Proc Natl. Acad Sci USA 1991;88:4626-30.
13. Correll PH, Colilla S, Karlsson S. Retroviral vector design for long-term expression in murine hematopoietic cells *in vivo*. Blood 1994;84:1812-22.
14. Kaleko M, Garcia JV, Osborn WRA, Miller AD. Expression of human adenosine deaminase in mice after transplantation of genetically-modified bone marrow. Blood 1990;75:1733.
15. Yu-SF, von Ruden T, Kantoff PW, et al. Self-inactivating retroviral vectors designed for transfer of whole genes into mammalian cells. Proc Natl Acad Sci USA 1986;83: 3194-98.
16. Guild BC, Finer MH, Houseman DE, Mulligan RC. Development of retrovirus vectors useful for expressing genes in cultured murine embryonal cells and hematopoietic cells *in vivo* J Virol 1988;62:3795-3806.
17. Miller DG, Adam MA, Miller AD. Gene transfer by retrovirus vectors occurs only in cells that are actively replicating at the time of infection. Mol Cell Biol 1990;10: 4239-42.
18. Springett GM, Moen RC, Anderson S, Blaese RM, Anderson WF. Infection efficiency of T lymphocytes with amphotropic retroviral vectors is cell cycle dependent. J Virol 1989;63:3865-69.
19. Hermonat PL, Muzyczka. Use of adeno-associated virus as a mammalian DNA cloning vector: Transduction of neomycin resistance into mammalian tissue culture cells. Proc Natl Acad Sci USA 1984;81:6466-70.
20. Kotin RM, Siniscalo M, Samulski RJ, et al. Site-specific integration by adeno-associated virus. Proc Natl Acad Sci USA 1990;87:211-15.
21. Walsh CE, Liu JM, Young N, Xiao X, Nienhuis AW, Samulski RJ. Regulated high level expression of a human g-globin gene introduced into erythroid cells by a novel adeno-associated virus (AAV) vector. Proc Natl Acad Sci USA 1992;89:7257-61.
22. Spangrude GJ, Heimfeld S, Weissman IL. Purification and characterization of mouse hematopoietic stem cells. Science 1988;24:58-62.
23. Correl PH, Kew Y, Perry LK, Brady RO, Fink JK, Karlsson S. Expression of human glucocerebrosidase in long-term reconstituted mice following retroviral-mediated gene transfer into hematopoietic stem cells. Hum Gene Ther 1990;1:277-87.
24. Craig JI, Turner ML, Parker AC. Peripheral blood stem cell transplantation. Blood Rev 1992;6:59-67.
25. Bodine DM, Karlsson S, Nienhuis AW. Combination of IL-3 and IL-6 preserves stem cell function in culture and enhances retrovirus-mediated gene transfer into hematopoietic stem cells. Proc Natl Acad Sci USA 1989;86:8897-8901.
26. Hogge DE, Humpries RK. Gene transfer to primary normal human hematopoietic progenitor cells using recombinant retroviruses. Blood 1987;69:611-17.
27. Dexter TM, Allen TD, Lajtha LG. Conditions controlling the proliferation of hemopoietic stem cells *in vitro*. J Cell Physiol 1977;91:335-44.

28. Abraham NG, Chertkov JL, Staudinger R, et al. Long-term bone marrow stromal and hemopoietic toxicity to AZT: Protective role of heme and IL-1. Exp Hematol 1993; 21:263-68.
29. Chertkov JL, Drize NJ, Gurevitch OA, Udalov GA. Cells responsible for restoration of hemopoiesis in long-term murine bone marrow culture. Leuk Res 1986;10:659-65.
30. Apperley JF, Williams DA. Gene therapy: Current status and future directions. Br J Haematol 1990;75:148-55.
31. Williams DA. Expression of introduced genetic sequences in hematopoietic cells following retroviral-mediated gene transfer. Human Gene Ther 1990;1:229-39.
32. Moritz T, Platel VP, Williams DA. Bone marrow extracellular matrix molecules improve gene transfer into human hematopoietic cells via retroviral vectors. J Clin Invest 1994;93:1451-57.
33. Luskey BD, Rosenblatt M, Zsebo K, Williams DA. Stem cell factor, IL-3 and IL-6 promote retroviral mediated gene transfer into murine hematopoietic stem cells. Blood 1992;80:396-402.
34. Moore KA, Deisseroth AB, Reading CL, Williams DE, Belmont JW. Stromal support enhances cell-free retroviral vector transduction of human bone marrow long term initiating cells. Blood 1992;79:1393-99.
35. Carter RF, Abrams-Ogg ACG, Dick JE, et al. Autologous transplantation of canine long-term marrow culture cells genetically marked by retroviral vectors. Blood 1991; 79:356-64.
36. Moore KA, Deisseroth AB, Reading CL, Williams DE, Belmont JW. Stromal support enhances cell-free retroviral vector transduction of human bone marrow long-term culture-initiating cells. Blood 1992;79:1393-99.
37. Molta JA, Hanley MB, Kohn DB. Sustained human hematopoiesis in immunodeficient mice by cotransplantation of marrow stroma expressing human IL-3: Analysis of gene transduction of long-lived progenitors. Blood 1994;83:3041-51.
38. Karlsson S, Bodine DM, Perry L, et al. Expression of the human β-globin gene following retroviral mediated transfer into multipotential hematopoietic progenitors of mice. Proc Natl Acad Sci USA 1988;85:6062-66.
39. Herrmann F, Brugger W, Kanz L, Mertelsmann. In vivo biology and therapeutic potential of hematopoietic growth factors and circulating progenitor cells. Seminars in Oncology 1992;19:422-31.
40. Janssen WE. Peripheral blood and bone marrow hematopoietic stem cells: Are they the same. Seminars in Oncology 1993;20:19-27.
41. Siena S, Bregni M, Brando B, Ravagnani F, Bonadonna G, Gianni AM. Circulation of $CD34^+$ hematopoietic stem cells in the peripheral blood of high dose cyclophosphamide treated patients. Blood 1989;74:1905-14.
42. Shimazaki C, Oku N, Ashihara E, et al. Collection of peripheral blood stem cells mobilized by high-dose Ara-C granulocyte-colony stimulating factor. Bone Marrow Transpl 1992;10:341-46.
43. Ahmed T, Wuest D, Ciavarella D. Peripheral blood stem cell mobilization by cytokines. J Clin Apheresis 1992;7:129-31.
44. Weaver CH, Buckner CD, Login K, et al. Syngeneic transplantation with peripheral blood mononuclear cells collected after administration of recombinant human granulocyte colony-stimulating factor. Blood 1993;82:1981-84.
45. Cassel A, Cottler-Fox M, Doren S, Dunbar CE. Retroviral-mediated gene transfer into CD34-enriched human peripheral blood stem cells. Exp Hematol 1993;21:585-91.

46. Bregni M, Magni M, Siena S, DiNicola M, Bonadonna G, Gianni AM. Human peripheral blood hematopoietic progenitors are optimal targets of retroviral-mediated gene transfer. Blood 1992;80:1418-22.
47. Bodine DM, Seidel NE, Gale MS, Nienhuis AW, Orlic D. Efficient retrovirus transduction of mouse pluripotent hematopoietic stem cells mobilized into the peripheral blood by treatment with granulocyte-stimulating factor and stem cell factor. Blood 1993;82:445-55.
48. Kerr WG, Mule JJ. Gene therapy: Current status and future prospects. J Leukocyte Biol 1994;56:210-24.
49. Gluckman E, Broxmeyer HE, Auerbach A, et al. Hematopoietic reconstitution in a patient with Fanconi's anemia by means of umbilical cord blood from an HLA-identical sibling. N Engl J Med 1989;321:1174-78.
50. Karson EM, Polvino W, Anderson WF. Prospects for human gene therapy. J Reproductive Med 1992;37:508-14.
51. Diukman R, Golbus MS. In utero stem cell therapy. J Reproductive Med 1992;37: 515-20.
52. Moritz T, Keller DC, Williams DA. Human cord blood cells as targets for gene transfer: Potential use in genetic therapies of severe combined immunodeficiency disease. J Exp Med 1993;178:529-36.
53. Bodine DM, Seidel NE, Gale MS, Nienhuis AW, Orlic D. Efficient retrovirus transduction of mouse pluripotent hematopoietic stem cells mobilized into the peripheral blood by treatment with granulocyte colony-stimulating factor and stem cell factor. Blood 1994;84:1482-91.
54. Sorrentino BP, Brandt SJ, Bodine D, et al. Selection of drug resistant bone marrow cells *in vivo* after retroviral transfer of human MDR-1. Science 1992;257:99-103.
55. Morgan RA, Cornetta K, Anderson WF. Applications of the polymerase chain reaction in retroviral-mediated gene transfer and the analysis of gene-marked human TIL cells. Hum Gene Ther 1990;1:135-49.
56. Topalian SL, Solomon D, Rosenberg SA. Tumor specific cytolysis by lymphocytes infiltrating human melanomas. J Immunol 1989;142:3714-25.
57. Rosenberg SA, Packard BS, Aebersold PM, et al. Use of tumor-infiltrating lymphocytes and interleukin-2 in the immunotherapy of patients with metastatic melanoma. A preliminary report. N Engl J Med 1988;319:1676-80.
58. Fisher B, Packard BS, Read EJ, et al. Tumor localization of adoptively transferred indium-111 labeled tumor infiltrating lymphocytes in patients with metastatic melanoma. J Clin Oncol 1989;7:250-61.
59. The N2-TIL human gene transfer clinical protocol. Hum Gene Ther 1990;1:73-92.
60. Rosenberg SA, Lotze MT, Muul LM, et al. A progress report on the treatment of 157 patients with advanced cancer using lymphokine-activated killer cells and interleukin-2 or high-dose interleukin-2 alone. N Engl J Med 1987;316:889-97.
61. Rill DR, Buschle M, Foreman NK, et al. Retrovirus-mediated gene transfer as an approach to analyze neuroblastoma relapse after autologous bone marrow transplantation. Hum Gene Ther 1992;3:129-36.
62. The University of Texas M.D. Anderson Cancer Center. Autologous bone marrow transplantation for CML in which retroviral markers are used to discriminate between relapse which arises from systemic disease remaining after preparative therapy versus relapse due to residual leukemia cells in autologous marrow: A pilot trial. Hum Gene Ther 1991;2:359-76.

63. Brenner MK, Rill DR, Holladay MS, et al. Gene marking to determine whether autologous marrow infusion restores long-term haemopoiesis in cancer patients. Lancet 1993;342: 1134-37.
64. Brenner MK, Rill DR, Moen RC, Krance RA, Mirro J, Anderson WF, Ihle JN. Gene-marking to trace origin of relapse after autologous bone-marrow transplantation. Lancet 1993;341:85-86.

TRANSLOCATION IN CANCER: MECHANISM OF ONCOGENIC CONVERSION AND IMPLICATIONS FOR THERAPY

R.S. Goodenow

The one universal characteristic of leukaemogenesis is the acquisition of specific chromosomal abnormalities with proven causality to oncogenes. Since the molecular characterization of the translocation involving the c-MYC gene in Burkitts lymphoma, our understanding of the pathways by which genetic translocations in haematologic malignancy lead to oncogenesis has increased dramatically. Molecular studies of the genes involved in these somatic rearrangements and the analysis of their function has elucidated their role in the initiation of tumorigenesis and the sustained cellular growth characteristic of the transformed cell. In global terms, the progression to the malignant state that accompanies translocations appears to proceed not through a single event but multiple steps including but not limited to : (1) the altered expression of DNA regulatory molecules that transcriptionally activate photo-oncogenes requisite for transformation; (2) the deregulation of gene products that control terminal differentiation; (3) the activation of growth factors or their receptors whose overexpression sustains unlimited cell growth; and/or (4) the activation of factors that prevent programmed cell death or apoptosis. Moreover, several preleukemic diseases show evidence of only one predisposing event, which by itself is insufficient to produce the complete immortalization of a cell. This has significant implications for the development of novel strategies for therapeutic intervention which may lead to new "fourth" generation modalities of treatment to reverse these changes through the use of recombinant biologics or gene therapy.

Molecular characterization of the translocations involved in the malignant haematological diseases and the role of altered DNA transcription on unregulated cell growth provide a unified picture of the means by which cells are ultimately transformed. Figure 1 depicts two major pathways associated with oncogenesis. First, translocation of an actively transcribed gene such as a recombined immunoglobulin or T cell receptor locus is brought into juxtaposition with a photo-oncogene, the net effect being to activate or render the oncogene transcriptionally deregulated by virtue of its physical association with the transcribed genetic element (Figure 2). Such translocations are thought to arise from errors caused by the V-D-J recombinase, active in lymphoid ontogeny, which appear sequence specific for heptamer-nanomer repeats [1]. Second, deregulation of an oncogene and/or independent secondary events affecting other loci (e.g., controlling dif-

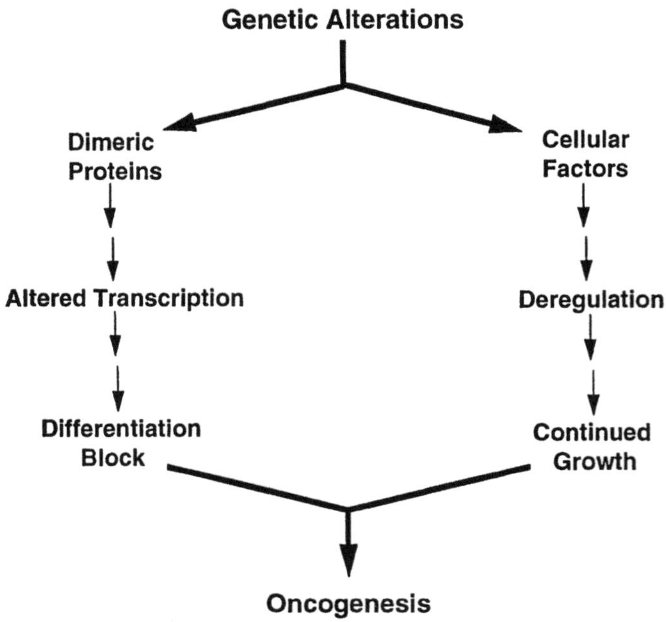

Figure 1. Molecular themes in leukaemogensis.

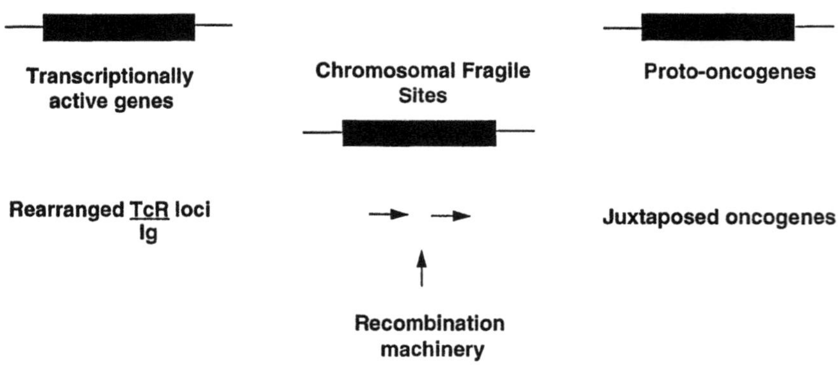

Figure 2. Chromosomal transductions in leukaemogenesis.

Table 1. Proto-oncogenes near chromosomal breakpoints in chronic and acute leukaemias.

Type	Translocation	Affected gene	Disease
Gene fusions	t(1;19)(q23;p13.3)	PBX-1 (1q23) E2A (19p13.3)	Acute pre-8 leukaemia
	t(9;22)(q34,q11)	c-ABL (9q34) BCR (22q11)	Chronic myelogenous leukaemia and acute leukaemia
	t(15;17)(q21;q11-22)	PML (15q21) RAR (17q21)	Acute myeloid leukaemia
	t(6;9)(p23;p34)	CAN (6p23) DEK (9q34)	Acute myeloid leukaemia
Basic-helix loop-helix proteins	t(6;14)(q24;q32) t(2;8)(q24;q24) t(8;22)(q24;q11)	c-MYC	Burkitts lymphoma, BI-AII
	t(8;14)(q24;q11)	c-MYC	Acute T cell leukaemia
	t(7;19)(q35;p13)	LYL-1	Acute T cell leukaemia
	t(1;14)(p32;q11)	TAL-1/SCL/TCL-5	Acute T cell leukaemia
	t(7;9)(q35;q34)	TAL-2	Acute T cell leukaemia
LIM proteins	t(11;14)(p15;q11)	Rhombotin 1/Tlg-1	Acute T cell leukaemia
	t(11;14)(p13;q11) t(7;11)(q35;p13)	Rhombotin 2/Tlg-2	Acute T cell leukaemia
Homeodomain proteins	t(10;14)(q24;q11) t(7;10)(q35;q24)	HOX-11	Acute T cell leukaemia
Others	t(14;18)(q32;21)	BCL-2	Follicular lymphomia
	t(14;19)(q32;q13.1)	BCL-3	Chronic B cell leukae-mia
	t(9;14)(q31;q32)	IL-3	Acute pre-B cell leukae-mia
	t(7;9)(q34;q34.3)	TAN-1	Acute T cell leukaemia

ferentiation or apoptosis) complete the progression of the cell to the transformed state.

While not all of the leukaemias exhibit evidence of translocations (only about 50% display changes that are represented in tumours of the same histologic type), there are nevertheless specific alterations that serve to distinguish tumours of similar lineage. In the acute leukaemia, the most frequent abnormalities appear to involve the direct effects of chromosomal alterations on DNA transcription factors, whose perturbation probably acts on multiple distal loci to account for oncogenic transformation (Table 1). Some of these DNA transcription factors are themselves important in differentiation and would normally be appropriately regulated if it were not for their activation via association with the actively transcribed gene sequences. In contrast, the chromosomal translocations associated

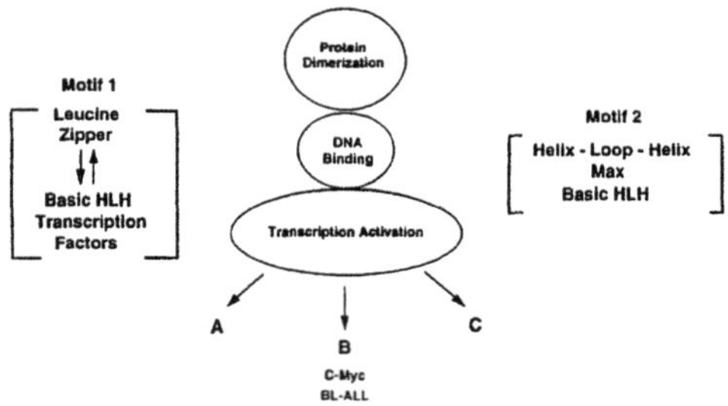

Figure 3. Master gene model for oncogenesis.

with chronic leukaemia and lymphomas appear to involve genes which do not encode transcription factors, per se, but products that control cell growth and division (See below).

The characterization of the gene products involved in translocations has revealed detailed information about the causality between translocations and the processes leading to malignant transformation. In some cases, the affected genes have been shown to be direct regulators of gene transcription such as c-MYC. The human c-MYC gene, which is associated with BL-ALL and T cell leukaemia, contains a DNA binding region of basic amino acids capable of dimerizing with other transcription factors (Table 2). Thus, the proteins may complex with other factors in dysequilibria to alter the transcriptional status of numerous responder genes leading to cellular transformation. For example, c-MYC has been shown to combine with MAX in regulating the transcription of other genes [2]. In these cases, the deregulation of the transcriptional activators has downstream effects on the expression of genes which in turn alter cellular growth (See below). In other cases, the translocation of a transcriptionally active gene may deregulate the expression of loci that directly affect cell growth or programmed cell death. As a result, the translocations can establish or support a cascade of events by which oncogenic transformation may occur through multiple and independent mechanisms.

The translocations that affect regulation of DNA transcription can be subdivided based on the molecular themes by which their affects are exerted. The Master Gene model for oncogenesis [1], involves protein dimerization that leads to DNA binding and transcriptional activation of other loci. There are two motifs that can be displayed in this model. The first motif (Figure 3) includes interactions between leucine zippers and basic helix-loop-helix specific transcriptional

Table 2. Master gene fusions.

T cell acute leukaemias and Burkitts lymphoma	t(8;14)
– c-Myc fused with IgJ segments/switch regions	t(2;8)
	t(8;22)
– DNA transcription perturbed through regulatory interactions with MAX etc.	
– Altered transcription of responder genes leads to oncogenesis	

factors. The second motif involves interactions of basic HLH sequences with the MAX protein. Another class of transcriptional deregulation that results from translocations involves the homeobox genes such as HOX-11 (Table 3). In this instance, the effect of deregulation is related to the activity associated with the LIM-domain of the homeobox which acts directly on its DNA binding activity to affect undefined loci causing oncogenesis [3-6]. Examples include the translocations characterized in several of the acute T cell leukaemia such as t(10;14)(q24;q11), t(1;14)(p32;q11), and t(11;14)(p13;q11) (See Table 1). Fusion between Master Genes has also been observed. Examples include the E2A-PBX fusion in pre-B cell acute leukaemia [7, 8], as well as the fusion of PML to the retinoic acid receptor α (RARα) gene in acute promyelocytic leukaemia [9, 10] characterized by the t(15;17) translocation (Table 4).

Table 3. Homeobox genes.

Acute T cell leukaemias (HOX-11)	t(10;14) t(7;10)
– LIM-domain leads to direct perturbation of DNA binding activity	t(1;14)
– Undefined target gene activation	

Table 4. Master gene fusion.

Promyelocytic leukaemia (RARα-PML)	t(15;17)
– Terminal differentiation block at the promyelocytic stage	
– Sensitive to differentiation via retinoic acid (RA)	
– RA receptor α (RARα) acts in transcriptional activation that induces differentiation	
– RA therapy reverses differentiation block	

For the chronic leukaemia and lymphomas, translocations often affect cellular growth properties through the aberrant expression of growth factors, their receptors, or products which control differentiation or programmed cell death [11]. The detailed characterization of the genotypic and phenotypic changes associated with the chronic leukaemia has elucidated the multi-step nature of the tumourigenic process in these neoplasms. For example, chronic myelogenous leukaemia or CML in the chronic phase is characterized by the clonal expansion of normally differentiated granulocytes and is essentially a benign myeloproliferative disorder until it evolves into full blown acute leukaemia with circulating myeloid or lymphoid blast cells. This disease is distinguished from non-leukaemic elevations in white blood cell count that result from excessive stimulation of normal haematopoiesis.

The Philadelphia chromosome is characteristic of the translocation that is common to the follicular lymphomas (Table 5). The t(14;18) translocation in the chronic B cell follicular lymphoma fuses the c-ABL gene with BCR, a transcriptional unit on chromosome 22 to produce a chimeric p210 protein that results has growth promoting tyrosine kinase activity [12]. p210 has been shown to have tumorigenic properties of inducing a CML-like disease in transgenic mice [13]. BCL-2 is thought to prevent programmed cell death similar to the mechanism by which EBV immortalizes but does not transform cells (See below). BCL-2 induction can therefore be viewed as an initializing step in transformation that culminated in prolonged cell survival. This in turn creates opportunities for additional mutations, such as the activation of c-MYC, to lead to tumorigenesis.

Table 5. Master gene fusion

Chronic myelogenous leukaemia (c-ABL-BCR)	t(9;22)
– Produces p210 a growth promoting tyrosine kinase activity – Prevents apoptosis similar to EBV	
Follicular lymphomas (BCL-2-IgH J chain)	t(14;18)
– Produces a mitochondrial product that inhibits apoptosis – Facilitates inheritance of secondary changes such as c-Myc	

Table 6. Biphenotypic leukaemias.

Early T cell ALL (TCL-5 + tal genes)	t(1;14)
– Lymphoblasts differentiated into myeloid cells after treatment with adenosine deaminase inhibitor – SCL expression increased in early myeloid and T cell lines due to translocation TcR locus to 3′ UT SCL	

Perturbations in differentiation, particularly blocks in terminal differentiation of haematopoiesis, also appear involved in transformations that accompany specific translocations. In acute promyelocytic leukaemia (APL), the haematopoietic precursors that give rise to the myeloid lineage are blocked in their terminal differentiation. This can be reversed by treatment with retinoic acid which induces blast formation both in vitro and in vivo [10]. APL is characterized by a 15;17 translocation with breakpoints within the RARα and the PML gene which encodes a putative transcription factor (Table 4). Remarkably, nearly 100% of APL is associated with this characteristic translocation [9]. The RARα gene product is a nuclear receptor that acts as a transcriptional enhancer in response to the binding of RA, a physiological metabolite of vitamin A [10]. Mutations that suppress RARα function in myeloid cells lead to the loss of terminal differentiation and growth arrest induced by RA. PML-RARα retains the RARα DNA and retinoid binding domains and therefore has the potential to antagonize RARα. Transcriptional activation of the RAR-PML fusion product results in acceleratedgrowth; however, this can be reversed by treatment with retinoic acid or RA consistent with a positive correlation between the expression of the chimeric receptor and sensitivity to RA [9]. Although treatment with retinoids is partially successful in treating APL, producing limited periods of remission, there is usually a breakthrough of RA resistant cells leading to relapse. Nevertheless, APL provides a striking example of a translocation that affects a gene product that controls differentiation and yet can serve as a target for therapeutic intervention. About 5-10% of the acute adult leukaemia cannot be characterized on the basis of lymphoid or myeloid markers and are therefore classified as biphenotypic based on their ability to differentiate into cells of either lineage (Table 6). This stems from the observation that certain committed bone marrow cell types can switch lineage upon exposure to certain growth factors/receptors and/or the activation of certain oncogenes [12]. For example, pre-B cells from Eμ-myc transgenics become macrophages after introduction of the serine/threonine kinase oncogene v-raf, while retaining their lymphoid immunoglobulin heavy chain gene rearrangements [14]. Another example involves the infection of normal bone marrow with a retrovirus expressing both v-myc and v-raf. This generates both pre-B and macrophage clones from the same progenitor cells and indicates that these cells demonstrate a certain degree of plasticity with regard to differentiation [15].

Table 7. Biphenotypic leukaemias.

5–10% adult acute leukaemias which cannot be classified as lymphoid or myeloid because of marker expression of both lineages
– Pre-B cells from Eμ-Myc transgenics + v-raf (serine threonine kinase) → → macrophages retaining IgG rearrangements
– Normal bone marrow transduced with retroviral v-Myc and v-raf generates pre-B and macrophages from the same lineage

The observation that blocks in differentiation, resulting from translocations, are associated with progression to malignancy stems from the analysis of the biphenotype leukaemia (Table 7). Recently, the SCL (stem cell leukaemia) gene (also called TCL5 and tal) was cloned from the t(1;14) translocation of a patient with biphenotypic leukaemia [12]. Although this patient appeared to have T cell ALL, the lymphoblasts differentiated into myeloid cells after treatment of this patient with an adenosine deaminase inhibitor. In this particular case, the translocation results from the fusion of the TCR receptor locus to the 3' untranslated region of the SCL gene causing the elevated expression of SCL. The SCL gene has homology with amphipathic helix-loop-helix DNA binding proteins such as c-MYC [reviewed in 16]. Thus, one possibility is that the SCL forms heterodimers with other HLH proteins that in turn regulate the activity of other HLH proteins that promote haematopoietic differentiation. Specifically, the overexpression of SCL may disrupt the balance between normal haematopoiesis and the arrest of cells at an early stage of development characterized by the production of leukaemic cells.

Another example of translocations affecting differentiation involves myelodysplastic syndrome (MDS) characterized by low numbers of circulating blood cells [12]. Morphologically, precursor cells show asynchronous maturation of the nucleus and cytoplasm as if their normal development has been arrested. Chromosomal abnormalities occur frequently in MDS, particularly the loss of chromosomes 5 and 7, with high predilection for leukaemogenesis. Although a specific gene in MDS has not been identified, the 5q chromosome region is located near several haematopoietic growth factor genes [17], e.g., IL-3, 4, 5, M-CSF, GM-CSF and IL-9 (Table 8). This suggests that perturbations in the expression of these growth factor genes contribute to the development of the disease, where a block in differentiation may be caused by the aberrant production of certain growth factors. However, attempts to induce differentiation through the administration of growth factors clinically has not been successful in reversing this disease.

Table 8. Myelodysplastic syndrome (MDS).

Preleukaemia
– Increased precursors in bone marrow that do not mature normally
– Asynchronous maturation nucleus and cytoplasm (normal differentiation arrested)
– Chromosomal abnormalities (CL 5&7) 5g between several haematopoietic growth factors IL 3/4/5/9, m-CSF; GM-CSF, PDGF, etc.

Another pathway for transformation involves the over-expression of growth factors that support continued or aberrant cell growth. Growth factor function normally exercises control over both growth and differentiation in vivo. The oncogenic potential of the aberrant expression of growth factors/receptor genes is well documented [11]. The incorporation of the PDGF B chain as the transforming oncogene in two retroviruses first suggested a relationship between the expression of growth promoting genes and virally induced cellular transformation [12]. Subsequently, the list of growth factors and their receptors that are aberrant expressed by tumour cells has increased significantly. The oncogenic potential of EGF, erbB, M-CSF (fms), and SLF (kit) receptors, each of which has been adopted as a viral oncogene represent a few additional examples [18]. In the case of translocation that activate growth factors or their cognate receptors, overstimulation of the cell through intracellular control processes is thought to constitute the predominant transforming signal.

Perturbations in normal proliferation and differentiation during tumorigenesis appear requisite for immortalization of the cell. However, the deregulation or overexpression of growth factors in autocrine fashion can also render the tumour independent of normal growth requirements. This is especially relevant where the tumour expresses the factors that can serve as a mitogenic signal so that it becomes independent of the normal growth environment supporting progression to metastasis. Under normal circumstances autocrine loops probably function to speed up responses or amplify cell numbers rapidly within limits that are established by internal programming or other external stimuli of cellular environment/interactions.

Translocations that affect growth factor genes have been reported in pre-B cell leukaemia [19], with a t(5;14) translocation characterized by the fusion of the Ig heavy chain gene from chromosome 14 to the promoter region of IL-3 upstream of the coding region (Table 9). This appears causally related to the overexpression of IL-3 in autocrine fashion that may account for the eosinophilia observed in patients with this class of haematologic disease. When the growth factors are overexpressed in the cells that also express the cognate receptors they appear to confer factor independence and sometimes tumorigenicity [11]. However, such growth factor independence alone appears insufficient to cause leukaemia.

Table 9. Proto-oncogenes as growth factors/receptors.

Acute pre-B cell leukaemia (IL-3)s	t(5;14)
– Ig heavy locus chromosome 14 to the promotor region IL-3 (upstream coding)	
– Results in leukaemia from an IL-3 autocrine loop	

The description of processes by which cells undergo programmed cell death or apoptosis and the deregulation of this process in oncogenesis provides yet another means by which deregulated DNA transcription accompanying translocations can lead to transformation. Programmed cell death is important to embryogenesis, neuronal development, and haematopoietic differentiation. Morphologically, apoptosis is characterized by premature chromatin condensation and cell shrinkage ending in cell death [20]. It is a process requiring protein synthesis and degradation of DNA and appears to be regulated by distinct gene products such as APO-1 [21]. The BCL-2 gene provides an example of a gene activated by translocation that may interfere with the normal apoptotic process leading to prolonged survival of cells associated with the malignant phenotype. First described in the translocation t(14;18), BCL-2 activation is found in 85% of follicular lymphomas [22]. Gene transfer experiments strongly support that BCL-2 expression in myeloid precursors and pre-B cells dramatically enhances the survival of these cells without proliferation upon withdrawal of growth factors [11]. Since these cells normally die by apoptosis, BCL-2 expression appears to inhibit programmed cell death as the oncogenic basis for the action of this gene product. In transgenics, BCL-2 expression results in the accumulation of follicular cell center B cells that have left the normal cell cycle to extend their life time in vitro [23]. Thus, the rate of cell death as opposed to cell proliferation appears to account for the pattern of human follicular lymphoma where B cells accumulate without evidence of marked cell division. Elevated BCL-2 expression may rescue antigen relative B cells as a part of the selective mechanism involved in antibody affinity maturation where B cells bypass their normal control mechanisms.

Interesting, aberrant BCL-2 expression represents a more direct means by which genetic rearrangements can lead to tumorigenesis by prolonging cell survival as the initial event in the progression to malignancy. Although BCL-2 activation alone is probably insufficient to induce transformation, it is probably analogous to the transformation of B cells with the EBV where the cells are immortalized but not transformed [23]. In fact, BCL-2-J_H translocations can be found in hyperplastic tonsillar B cells [24], suggesting that such rearrangements are in fact common but do not always lead to the production of malignant cells. In addition to changes in programmed cell death, translocations may impact the normal ability to the cell to regulate cell division. BCL-3 in B cell chronic leukaemia is one such example where the protein product associated with transformation has homology with a CD10 motif and may be involved in altering cell-cell interactions or the cell cycle directly leading to tumorigenesis [25].

BCL-2 may exert effects similar to EBV where apoptosis is inhibited through the action of the EBV latent gene products. Expression of Latent Membrane Protein 1 has been shown to suppress apoptosis and correlates with the induction of endogenous BCL-2. Initial studies suggested that the BCL-2 product was a GTP-binding protein located on the cytoplasmic side of the cellular membrane [26]. However, it now seems more likely to be a mitochondrial protein located in the inner membrane [27]. Rearrangements joining BCL-2 at the 3' untranslated region to the Ig J chain element are characteristic of Burkitts lymphoma and the fusion product appears to promote cell survival without cell proliferation in growth factor independent cell lines [28-31]. BCL-2 transgenics show disease similar to follicular lymphoma with polyclonal expansion of mature B cells [23].

The tumour suppressor gene p53, while not directly associated with translocations in haematologic disease, provides additional insights into the means by which perturbation in programmed cell death can be accomplished through genetic abnormalities. The p53 gene was discovered because it complexes to the large T transforming protein of SV20 [32]. Sequence analysis of the p53 mRNA from tumours that had undergone the loss of one p53 allele showed the presence of point mutations in the remaining expressed gene corresponding to regions that had been identified as sites of mutations in p53 cDNAs cloned from tumour cell lines [33]. Mutations in the p53 from tumour lines showed that the altered regions occur within stretches of evolutionary conserved blocks of amino acids shown to increase the stability of p53 or to alter the conformation of the protein to affect its function [33].

Some murine cell lines contain insertions or deletions at the p53 locus which result in the complete loss of the expression of wild type p53 [34]. This suggested that p53 might be a tumour suppressor gene; and wild type p53 was in fact shown to be capable of suppressing cellular transformation in vitro using the ras gene [35-37]. All the p53 mutations characterizedto date appear to have lost the ability to suppress transformation in vitro [32]. While the function of p53 and the mechanisms underlying its role in malignancy remain unclear, p53 is probably a nuclear protein which is involved in the transcriptional regulation of other loci controlling cell proliferation or differentiation. One hypothesis is that p53 controls DNA synthesis as the cell proceeds through cell division and that the mutant forms of the gene product block this process in such a way that the chance for mutational events leading to tumorigenesis increase.

Although altered p53 expression is linked to the production of solid tumours, attempts to reverse the malignant phenotype through the restoration of normal p53 expression have piloted genetic intervention in treating p53 related malignancy. Experiments with gene transfer of wild type p53 into tumours has been shown to reverse the malignant phenotype of certain solid tumours both in vitro as well as in vivo [32]. Clinical attempts to deliver wild type p53 to tumours in patients with lung and head and neck carcinoma may establish the validity of this approach as a mode of treatment. If successful, the introduction of genes into tumour cells to alter the growth promoting properties associated with malignancy would be a positive indication of the potential of gene therapy to intervene in specific cellular disease processes.

Prospects for the future development of novel cancer therapies will most likely include combinations of drug as well as gene therapies (Table 10). Drugs that may reverse the effects of translocations would target the induction of differentiation or apoptosis. The use of RA points to the potential of drugs to reverse differentiation blocks. For apoptosis, the use of antibodies recognizing the APO-1 cell surface molecule [21] represents another approach for inducing apoptosis in tumour cells that have lost the capacity to appropriately regulate programmed cell death. Although the clinical use of p53 or antisense sequences to reverse malignant processes may afford some therapeutic benefit, the requirement to target each tumour cell in vivo will undoubtedly present a significant limitation to this form of therapy. However, these genetic approaches may prove efficacious in combination with other drug or immune based therapies.

Table 10. Future prospects for therapy.

	Drugs	**Genes**
– Induce apoptosis	Yes	Yes
– Reverse differentiation block	Yes	Yes
– Increase genomic instability	Yes	Yes

Thus, the increased understanding of cellular transformation in haematological malignancy will be critical in designing future therapeutic strategies for clinical intervention in these diseases.

References

1. Rabbits T. Translocations, master genes, and differences between the origins of acute and chronic leukemias. Cell 1991;67:641-44.
2. Cole M. Myc meets Hs max. Cell 1991;65:715-16.
3. Dube' ID, Kamel-Reid S, Yuan CC, et al. A novel human homeobox gene lies at the chromosome 10 breakpoint in lymphoid neoplasias with chromosomal translocation t(10;14). Blood 1991;78:2996-3003.
4. Hatano M, Roberts CWM, Minden M, Crist A, Korsmeyer SJ. Deregulation of a homeobox gene, HOXII, by the t(10;14) in T cell leukemia. Science 1991;253:79-82.
5. Kennedy MA, Gonzalez-Sarmiento R, Kees UR, et al. HOXII, a homeobox-containing T cell oncogene on human chromosome 10q24. Proc Natl Acad Sci USA 1991;88: 8900-04
6. Lu M, Gong Z, Shen W, Ho AD. The tcl-3 proto-oncogene altered by chromosomal translocation in T cell leukemia codes for a homeobox protein. EMBO J 1991;10:2905-10
7. Kamps MP, Murre C, Sun X-H, Baltimore D. A new homeobox gene contributes the DNA binding domain of the DNA t(1;19) translocation protein in pre-B ALL. Cell 1990;60:547-55.
8. Nourse J, Mellentin JD, Galili N, et al. Chromosomal translocation t(1;19) results in synthesis of a homeobox fusion mRNA that codes for a potential chimeric transcription factor. Cell 1990;60:535-45.
9. Kakizuka A, Miller WH, Umesono K, et al. Chromosomal translocation promyelocytic leukemia fuses RARx with a novel putative transcription factor, PML. Cell 1991;66:663-74.
10. De The' H, Laveau C, Marchio A, Chomeinne C, Degos L, Dejean A. The PML-RARx fusion mRNA generated by the t(15;17) translocation in acute promyelocytic leukemia encodes a functionally altered RAR. Cell 1991;66:675-84.
11. Cross M, Dexter T. Growth factor in development, transformation, and tumorigenesis. Cell 1991;64:271-80.
12. Sawyers CL, Denny CT, Witte ON. Leukemia and the disruption of normal hematopoiesis. Cell 1991;64:337-50.
13. Heisterkamp N, Jenster G, Hoeve JT, Zovich D, Pattengale PK, Groffen J. Acute leukemia in bcr/abl transgenic mice. Nature 1990;344:251-53.
14. Klinken SP, Alexander WS, Adams JM. Hemopoietic lineage switch -v-raf oncogene converts Eu-myc transgeneic B cells into macrophages. Cell 1988;53:857-67.
15. Principato M, Cleveland JL, Rapp UR, et al. Transformation of murine bone marrow cells with combined v-raf-v-myc oncogenes yields clonally related mature B cells and macrophages. Mol Cell Biol 1990;10:3562-68.
16. Cline T. The affairs of daughterless and the promiscuity of developmental regulators. Cell 1989;59:231-34.
17. Groopman JE, Molina J-M, Scadden DT. Hematopoietic growth factors: Biology and clinical applications. N Engl J Med 1989;321:1449-59.
18. Cantley L, Auger K, Carpenter C, et al. Oncogenes and signal transduction. Cell 1991;64:281-302.
19. Meeker TC, Hardy D, Willman C, Hogan T, Abrams J. Activation of the Interleukin-3 gene by chromosome translocation in acute lymphocytic leukemia with eosinophilia. Blood 1990;76:285-89.

20. Williams T. Programmed cell death: Apoptosis and oncogenesis. Cell 1991;65:1097-98.
21. Trauth BC, Klas CM, Peters AMJ, et al. Monoclonal antibody-mediated tumor regression by induction of apoptosis. Science 1989;245:301-45.
22. Fukuhara S, Rowley JD, Varrakujis D, Golomb HM. Chromosome abnormalities in poorly differentiated lymphocytic lymphoma. Cancer Res 1979;39:3119-31.
23. McDonnell TJ, Deane N, Platt FM, et al. Bcl-2-immunoglobulin transgenic mice demonstrateextended B cell survival and follicular lymphoproliferation. Cell 1989;57: 79-88.
24. Limpens J, de Jong D, van Krieken JHJM, et al. Bcl-2/J_H rearrangements in benign lymphoid tissues with follicular hyperplasia. Oncogene 1991;6:2271-76.
25. Ohno H, Takimoto G, Mckeithan TW. The candidate proto-oncogene bcl-3 is related to genes implicated in cell lineage determination and cell cycle control. Cell 1990; 60:991-97.
26. Halder S, Beatty C, Tsujimoto Y, Croce CM. The bcl-2 gene encodes a novel G protein. Nature 1989;342:195-98.
27. Hockenbery D, Nunez G, Millman C, Schreiber RD, Korsmeyer S. Bcl-2, an inner mitochondrial membrane protein blocks programmed cell death. Nature 1990;348:334-36.
28. Tsujimoto Y, Gorham J, Cossman J, Jaffe E, Croce C. Chromosome translocation involved in B-cell neoplasms results from mistakes in VDJ cloning. Science 1985; 229:390-93.
29. Bakshi A, Jensen JP, Goldman P, et al. Cloning the chromosomal breakpoint of t(14;18) human lymphomas; clustering around J_H on chromosome 14 and near a transcriptional unit on 18. Cell 1985;41:899-906.
30. Cleary ML, Sklar J. Nucleotide sequence of a t(14;18) chromosomal breakpoint in follicular lymphoma and demonstration of a breakpoint cluster region near a transcriptionally active locus on chromosome 18. Proc Natl Acad Sci USA 1985;82:7439-43.
31. Nunez G, London L, Hockenbery D, Alexander M, McKearn JP, Korsmeyer S. Deregulated bcl-2 gene expression selectively prolongs survival of growth factor-deprived hemopoietic cell lines. J Immunol 1990;144:3602-10.
32. Marshall C. Tumor supressor genes. Cell 1991;64:313-26.
33. Finlay CA, Hinds PW, Tan T-H, Eliyahu D, Oren M, Levine AJ. Activating mutations for transformation by p53 produce a gene product that forms an hsc70-p53 complex with an altered half-life. Mol Cell Biol 1988;8:531-39.
34. Gannon JV, Greaves R, Iggo R, Cane DP. Activating mutations in p53 produce a common conformational effect. A monoclonal antibody specific for the mutant form. EMBO 1987;39:1595-1602.
35. Eliyahu D, Raz A, Gruss P, Givol D, Oren M. Participation of p53 cellular tumor antigen to transformation of normal embryonic cells. Nature 1984;312:646-49.
36. Jenkins JR, Ruge K, Currie GA. Cellular immortalisation by a CDNA clone encoding the transformation-association phosphoprotein p53. Nature 1984;312:651-54.
37. Parada LF, Land H, Weinberg RA, Wolf D, Rotter V. Cooperation between gene encoding p53 tumor antigen and ras in cellular transformation. Nature 1984;312:649-51.

ROLE OF TOPOISOMERASE II α AND β ISOZYMES IN DETERMINING DRUG RESISTANCE *in vitro* AND *in vivo*

S. Davies, M. Sandri, S. Houlbrook, A. Harris and I. Hickson

Introduction

Chemotherapeutic agents which target the nuclear enzyme topoisomerase II (topo II) play a major role in the treatment of acute leukaemias and lymphomas. Treatments commonly include an anthracycline (e.g. doxorubicin) or anthracenedione (e.g. mitoxantrone), and, more recently, regimens have also included amsacrine (m-AMSA) [1] or etoposide [2]. Complete responses occur in 50-57% of patients. However, the underlying biochemical factors which distinguish the cancer cells of responsive from non-responsive patients remain unknown. A common problem limiting the clinical utility of these agents is the emergence of drug resistant tumour cells. Resistance to therapy can either be intrinsic (*de novo*) or acquired in response to the therapy. Intrinsic resistance is most likely to be conferred by the general defense mechanisms of the body against cytotoxic insults. For example, cells derived from melanomas, hypernephromas and colon carcinomas are highly drug resistant. In contrast some tumour types initially respond to treatment but subsequently recur in a form which is no longer drug responsive. This phenomenon is presumably a reflection of the selection of resistant cell subgroups, that either pre-existed or were induced by therapy [3].

The phenomenon of acquired drug resistance has been extensively studied *in vitro*, using cell line models [4, 5]. The identification and characterization of cellular factors mediating drug resistance in these cell lines should facilitate the identification of the relevant factors determining drug resistance in tumour samples.

Cellular factors determining drug resistance

For convenience, drug resistance can be subdivided into three separate categories. First, classical multidrug resistance (MDR) which is characterized by cross resistance to many structurally unrelated drugs and the overexpression of the transmembrane efflux pump p-glycoprotein [6, 7]. More recently, a non-pgp mediated form of MDR associated with the overexpression of a novel gene called MDR related protein (MRP) had been described [8]. This gene codes for a protein of 1522 amino acids that belongs to the same ATP-binding cassette superfamily of membrane proteins as the MDR gene product. MRP is thought to act as a transporter and may confer drug resistance in small cell lung carcinoma (SCLS) and possibly other malignancies [9]. A third form of resistance called atypical MDR [10] is associated with alterations in the nuclear enzyme topo II. In this case, cross resistance is restricted to topo II targeting drugs, with no change in transport mechanisms.

A number of factors influencing the cytotoxicity of topo II-directed agents have been identified. The most common observation is that topo II content correlates with drug sensitivity. Cells expressing low levels of topo II accumulate fewer topo II-mediated DNA strand breaks and are therefore less sensitive to topo II directed agents, whereas cells expressing high levels of topo II accumulate more topo II mediated strand breaks and are therefore more sensitive [11, 12].

Mechanisms of action of topo II

Many DNA-associated activities, including transcription, recombination and replication, require alterations in DNA topology. DNA topoisomerases are enzymes that regulate chromosome structure through their ability to catalyse the interconversion of topological isomers of DNA. Depending upon their mechanism of action, topoisomerases are classified as either type I or type II; the former making single strand cleavage in DNA and the latter double strand cleavages. The transient breakage of a double strand of DNA by topo II is followed by passage of a second duplex of DNA. The DNA is then religated, hydrolysis of ATP enables enzyme turnover and a further round of enzyme activity to occur [13-15].

Mammalian cells have been shown to contain two drug-sensitive topo II isozymes [16], topo IIα (relative molecular mass [M_r]~170 000) and topo IIβ ([M_r]~180,000). The two isozymes are encoded by separate genes mapping to chromosomes 17q 21-22 (topo IIα) and chromosome 3p 24 (topo IIβ) [17, 18]. Differential regulation of these two isozymes has been reported in certain model systems, with the topo IIα isozyme decreasing and the topo IIβ form increasing as cells become quiescent [19].

Topoisomerase II has been localised to the base of chromatin loop domains where it is proposed to play a structural role as part of the chromosomal scaffold or matrix [20]. The enzyme has been shown to be vital for normal cell cycle progression, as yeast temperature-sensitive mutants are unable to traverse mitosis properly due to a failure to segregate newly-replicated chromosomes [21, 22]. Other functions of topoisomerase II include the suppression of recombination in the highly repetitive ribosomal DNA cluster, maintenance of DNA supercoiling status during DNA replication, and possibly transcription [13-15].

Role of topo II in drug resistance

A wide variety of topo II-directed agents can influence the catalytic cycle of topo II. Intercalating agents such as doxorubicin, mitoxantrone and m-AMSA and the non-intercalating epipodophyllotoxins, etoposide (VP-16) and teniposide (VM-26) stabilize a reaction intermediate called the "cleavable complex". In general, topo II-DNA complexes accumulate in drug-treated cells because the drug permits DNA cleavage but shows down the DNA religation step [15]. The build up of

Table 1. Examples of topo II mediated changes in drug resistance

Alteration in topo II	Effect	Cell line	Reference
Decreased activity	Adriamycin resistant	P388 human leukaemic	[12]
Increased activity	Topo II inhibitor sensitive	CHO ADR-1	[11]
Increased phosphorylation	Etoposide resistant	KB human epidermoid carcinoma	[24]
Loss of nuclear localisation signal	Etoposide resistant	Human SCLC	[25]

these DNA adducts initiates a series of events which culminate in cell death [23]. A further class of topo II-directed agents exert their effect without the formation of cleavable topo II-DNA complexes. These compounds include the dioxopiperazine derivatives such as ICRF-159. In this case the drug acts as a catalytic inhibitor by blocking the interconversion of the open and closed clamp forms of the enzyme. (See [24, 25] for a detailed description of the mechanism of topo II action.) In the absence of active topo II, tangled DNA will be pulled apart and can be broken during chromosomal segregation in mitosis.

Regulation of topo II activity in cells

Topo II activity can be regulated in many different ways:

- by transcriptional regulation of the expression of each gene;
- the degree of phosphorylation can determine both the specific activity and regulate the mitotic functions of the enzyme;
- the subcellular localisation of the two isoforms may affect their function, since nuclear localisation is generally thought to be essential.
- a splice variant form of topo IIβ has been reported [26], however the functional distinction, if any, between these two forms remains to be determined;
- topo IIα expression and its phosphorylation are both regulated in a cell cycle dependent manner;
- the C-terminal domains of topo IIα and β are the regions of greatest sequence diversity, both between isozymes and between species. This region contains many phosphorylation sites, some nuclear localisation signals and possibly the dimerization domain and thus represents the area of greatest regulatory potential [14].

Results and discussion

Changes in topo II identified in drug resistant cell lines

Cell line studies have linked several different changes in topo II activity to the development of drug resistance (Table 1) [11, 12, 27, 28]. In general low levels of topo II activity confer drug resistance, while high levels confer relative

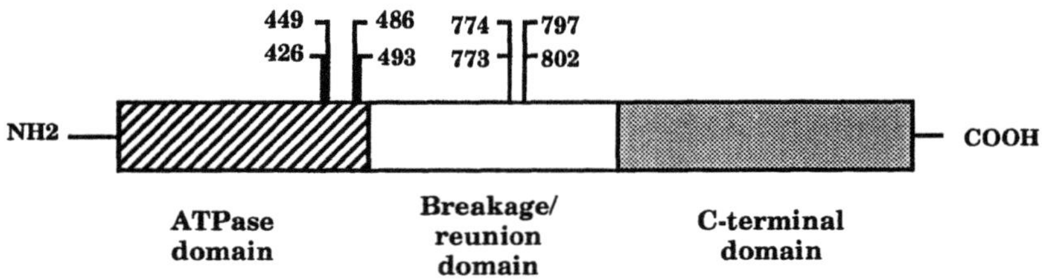

Figure 1. Topoisomerase II mutants and drug resistance.
The topoisomerase II protein is shown graphically as comprising three domains (not to scale): an N-terminal domain (cross hatched), a central breakage/reunion domain (open box) and a C-terminal domain (shaded grey). The positions of amino acid substitutions associated with drug resistance are indicated above the boxes.

sensitivity. Clearly, these changes can be mediated in many different ways (see previous section on topo II regulation). For example, downregulation of topo II gene expression in a Chinese hamster ovary cell line has been reported [29]. The etoposide resistance of a KB cell line was associated with a fifteen fold increase in the phosphorylation of topo IIα [27], suggesting that either phosphorylation directly mediates drug resistance or it provides a compensatory change in topo II activity, required in cells which downregulate their enzyme levels. An etoposide-resistant SCLC cell line has been shown to be missing part of the C-terminal domain of its topo IIα protein [28]. The truncated protein was localised in the cytoplasm, suggesting that the missing region is the site of at least one of the proposed topo II nuclear localisation signals.

Mutation within the topo IIα gene associated with drug resistance

Several sites of mutation have been identified in drug resistant mammalian cell lines [30]. The mutations appear to cluster at two distinct sites (Figure 1): one within the ATPase domain and the other in the breakage reunion domain of the protein, adjacent to the active site tyrosine residue. In yeast systems mutations, conferring drug resistance, have also been located in the C-terminal "regulatory" domain. The *in vivo* significance of these results is unclear since no mutations have been reported in primary tumour samples to date.

These observations pose several questions concerning the respective roles of the two isozymes in contributing towards the drug resistance phenotype. The majority of studies have concentrated on the α isozyme, but the β isozyme could equally be critical determinant of drug resistance *in vivo*. In differential expression of the two isozymes is observed in tumours versus normal tissues, then it is possible that drugs which target a specific isozyme could be of clinical value.

We have taken several different approaches to determine the relationship between topo II isozyme expression and drug resistance in mammalian cells. *In*

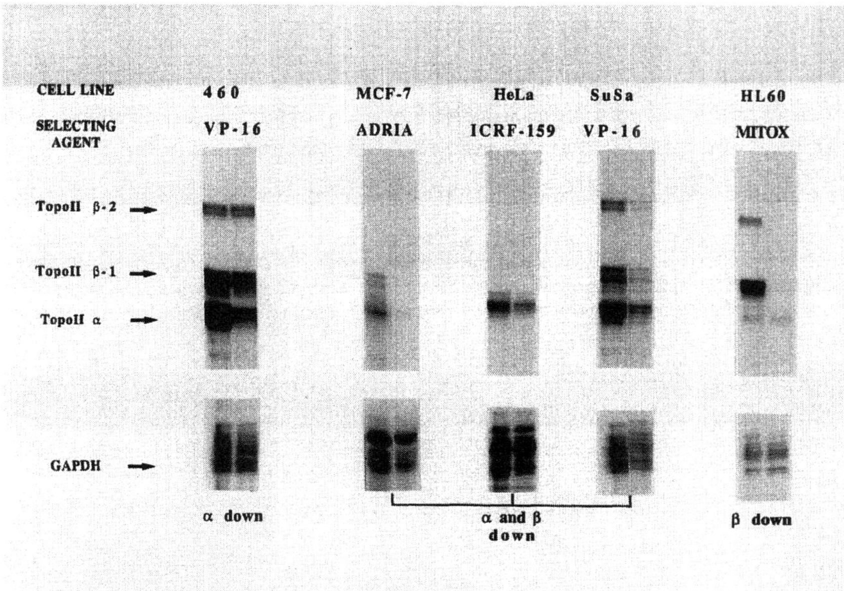

Figure 2. RNase protection analysis of topoisomerase IIα and β mRNA levels in human tumour cell lines (as indicated above each pair). In all cases the sample on the left hand side represents the drug sensitive parent and the resistant counterparts are on the right hand side. The RNA samples were prepared and the RNase protection assays carried out as described by Jenkins et al [18]. The positions of the 296 and 228 bp topo IIβ protected fragments, the 215 bp topo IIα protected fragment and the GAPDH internal loading control are shown on the left.

vitro transcription studies have been carried out using the RNase protection assay to determine mRNA levels of topo IIα and β isozymes in a group of drug resistant cell lines and their sensitive parental cells. Figure 2 shows that in five matched pairs of drug resistant/sensitive cell lines there was a reduction in the level of expression of one or other or both of the mRNAs for the topo IIα and β isozymes. In addition topo IIα and β protein levels have been analysed in a panel of breast cancer cell lines and expression levels for one or other isozyme correlated with sensitivity of different classes of topo II inhibitor. For example, mAMSA sensitivity correlated with expression of the topo IIα isozyme (data not shown).

It is always difficult to dissect the role of one particular factor in drug resistant cell lines, as many changes can occur during selection for these variants. Thus,

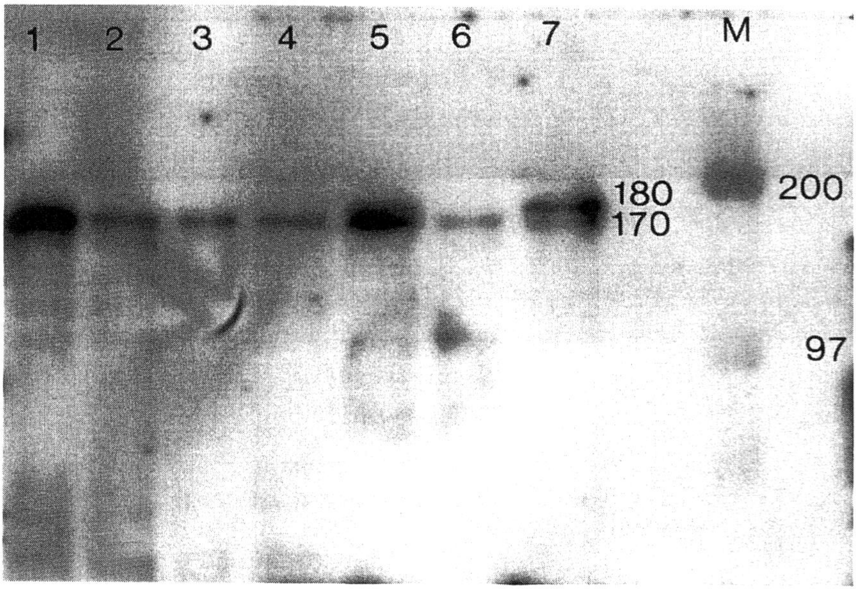

Figure 3. Western blot of nuclear extracts (32) from different AML patient biopsies (lanes 1-7), equalized in terms of total protein content and probed with topo IIα and β-specific antibodies. Positions of the 170 kD topo IIα isoform, the 180 kD topo IIβ isoform and the molecular weight standards are shown on the right.

to provide a more direct assessment of the role of each isozyme in drug resistance, topo IIα and β cDNAs were transfected into CHO cell lines to increase expression of the individual topo II isozymes. These overexpressing clones were then analysed for changes in sensitivity to different topo II antagonists and inhibitors. Preliminary data suggest that overexpression of either isozyme can confer a drug sensitive phenotype (data not shown).

One strategy for circumventing drug resistance developed *in vivo* could be to switch to drugs that target a different enzyme or the same enzyme but by a different mechanism. In a preliminary study of the different drug resistant/sensitive paired cell lines described earlier, no cross resistance could be found to the catalytic inhibitor of topo II ICRF-159. This suggests that the resistance to the dioxopiperazine derivative, ICRF-159, is mediated by mechanisms different from those relevant to cleavable complex forming topo II inhibitors. We have analysed the expression of topo IIα and β in biopsies from patients with AML. A wide variation in expression of both isozymes is apparent (Figure 3). However, in neither case did expression correlate with drug responsiveness as determined by *in vitro* drug sensitivity measurements. These data are in agreement with those reported by Kaufmann et al [30]. The suggestion from these findings is that the sensitivity/resistance of AML cells to topo II targeting drugs is determined by mechanisms other than, or in addition to, the level of topo II expression.

Future studies should determine the respective roles of topo IIα and β in drug sensitivity in clinical samples. Topo IIα promoter studies will indicate whether it is possible to upregulate the gene *in vivo* which should sensitize tumours to topo II targeting drugs. Thus drugs modifying topo II activity or upregulating topo II expression may provide novel therapeutic strategies.

References

1. Jehn U, Heniemann V. New drugs in the treatment of acute and chronic leukemia with some emphasis on m-AMSA. Anticancer Res 1991;11:705-11.
2. Bishop J. Etoposide in the treatment of leukemias. Sem Oncol 1992;19:33-38.
3. Carmichael J, Hickson ID. Mechanism of cellular resistance to cytotoxic drugs and x-irradiation. Int J Rad Oncol Biol Phys 1991;20:197-202.
4. Endicott J, Ling V. The biochemistry of p-glycoprotein-mediated drug resistance. Ann Rev Biochem 1989;58:137-71.
5. Pastan I, Gottesman M. Multiple drug resistance in human cancer. N Engl J Med 1987;316:1388-93.
6. Roninson IB (ed). Molecular and cellular biology of multidrug resistance in tumour cells. Plenum Press, New York 1991:406-14.
7. Schinkel A, Borst P. Multidrug resistance mediated by P-glycoproteins. Sem Cancer Biol 1991;2:213-26.
8. Cole S, Chanda ER, Dickie FP, Gerlach JH, Mirski SEL. Non-P-glycoprotein-mediated multidrug resistance in a small cell lung cancer cell line: Evidence for a decreased susceptibility to drug induced DNA damage and reduced levels of topoisomerase II. Cancer Res 1991;51:3345-52.
9. Zaman G, Versantvoort CHM, Smit JJM, et al. Analysis of the expression of MRP, the gene for a new putative transmembrane drug transporter, in human multidrug resistant lung cancer cell lines. Cancer Res 1993;53:1747-50.
10. Beck W. Unknotting the complexities of multidrug resistance: The involvement of DNA topoisomerases in drug action and resistance. J Natl Cancer Inst 1989;81:1683-85.
11. Davies SM, Robson CN, Davies SL, Hickson ID. Nuclear topoisomerase II levels correlate with the sensitivity of mammalian cells to intercalating agents and epipodophyllotoxins. J Biol Chem 1988;263:17724-29.
12. Deffie A, Batra JK, Goldenberg GJ. Direct correlation between DNA topoisomerase II activity and cytotoxicity in Adriamycin-sensitive and resistant P388 leukemia cell lines. Cancer Res 1989;49:58-62.
13. Wang J. DNA topoisomerases. Ann Rev Biochem 1985;54:665-97.
14. Watt P, Hickson ID. Structure and function of type II DNA topoisomerases. Biochem J 1994;303:681-95.
15. Osheroff N, Zechiedrich EL, Gale KC. Catalytic function of DNA topoisomerase II. BioEssays 1991;13:269-75.
16. Drake FH, Hoffmann GA, Bartus HF, Mattern MR, Crooke ST, Mirabelli CK. Biochemical and pharmacological properties of p170 and p180 forms of topoisomerase II. Biochem 1989;28:8154-60.

17. Tan KB, Dorman TE, Falls KM, et al. Topoisomerase IIα and topoisomerase IIβ genes: Characterization and mapping to human chromosomes 17 and 3 respective. Cancer Res 1992;52:231-34.
18. Jenkins J, Ayton P, Davies SL, et al. Isolation of cDNA clones encoding the β isozyme of human DNA topoisomerase II and localisation of the gene to chromosome 3p24. Nucl Acids Res 1992;20:5587-92.
19. Woessner RD, Mattern MR, Mirabelli CK, Johnson RK, Drake FH. Proliferation and cell cycle dependence differences in expression of the 170 kilodalton and 180 kilodalton forms of topoisomerase II in NIH-3T3 cells. Cell Growth Differ 1991;2: 209-14.
20. Gasser S, Laemmli UK. The organisation of chromatin loops: Characterization of a scaffold attachment site. EMBO J 1986;5:511-18.
21. DiNardo S, Voekel K, Sternglanz R. DNA topoisomerase mutant of *Saccharomyces cerevisiae*: topoisomerase II is required for the segregation of daughter molecules at the termination of DNA replication. Proc Natl Acad Sci USA 1984;81:2616-20.
22. Holm C, Goto T, Wang JC, Botstein D. DNA topoisomerase II is required at the time of mitosis in yeast. Cell 1985;41:553-63.
23. D'Arpa P, Beardmore C, Liu LF. Involvement of nucleic acid synthesis in cell killing mechanisms of topoisomerase poisons. Cancer Res 1990;50:6921-24.
24. Ischida R, Miki T, Narita, et al. Inhibition of intracellular topoisomerase II by antitumour bis(2,6-dioxopiperazine) derivatives: Mode of cell growth inhibition distinct from that of cleavable complex-forming type inhibitors. Cancer Res 1991;51:4909-16.
25. Tanabe K, Ikegami Y, Andoh T. Inhibition of topoisomerase II by antitumour agents bis(2,6-dioxopiperazine) derivatives. Cancer Res 1991;51:4903-08.
26. Davies S, Jenkins JR, Hickson ID. Human cells express two differentially spliced forms of topoisomerase IIβ mRNA. Nucl Acids Res 1993;21:3719-23.
27. Takano H, Kohno K, Ono M, Uchida Y, Kuwano M. Increased phosporylation of DNA topoisomerase II in etoposide-resistant mutants of human cancer KB cells. Cancer Res 1991;51:3951-57.
28. Feldhoff P, Mirski SEL, Cole SPC, Sullivan DM. Altered subcellular distribution of topoisomerase IIα in a drug resistant human small cell lung cancer cell line. Cancer Res 1994;54:756-62.
29. Webb C, Latham MD, Lock RB, Sullivan DM. Attenuated toposiomerase II content directly correlates with a low level of drug resistance in a Chinese hamster ovary cell line. Cancer Res 1991;51:6543-49.
30. Carron P, Wang JC. Alignment of primary sequences of DNA topoisomerases. In: Liu LF (ed). Advances in pharmacology. Academic Press, New York 1994;Vol 298:271-97.
31. Kaufmann S, Karp JE, Jones RJ, et al. Topoisomerase II levels and drug sensitivity in adult acute myelogenous leukemia. Blood 1994;83:517-30.
32. Fry A, Cresta CM, Davies SM, et al. Relationship between topoisomerase II level and chemosensitivity in human tumour cell lines. Cancer Res 1991;51:6592-95.

IMPACT OF CELL CULTURE TECHNOLOGY ON TRANSFUSION MEDICINE

G.T. Roberts, R.A. Sacher

Introduction

Understanding of the processes of haematopoiesis took a major leap forward when it was shown by Till and McCullouch in the 1960's that splenic cell from normal mice could re-instate haematopoiesis in lethally irradiated mice [1]. The concepts of a multipotent haematopoietic cell emerged from these early experiments, and led to the development of *in vitro* investigative tools to help identify the cell(s) responsible for initiating and maintaining haematopoiesis.

Progress was marked by the *in vitro* demonstration that putative haematopoietic stem cells (HSC), simulated by various growth factors, developed into differentiating clusters of blood cells in various culture milieu. To date, intensive study has identified multiple growth factors together with their receptors, as well as some of their effects in various putative stem cells.

With these developments, it has been anticipated that pure stem cells could be grown and expanded *in vitro* levels sufficient to repopulate the bone marrow (BM) or provide blood product support for patients with cytopenias.

Definition of human stem cells

It has been difficult to characterize the nature and origin of HSC, although they are conceptually, haematopoietic progenitor cells capable of self-renewal, proliferation and differentiation into the mature cell present in the peripheral blood and other sites. They are present not only in the BM, but also circulate in peripheral blood and are found in cord blood. As a pre-requisite toward ex-vivo expansion it would be desirable to identify and harvest and purify these cells.

When BM cells are plated on appropriate medium and supplied with relevant growth factors, they give rise to colonies of erythroid cells, granulocytic-monocytic or megakaryocytic progeny, usually over a period of about 7-14 days.

However, the cells that give rise to these colonies are considered to be the progenies of earlier cells that are the true HSC, and which, in fact, require long term culture in order to emerge slowly from their quiescent state. These HSC give rise, in 5-6 weeks, to colonies that consist of mixed populations of erythroid, granulocytic, monocytic and megakaryocytic forms [2].

Table 1. Expression of CD45RO on directly clonogenic cells and ITC-IC.

Clonogenic and LTC-I cells		Unsorted	CD34^{+}	
			CD45RO^{-}	CD45RO^{+}
BFU-E1	1	416	11,000	0
(per 10^5)	2	93	2,550	0
	3	132	4,930	0
CFU-GM	1	358	5,680	12,000
(per 10^5)	2	86	849	4,200
	3	140	2,670	15,700
LTC-IC	1	371	24,100	3,220
(per 2×10^6)	2	630	21,300	100
	3	204	19,400	12,705

Table 2. Generation of secondary CFU-GM from 4-HC^{resistant}/CD34^{+} human BM following cytokine treatment in suspension cultures.

Cytokine	D_0CFU-GM	Secondary CFU-GM
G-CSF	1.5 1.5	26.3 ± 11.2
GM-CSF	1.5 1.5	24.4 ± 9.0
IL-3	1.5 1.5	66.0 ± 16.6
M-CSF	1.5 1.5	2.8 ± 1.7
IL-1	1.5 1.5	12.1 ± 4.3
IL-6	1.5 1.5	11.4 ± 5
IL-1 + G-CSF	1.5 1.5	52.5 ± 26.4
IL-1 + GM-CSF	1.5 1.5	31.0 ± 19.4
IL-1 + IL-3*	1.5 1.5	119.3 ± 18.3*
IL-1 + M-CSF	1.5 1.5	21.9 ± 3.3
IL-6 + IL-3	1.5 1.5	66.3 ± 25.3

Values are mean standard errors of three separate experiments. GM-CSF (1,000 U/mL) was used in all CFU-GM assays. IL-1 + IL-3 secondary CFU-GM mean was greater than all other cytokine treatments at $P < 0.5$ except IL-3 alone ($P < 0.85$) and IL-1 + G-CSF is due to the large IL-1 + C-CSF standard deviation. In all experiments analyzed to date, IL-1 + IL-3 has consistently generated more secondary CFU than IL-1 + G-CSF. Adapted from Smith, et al [4].

Over the last decade or so, work in a number of laboratories has shown that they belong to a small fraction of bone marrow cells that are present among the 3-5% of light density marrow mononuclear cells, and which are also Rhodamine 123 (Rhod123)-dull and CD34^{+}. Such cells can be further classified into CD45RO^{+} or CD45RO- sub-sets. It is within these groups that different levels of stem cells reside. Lansdorp et al [3] showed that the CD34^{+}/CD45RO^{+} subset gives rise to BFU-E in *in vitro* culture, and can also give rise to mixed erythroid granulocytic

colonies after 5 weeks of culture. On the other hand, the $CD34^+$/CD45RO-cells give rise to predominantly granulocytic colonies (Table 1). This issue has been addressed by a number of other authors including Smith et al [4] who also showed that 4-hydroperoxycyclophosphamide (4HC)-resistant ($4HC^{res}$) $CD34^+$ cells are capable of long term culture initiating cells (LTC-IC) activity. In this study they used a variety of cytokines, both singly and in combination, to stimulate $4HC^{res}$ $CD34^+$ cells, and showed that the most powerful combination was IL-1/IL-3 (Table 2). The differential characteristics of early precursors in culture and their responses to combinations of cytokines are important factors influencing the potential large scale ex-vivo expansion of these cells.
There are also differences between bone marrow precursors and those present in peripheral blood (steady state and mobilized) and cord blood.
Peripheral blood also contains LTC-IC at very low concentration, probably at two orders of magnitude less than in the bone marrow. These LTC-IC are also Rhod123 dull, $CD34^+$, HLA-DR- and $4HC^{res}$, and are present in the light density fraction (<1.077 gm/mL) of peripheral blood at a concentration of about 3.0 cell/ml of blood [5] (Table 2a). But in spite of all these investigations, the precise morphological, phenotypic and functional attributes of the pluripotent HSC have not been ascertained. Operationally, they are considered $CD34^+$, $CD33^-$, $CD71^-$, $CD77^-$, $CD15^-$, $CD38^-$, HLA-DR^-, $CD45RA^-$, Rhod 123 dull, and $4HC^{res}$ [6]. Such LTC-IC are thought to be identical to the cells capable of repopulating an ablated bone marrow (marrow repopulating cells -MRC) [2, 7].

Sources of stem cells

Whilst stem cells have traditionally been obtained from adult bone marrow and more recently peripheral blood, one promising new resource is human umbilical cord (HUC) and placental blood [8, 9]. HUC-placental blood is a rich source of HSC, which has now been used in BM reconstitution in the treatment of paediatric patients with haematological malignancies and other life-threatening haematological disease [9].

The number and nature of stem cells in a cord blood sample though generally similar, in relative terms, to those in normal BM (Table 4-5), is finite and may be insufficient for bone marrow repopulation in adult patients. However, it is potentially expandable [10, 11]. For example, Gabutti et al were able to effect a greater than 30-fold increase in haematopoietic progenitors when stimulated by SCF and other cytokines [11]. Their results also showed that the number of early progenitors is higher in HUC-placental blood.

HUC-placental blood has a number of distinct advantages over adult bone marrow or peripheral blood as a means of haematopoietic reconstitution. These include: (Table 6)
- Unlimited availability;
- Reduced immunogenicity, and, therefore, less likely to cause GvHD;
- Potentially markedly improved genetic and ethnic diversity;
- Potentially less likely to carry pathogenic viruses such as CMV [10, 12].

Table 2a. Quantitative of LTC-IC and clonogenic cells in normal PB.

Cell type	Concentration (per mL)
BFU-E	170 ± 20
CFU-GM	51 ± 5
CFU-GEMM	4.6 ± 0.6
LTC-IC	2.9 ± 0.5

Values for individual patients were calculated by multiplying the progenitor frequency per 10^5 cells by the nucleated cell recovery after both the T-cell-depletion and FH density centrifugation steps and then again by the blood cells per milliliter. Values shown are the mean SEM of data obtained from 23 different normal individuals.
Adapted from Udomsakdi, et al [5].

Table 3. Characteristics of human haemopoietic stem cells.

$CD34^+$
$CD33^-$, $CD71^-$, $CD77^-$, $CD15^-$, $CD38^-$, HLA-DR^-, $CD45RA^-$
Rhodamine dull
4HC resistant

Adapted from Nicol, et al [6].

Moreover, use of allogeneic cord blood, collected at no risk to infant or mother, avoids the discomfort and potential hazards of general anaesthesia in unrelated allogeneic donors [13].

Because of its potential as a haematopoietic stem cell resource, it has now become appropriate to devise protocols for collecting, harvesting and storing stem cells from HUC-placental blood. The ultimate objective would be to have serial banks of harvested umbilical blood that would be available, as in current allogeneic unrelated bone marrow registries, for patients in need of bone marrow reconstitution. Unlike paper registries, however, the inoculum would be readily available for use, bypassing the time-consuming process of bringing the registry donor into the hospital for final testing and harvesting. One obvious difficulty is that of volume reduction so that storage space requirements would be reduced to a minimum. Other long-term objectives in HUC-placental blood, as well as for BM and PB manipulation, include isolation of the stem cells for the purpose of gene transfer in order to correct genetic abnormalities [8, 14].

Isolation or purification of stem cells

Although it is not necessary to have a pure fraction of stem cells or MRC in order to grow them, it is nevertheless highly desirable to secure some for the purpose of direct manipulation, in for example, experiments aimed at inserting genes into cells for the purpose of gene therapy.

There are many *in vitro* methods for separating and enriching stem cells, both from marrow and peripheral blood (see Table 7). They depend on two primary modalities [15].

- Negative selection;
- Positive selection.

In negative selection, passenger cells are actively removed from a population by means of some physical attribute such as cell density or inability to withstand osmotic lysis. In many systems, this primary mode results, not only in removing unwanted nucleated cells, but also in volume reduction as well. By positive selection, HSC are actively recruited through the means of some biological or physical attribute of the cell that enables them to be sequestered from the other cell components in the sample.

Negative selection:

- a) Density gradient, single (Ficoll), or dual (Percoll) state;
  b) Mechanical adherence to plastic or glass.
- Immunoadsorption by antibody directed against epitope on accessory cells followed by either mechanical extraction or killing by attached toxin or added complement.
- Sheep red blood cell adherence.
- Immunomagnetic selection [16].
- 4HC treatment, which will kill all cells apart from non-cycling progenitor cells [4, 17].

Positive selection:
Immunoadsorption of stem cells, using monoclonal antibodies directed against epitodes on the cells of interest [18]. This is most often directed to the most reliable marker of early progenitors, the CD34 antigen, which may be preferentially removed and concentrated as described below.

Practical considerations

There are many protocols by which stem cells can be separated, but virtually all use modifications or refinements of the sequence described in the preceding section. Practical considerations include whether a process of negative selection could be performed in a primary collection receptacle such as a plastic blood donation bag, or whether the selection should be done in secondary vessels such as centrifuge tubes. The adherence technique is performed in flat-bottomed or other type vessel with sufficient surface area, exploiting the natural property of plastic and glass to firmly bind mononuclear cells; or alternatively, making use of specific binding by MoAb fixed to the vessel surface. In positive selection, the HSC is selected by:

- Immunoadsorption to MoAb fixed to a solid phase such as glass or plastic beads followed by removal either by mechanical agitation, or eluted off with the aid of buffer, tissue culture fluid or enzymatic cleavage [19].

Table 4. Comparison of stem cells in cord blood and normal bone marrow by colony assays.

	HUC	Bone marrow	% Difference
	Mean±SEM	Mean±SEM	
Nucleated cells $\times 10^9$	1.8±0.2	12.8	14.1
CFU-GM, GM-CSF	4.4±0.8	4.8	96.1
CFU-GM, GM-CSF + SLF	9.8±1.8	12.5	78.4
BFU-E, EPO + IL-3	13.1±1.6	45.1	29
CFU-GEMM, EPO + SLF	10.1±1.9	43.0	23.5
CFU-GEMM, EPO + SLF + IL-3	14 ±2.4	57.6±15.1	24.3

Adapted from Broxmeyer, et al [10].

Table 5. Mean (SE) cell colonies in HUC blood and normal bone marrow measured in clonogenic assays for committed haemopoietic progenitor cells.

Colony type	HUC blood		Normal bone marrow	
CFU-GM*	70	5.3	80	(5.2)
CFU-mix*	2.1	(0.4)	1.9	(0.31)
BFU-E*	47	(5.3)	30	(2.5)
CFU-E*	32	(4.7)	49	(5.5)
Megakaryocytes				
Total	19	(3.9)	24	(6.0)
20 cells	7.5	(1.6)	17	(1.9)
20-200 cells	9	(1.8)	7	(2.0)
200 cells	3	(0.94)	1	

Numbers are mean (SE) colonies derived from 5×10^4 mononuclear cells.
* Results calculated from 36 experiments with HUC blood and 34 with normal bone marrow, or from 10 with HUC blood and 13 with normal bone marrow.
Adapted from Nicol, et al [6].

Table 6. CBSCs: Potential advantages.

- Ease and safety of collection
- Low risk of viral contamination (CMV, EBV, hepatitis B, HIV)
- Reduced graft-versus-host reactivity (not proven)
- Enriched for long-term bone marrow culture initiating cells

Adapted from Wagner [9].

- Immunoadsorption to MoAb fixed to magnetic beads which are then extracted with a magnet [19]. The HSC are then separated from the beads by proteolytic enzyme action. Alternatively, magnetic wool could be used as the solid phase.

- HSC, treated with MoAb conjugated with fluorescein or other fluorochrome can be separated in a fluorescence activated cell sorter (FACS) [18]. This method, because of its time-consuming nature, is the least efficient for collecting purified cells for direct use in haematopoietic grafting.

Cultural selection can also be performed, based on the principle that, in a mixture of normal stem cells and leukaemic cells, the latter will fail to grow in long-term culture, whereas the former will multiply sufficiently to secure autologous engraftment in patients with chronic and acute myeloid leukemias [20].

A practical approach is to use the CD34 affinity CellPro® column (Bothell, WA) where the cell mixture with CD34 cells are incubated with biotinylated anti-CD34 MoAb. The sample containing the HSC is run through a column filled with avidin-coated beads, during which process, the target cells adhere to the beads and may then be subsequently eluted from the column, yielding a considerably enriched harvest.

Investigators at Applied Immune Sciences (Santa Clara, CA) have developed a strategy that recovers an enriched fraction of $CD34^+$ progenitor cells from BM harvests after low density separation of the BMMC. The system goes through a series of steps of:
- purification;
- enrichment;
- isolation by positive selection.

In their technique, they used polystyrene flasks, modified so as to enhance surface immobilization of soy bean agglutinin for the enrichment step by negative selection; this was followed by positive selection in flasks with immobilized anti-CD34 MoAb. By this method, they were able to obtain a 10-50 fold enrichment of $CD34^+$ cells which were 97.5 to >99.5% pure, and which were free of deliberately introduced malignant cells [21]. Holyoake et al have confirmed that $CD34^+$ adherent cells, obtained in this system are most efficient in producing multipotential colony-forming units, Type A [22].

In vitro manipulation of purified stem cell fractions

One of the challenges that now face biologists and clinical scientists is to perform either *in vitro* or *in vivo* expansion of these haematopoietic progenitor cells (HPC) to levels adequate for adult transplantation, and perhaps effect differentiation on a scale that would be large enough to provide mature RBC, leukocytes and platelets for realistic clinical transfusion. A number of workers have used various culture conditions in which increases in CFUe and other committed stem cells have been achieved (Table 8, 8a, 8b) [10, 11, 23].

Table 7. Methods used in the purification of CD34$^+$ cells.

Positive selection

Monoclonal antibodies to 115 kD

Membrane glycoprotein on all precursor cells

Negative selection (purging)

Non-antibody mediated:

- Durgs, density separation
- Lectins, chemical (e.g. ether)
- Long term culture

Antibody mediated:

- Complement lysis
- Immunotoxins
- Immunomagnetic techniques
- immunorosettes

Table 8. Fold changes in detection of myeoloid progenitor cells with added SLF.

		Human umbilical cord	**Adult bone marrow**
CFU-GM	CM	+ 8.2 (1.))	+2.1 (0.2)
	CSF	+10.7 (1.2)	+3.6 (0.3)
CFU-GEMM	EPO + CM	+11.3 (1.2)	ND
	EPO + IL-3	+10.5 (1.1)	+5.6 (0.6)
BFU-E	EPO	− 8.8 (1.3)	+3.4 (0.6)
	EPO + CM	−13.0 (2.4)	+3.4 (0.6)
	EPO + IL-3	−18.2 (2.8)	+1.6 (0.2)

Numbers indicate mean (SEM) changes in detection of progenitor cells when stem cell factor (SLF) is added together with the cytokines cited. CM = conditioned medium. Adapted from Broxmeyer, et al [10].

Part of the difficulty is that the MRC cannot, as yet, be easily assayed *in vitro*. Yet the studies of Abboud et al [23] clearly indicate that a primitive cell can be induced in a two-stage *in vitro* assay, to produce clonogenic cells which, in turn, give rise to CFUs, BFU-E, CFU-GM and CFU-Mix (Table 9). In these experiments, CD34$^+$ cells, isolated from HUC-placental blood, have had greater *in vitro* expansion potential than adult marrow and peripheral blood [24].

Potential Danger of stem cell "exhaustion"

The process of *in vitro* expansion of stem cells has to be exquisitely controlled if irreversible uni-directional differentiation of the stem cells is not to occur. Likewise, there has also been concern that a similar "exhaustion" of stem cells could occur *in vivo* on repeated stimulation by cytokines [25], although some of

Table 8a. Expansion of cord blood CD34$^+$ cells in weekly delta cultures stimulated with IL-1 + IL-3 + KL EPO*.

Delta IC No. increase	Cells $\times 10^6$	Fold fold in-crease	CFU/BFU $\times 10^5$	Fold LTC increase
0	0.04	1	0.03	13001
1	3.5	88	2.2	725,00017
2	110.6	2,800	19.0	6145,53018+
3	1,507	38,000	73.2	2,364NDND
4	2,778	69,000	10.0	323-----
5	4,036	101,000	3.2	104-----

* CFU/BFU stimulated by IL-1 + IL-3 + KL + EPO.
ND = not detected.
LTC-IC = long-term culture-initiating cells assayed at 5 weeks on irradiated SV40-transformed human bone marrow fibroblasts.
Adapted from Moor [8].

Table 8b. Cumulative production of CFU-GM* in cultures initiated with 4×10^4 CD34$^+$ cells from cord blood and passaged weekly with 4×10^4 cells and cytokines.

Stimulus	Peak CFU-GM number	Fold increase	Days	
IL-6 + KL + IL-3	1.39×107	3.73×10^3	34	0.3
IL-6 + KL + IL-3	5.3 ×106	3.43×10^3	21	
IL-6 + KL + IL-3 + EPO**	2.7×10^6	1.7×10^3	28	
IL-1 + KL + IL-3	6.3×10^6	2.8×10^3	25	1
IL-1 + KL + IL-3 + EPO	4.1×10^6	2.0×10^3	25	4
IL-1 + KL + IL-6	0.4×10^6	0.4×10^6	28	
IL-1 + KL + IL-6 + EPO	0.5×10^6	0.3×10^3	14	

* Stimulus for CFU-GM, IL-1 or IL-6 + KL + IL-3 + EPO.
** Cocultured for the first week with mouse fibroblast line AM-12.
Adapted from Moore [8].

the experimental evidence suggests that there is no loss of proliferative potential in *ex vivo* treatment of stem cells with IL-1 plus Kit-ligand [26].

Other *in vitro* manipulation of stem cells

Expansion of stem cells is not the only *in vitro* procedure that may have utility in haematopoietic reconstitution. Purging of autologous marrow of malignant cells, and allogeneic marrow of immune reactive cells has been commonly performed.

Table 9. Colonies developing from CD34$^+$/4HC^{res} cord blood cells.

	Day 0	IL-3	IL-1	IL-3/IL-1	IL-6	IL-3/IL-6
BFU-E	5 (3)	68 (35)	9 (1)	116 (30)	10 (0.5)	99 (32)
CFU-GM	13 (6)	302 (105)	20 (1)	391 (200)	25 (9.8)	335 (170)
CFU-mix	0 (0)	9 (5)	0 (0)	20 (5)	0 (0)	13 (5)
Cell #	100 (0)	128 (21)	95 (15)	124 (21)	50 (5)	134 (25)

Mean (SEM) of colonies developing from CD34$^+$/4HC^{res} cells plated directly (Day 0), and after 7 days in suspension with the different cytokines cited.
Adapted from Abboud et al [23].

Table 10. Ex-vivo haematopoietic expansion.

Potential applications

Expansion of stem cells for haematopoietic cell reconstitution:
- Alternative to bone marrow
- Alternative to leukapheresis

Gene transfer:
- Genetic labeling
- Gene therapy

Target cell expansion:
- Immunotherapy
- Tumour cell purging
- Cellular reservoirs

Reduction of immune reactive cells

This is aimed at reducing cells that can cause clinically troublesome reactions such as GvHD [27-29] reaction that are mediated by T cells and their cytokine secretions.

The procedure of T-cell purging has now been a well-established modality for reducing immune reactive T-cells in allogenic marrow transplants. Numerous protocols exist, including E-rosetting, MoAb directed against T-Cells, use of various lectins, immunotoxins [30], etc. However, in the setting of the treatment of acute leukemias, depletion of T-cells renders the inoculum unable to exert a graft vs leukaemia effect that is essential for holding the disease at bay.

Recently, the ability of autologous T-cell to exert anti-tumour effects has been exploited by lymphokine activation of autologous marrow or peripheral blood [31-33].

Bone marrow purging

Autologous BM purging is used in some protocols when allogeneic donors are unavailable for the radical treatment of patients with malignant disease. This approach has been used for non-haematologic malignancies as well as for the haematologic malignancies. In these settings, monoclonal antibodies directed against epitodes on malignant cells, may be used to selectively remove the malignant cells from marrow or alternatively demo therapeutic purging may be attempted (as described earlier).

It has been expected that peripheral stem cell harvests could be used for bone marrow reconstitution in patients with haematologic and non-haematologic malignancies without the risks of tumour cell contamination attendant in bone marrow harvests, but is has recently become evident that micrometastases may be present in peripheral blood stem cell harvests also, potentially limiting their usefulness in restoring marrow ablated for radical cure. Purging the malignant cells is desirable for minimizing the chances of disease recurrence.

Methods for purging malignant cells

There is a variety of methods for purging bone marrow or PB of malignant cells. Techniques include:

- Use of MoAb directed against tumour cell antigen. The lever for removing antibody coated cells include:
  a) Magnetic bead conjugate.
  b) Conjugates involving immunotoxins as shown by Meyer et al [34], who used a streptavidin-biotin-ricin conjugate to kill target cells sensitized with biotinylated MoAb.
- Use of either endogenous or exogenous cytokines to activate autologous T cells, thus producing lymphokine activated killer cells, or LAK.

In addition to their by now well-established role in haematopoietic cell differentiation, cytokines are also partly responsible for enhancing the functional activity of immune reactive cells. The most relevant area in this respect is that of enhancement of lymphocyte killer cell activity inducible by interleukin 2 (IL-2) [31, 32]. For example, Charak et al demonstrated that BM could purge itself of haematologic tumour cell lines such as K-562, CEM or Daudi, when incubated with added IL-2 [31]. This cytokine is also able to activate marrow to purge itself of autologous acute myeloid or lymphoid leukaemia. This method has now been upscaled in our laboratory and we now have several clinical protocols for activating cytotoxic lymphocytes in both autologous marrow and G-CSF mobilized peripheral blood stem cells transplantation. The preliminary results appear promising but it is too early to evaluate long term disease free survival. Interferon-gamma (IFN-γ) is also effective in purging BM of CML cells in patients with chronic myeloid leukaemia. Twenty-four hour incubation *in vitro* with IFN-γ, followed by long-term liquid culture, showed by PCR, that bcr/ABL II RNA transcripts became undetectable in the culture after 4 weeks. In this experiment by Becker et al, there was, however, a 75% inhibition of CFU-GM production [35]. Cytokines are also active against epithelial cells. Other modalities for purging tumour cells from marrow and peripheral blood include the use of chemotherapeutic agents such as 4HC, by which Passos-Coelho et al were able to effect a 100% sterilization of BM harvests contaminated with metastatic breast carcinoma [36]. There are clinical trials in progress to determine whether these *in vitro* and animal studies can be replicated in the therapy of human malignant disease.

Storage and preservation of haematopoietic cells

As previously mentioned, storage of HUC-placental blood stem cells could expand the possibilities for transplanting a wide range of ethnically diverse patients. Thawed cryopreserved HUC-placental blood has been used at least once in the transplant treatment of a child with acute leukaemia (J. Kurtzberg, personal communication). The opportunities for expansion of HSC are listed in Table 10 and are clearly exciting avenues of cellular therapy. These also include the opportunity for expansion of differentiating cells and ultimately cellular component factories. As an example, partially differentiated myeloid precursors expanded ex-vivo by cytokine and growth factor stimulation, and could be given with autologous mobilized PBSC to abroage the "obligatory period" of neutropenia (8-10 days) after transplantation. The promyelocytes would have to be expanded 100 fold. Juttner has estimated that to achieve this 6.25×10^9 promyelocytes derived from 5×10^7 $CD34^+$ stem cells [40] would be needed to differentiate into 2×10^{11} neutrophils.

Outlook for clinical haematopoietic stem cell reconstruction

The significance of these new approaches is that blood banks and transfusion services are now becoming blood and cell culturing laboratories in which the management of cell culture, live storage and manipulation of viable bone marrow, peripheral blood, HUC and human cord blood harvests would become standard. Transfusion Medicine specialists and Blood Banks are natural areas for necessary expertise to ensure quality control and continuous good manufacturing practices.

References

1. Till JE, McCulloch EA. A direct measurement of radiation sensitivity of normal mouse bone marrow cells. Radiat Res 1961;14:213-22.
2. Gartner S, Kaplan HS. Long term culture of human bone marrow cells. PNAS USA 1980;77:4756-59.
3. Lansdorp PM, Sutherland JH, Eaves CJ. Selective expression of CD45 isoforms on functional subpopulations of CD34+ hemapoietic cells from human bone marrow. J Exp Med 1990;172:363-66.
4. Smith C, Gasperetto C, Collins N, et al. Purification and partial characterisation of a human hematopoietic precursor population. Blood 1991;77:2122-28.
5. Udomsakdi C, Lansdorp PM, Hogge DE, Reid DS, Eaves AC, Eaves CJ. Characterization of primitive hematopoietic cells in normal human peripheral blood. Blood 1992;80:2513-21.

6. Nicol AJ, Hows JM, Bradley BA. Cord blood transplantation: A practical option? Annotation: Brit J Haematol 1994;87:1-5.
7. Lansdorp PM, Dragowska W. Long-term erythropoiesis from constant numbers of CD34+ cells in serum-free cultures initiated with highly purified progenitor cells from human bone marrow. J Exp Med 1992;175:1501-09.
8. Moore MAS. Ex vivo expansion and gene therapy using cord blood CD34+ cells. J Hematotherapy 1993;2:221-24.
9. Wagner JE, Kernan NA, Broxmeyer HE, Gluckman E. Allogeneic umbilical cord blood transplantation: A report of results in 26 patients. Blood 1993;(Suppl)82:86a.
10. Broxmeyer HE, Hangoc G, Cooper S, et al. Growth characteristics and expansion of human umbilical cord blood and estimation of its potential for transplantation in adults. Proc Natl Acad Sci USA 1992;89:4109-13.
11. Gabutti V, Timeus F, Ramenghi U, et al. Expansion of cord blood progenitors and use for hematopoietic reconstitution. Stem Cells 1993;(Suppl 2)11:105-12.
12. Rubinstein P, Rosenfield RE, Adamson JW, Stevens CE. Stored placental blood for unrelated bone marrow reconstitution. Blood 1993;81:1674-90.
13. Stroncek DF, Holland PV, Bartch G, et al. Experiences of first 493 unrelated marrow donors in the National Marrow Donor Program. Blood 1993;81:1940-46.
14. Lu M, Maruyama M, Zhang N, Levine F, Friedman T, Ho AD. High efficiency retroviral-mediated gene transduction into CD34+ cells purified from peripheral blood of breast cancer patients primed with chemotherapy and granulocyte-macrophage colony-stimulating factor. Hum Gene Ther 1994;5:203-8.
15. Gabbianelli M, Sargiacomo M, Pelosi E, Testa U, Isaachi G, Peschle C. "Pure" human hematopoietic progenitors: Permissive action of basic fibroblast growth factor. Science 1990;249:1561-64.
16. Egeland T, Albrechtsen D, Martin PJ, Hansen JA. Immunomagnetic depletion of CD6+ cells from bone marrow and peripheral blood. Bone Marrow Transplant 1990;5:193-98.
17. Yeager AM, Kaizer H, Santos GW, et al. Autologous bone marrow transplantation in patients with acute nonlymphocytic leukemia, using ex vivo marrow treatment with 4-hydroperoxcyclophosphamide-purged bone marrow. N Engl J Med 1986;315:141-47.
18. Sowala H, Wunder E, Herron PH. Purification and characterization of the CD34+ hematopoietic precursor cell population by flow cytometry. Bone Marrow Transplant 1990;(Suppl 1)5:9-10.
19. Grimsley PG, Amos TA, Gordon MY, Greaves MF. Rapid positive selection of CD34+ cells using magnetic macrospheres coated with monoclonal antibody QBEND/10 linked via a cleavable disulphide bond. Leukemia 1993;7:898-908.
20. Ozsahin H, Fabrega S, Douay L, Barbu V, Gorin NC. Application of serum-free liquid bone marrow cultures to bone marrow purging for autologous bone marrow transplantation in acute lymphoblastic leukemia. Nouv Rev Fr Hematol 1990;32:353-55.

GENE THERAPY FOR PRIMARY IMMUNE DEFICIENCIES

K.I. Weinberg

Historically, severe combined immune deficiency (SCID) has been a model disease for the development of innovative transplantation procedures, e.g., the first successful histocompatible bone marrow transplants (BMT), haploidentical T-cell depleted BMT, or matched unrelated donor BMT [1]. Because patients with SCID have defective immunity, their ability to reject transplanted marrow is limited. This characteristic has made it possible to achieve engraftment from a variety of sources. In histocompatible BMT, pre-transplant cytotoxic conditioning is not required to ensure engraftment, although conditioning is usually needed for histoincompatible BMT [2]. Transplants without conditioning result is a state of chimerism with donor T lymphocytes, donor or recipient B lymphocytes, and recipient haematopoietic cells being found after BMT. The engraftment of only recipient T lymphocytes in patients with SCID, who did not receive pre-transplant conditioning, establishes that normal donor T lymphocyte progenitors have a proliferative advantage over the recipient SCID T lymphocyte progenitors.

The definition of mutations responsible for the human SCID phenotype has allowed consideration of a novel treatment modality, gene therapy with modified autologous haematopoietic stem cells [3]. Gene therapy offers theoretical advantages over haploidentical T cell depleted or matched unrelated bone marrow transplants, the usual treatments for SCID patients lacking a sibling matched donor. Gene therapy for SCID might avoid a number of immunologic problems. The risks of non-engraftment, pre-transplant chemotherapy, and GvHD currently limit the success of non-sibling matched BMT [2].

Absence of the enzyme adenosine deaminase (ADA) was the first genetic basis for SCID to be defined, and accounts for about 25% of all cases. In ADA deficiency, deoxyadenosine metabolites accumulate, which are toxic to lymphocytes. ADA deficiency can be successfully treated with either BMT or with replacement therapy with PEG-ADA, a chemically modified form of ADA [4]. In the past five years, several other genes which are mutated in a variety of SCID syndromes have been identified. Among the loci responsible for SCID are those encoding the IL-2 receptor γ chain (X-SCID), ZAP-70 (CD8 lymphopaenia), CD3 components, and a Class II trans-activator (bare lymphocyte syndrome, MHC deficiency) [5-9].

Gene therapy with retroviral vectors has been attempted for ADA deficiency, using peripheral blood T lymphocytes, and progenitors derived from bone marrow, umbilical cord blood, and peripheral blood as targets [10-13]. Some features of ADA deficiency that have made it an attractive target for experimental gene therapy include recessive mode of inheritance, ubiquitous expression of the ADA gene in all cell types and stages of differentiation, a broad range of acceptable levels of expression, selective advantage to transduced cells, and availability of enzyme replacement as an adjunctive therapy. The ADA gene therapy trials to date have demonstrated the need to efficiently transduce long-lived cells. T cells can be used as a target if enzyme replacement is used prior to gene therapy. Otherwise, the target for gene therapy must be the pluripotent haematopoietic stem cell (HSC). In the absence of ablative chemotherapy, transduction of a limited number of cells can only be successful if there is a selective advantage to the genetically normal T lymphocytes.

In May and June, 1993, three infants were born with ADA deficiency after prenatal diagnosis had been performed [13]. At the time of birth, umbilical cord blood was obtained and transported to Childrens Hospital Los Angeles for transduction with LASN, a retroviral vector containing the normal ADA cDNA. $CD34^+$ cells were isolated from the cord blood, using the CellPro® apparatus. The cells were stimulated with IL-3, IL-6 and SCF, and cultured for 3 days with supernatant containing LASN. 12-20% of the cells were transduced, using G418 resistance to measure LASN-transduced colonies. After testing for sterility, the transduced cells were transported back to the patients' hospital and infused into the patients without incident. The patients have been maintained on PEG-ADA enzyme replacement therapy. They have developed normal immune function, probably because of the PEG-ADA treatment [4]. With follow-up of >400 days, there are circulating LASN-transduced mononuclear cells at a frequency of 1:3000-1:100,000, indicating that long-lived progenitor cells from the umbilical cord blood were transduced. The selective advantage that the transduced cells have over the patients' ADA-cell may be blunted by the PEG-ADA therapy.

The knowledge gained from the ADA gene therapy trials, while still preliminary, provides a framework for designing gene therapy for non-ADA deficient SCID. The problems of stem cell isolation and manipulation, and transduction efficiency need to be overcome before gene therapy can be considered to be a routine procedure. The rest of this presentation will be on problems to be solved in the use of gene therapy for X-SCID and ZAP-70 deficiency.

Gene therapy for X-SCID will require the genetic reconstruction of complex multimeric receptors, which use the common γ chain. The γ_c protein is a component of the IL-2, IL-4, IL-7, IL-15 receptors, and probably the IL-13 receptor [14, 16]. Analysis of heterozygous female carriers indicates that, as in ADA deficiency, there is a selective advantage to genetically normal cells [17]. However, unlike ADA deficiency, the levels of expression of the normal gene needed to reconstitute deficient cells is not known. The stoichiometry of the receptor subcomponents may require a tighter control of the level of expression than the current retroviral vectors allow. The pattern of expression of γ_c is much more restricted than for ADA deficiency, raising the question of whether ectopic expression in normally non-expressing cells will have untoward consequences. Analysis of cell lines and the known patterns of IL-2, IL-4 and IL-7 receptor expression indicates that the gene is normally expressed in a variety of haematopoietic lineages, and at early stages of differentiation. The X-linked pattern of inheritance means that dominant-negative mutations are theoretically possible. Such mutations would require gene replacement therapy, rather than the gene addition currently being envisioned.

A number of models for the preclinical evaluation of gene therapy for X-SCID exist. EBV-transformed lymphoblastoid cell lines from patients with X-SCID can be used to test the function of the IL-4R. Unfortunately, T cell lines generally require a functional IL-2R to be established, making it difficult to evaluate the direct effects of γ_c transduction on X-SCID T cells. Several systems now exist that allow $CD34^+$ progenitor cells to differentiate in vitro into thymocyte-like cells. Adaptation of these culture techniques for transduction of γ_c into normal and X-SCID progenitors may be an in vitro model of the effects of X-SCID gene therapy on thymopoiesis. Ultimately, in vivo models will be required to test the feasibility of gene therapy. The X-SCID dog has a γ_c mutation, and is immunologically similar to that of the human disease, although maternal graft-versus-host disease is not observed in the canine model. Reagents are being developed to isolate pluripotent canine HSC, which will facilitate the use of the dog model for gene therapy. Murine knockout models of X-SCID may also be useful, but many of the technical issues is gene therapy, e.g., transduction of HSC, are best addressed in large animal models.

ZAP-70 deficient SCID is another candidate for gene therapy [7]. ZAP-70 is a protein tyrosine kinase, which associates with the T cell receptor-associated $CD\zeta$ chain after receptor engagement with the antigen-MHC complex. Patients with ZAP-70 deficiency have abnormal levels of mature CD8 T lymphocytes due to a defect in thymopoiesis. Although $CD4^+$ cells are generated in normal numbers, signalling through the TCR is abnormal and sub-optimal levels of IL-2 are generated. Thus, ZAP-70 deficiency results in a failure of ontogeny of $CD8^+$ cells, and defective function in $CD4^+$ cells. Like X-SCID, ZAP-70 deficiency involves the reconstruction of a complex receptor that may require tighter levels of control than current retroviral technology allows. ZAP-70 is expressed in a T cell-specific manner; and the effects to ectopic expression in non-T cells are unknown. There is evidence that the ZAP-70 and syk genes can complement each other and it is not known whether expression of ZAP-70 in cell lineage that normally express syk, but not ZAP-70, could be deleterious.

Models for testing gene therapy for ZAP-70 deficiency are limited by the absence of an animal model. Our laboratory has HTLV-I transformed T cell lines from peripheral blood and thymus of ZAP-70 deficient patients, which are being used to test the effect of ZAP-70 transduction on TCR-mediated signalling. A thymic stroma system for the growth of thymocytes from $CD34^+$ cells may be useful in the evaluation of whether the defect in CD8 ontogeny can be corrected.

A major problem with T cell depleted BMT has been the observed delay in immune reconstitution, due primarily to the long time, e.g., 6-12 months, required for differentiation of haematopoietic stem cells into functional T lymphocytes. Gene therapy approaches that target the HSC, a necessity for X-SCID of ZAP-70 deficiency, are likely to suffer from the same delays in immune reconstitution. Therefore, the ability to manipulate thymic differentiation in vivo would be very useful for both T cell depleted BMT and stem cell gene therapy. The identification of thymopoietic cytokines (IL-7 and SCF) will allow us to test whether thymic differentiation can be stimulated in vivo [18].

Clinical gene therapy trials for X-SCID of ZAP-70 deficiency would involve more risk to the patient than the current ADA trials. The selective advantage of transduced cells may allow clinical benefit even if the efficiency of stem cell transduction is limited. The availability of palliative ADA enzyme replacement therapy has made it ethically justifiable for patients with ADA deficiency to receive gene therapy. In diseases such as X-SCID or ZAP-70 deficiency where such options do not exist, gene therapy would be performed instead of bone marrow transplant. Certainly, for all SCID patients with an HLA-matched sibling, allogeneic transplant should be performed. For patients lacking a sibling donor, the choice of treatment options is less clear-cut. The efficacy of gene therapy is still unknown, and it may be prudent to reserve this experimental treatment for neonates or uninfected young infants who lack a sibling donor. Such patients could be kept in a pathogen-free environment until either gene therapy is successful or a bone marrow transplantation is performed.

References

1. Parkman R. The application of bone marrow transplantation to the treatment of genetic diseases. Science 1986;232:1373-78.
2. O'Reilly RJ, Keever CA, Small TN, Brochstein J. The use of HLA-non-identical T-cell depleted marrow transplants for correction of severe combined immunodeficiency disease. Immunodefic Rev 1989;1:273-309.
3. Anderson WF. Prospects for human gene therapy. Science 1984;226:401-9.
4. Weinberg K, Hershfield MS, Bastian J, et al. T lymphocyte ontogeny in adenosine deaminase-deficient severe combined immune deficiency after treatment with polyethylene glycol-modified adenosine deaminase. J Clin Invest 1993;92:596-602.
5. Noguchi M, Yi H, Rosenblatt HM, et al. Interleukin 2 receptor γ chain mutation results in X-linked severe combined immunodeficiency in humans. Cell 1993;73:147-57.
6. Arpaia E, Shahar M, Dadi H, Cohen A, Roifman CM. Defective T cell receptor signaling and CD8+ thymic selection in humans lacking Zap70 kinase. Cell 1994;76:947-58.
7. Elder ME, Lin D, Clever J, et al. Human severe combined immunodeficiency due to a defect in ZAP-70, a T cell tyrosine kinase. Science 1994;264:1596-99.
8. Arnaiz-Villena A, Timon M, Corell A, Perez-Aciego P, Martin-Villa JM, Regueiro JR. Primary immunodeficiency caused by mutations in the gene encoding the CD3-γ subunit of the T-lymphocyte receptor. N Engl J Med 1992;327:529-33.
9. Steimle V, Otten LA, Zuffery M, Mach B. Complementation cloning of an MHC Class II transactivator mutated in hereditary MHC Class II deficiency (or bare lymphocyte syndrome). Cell 1993;75:135-46.

10. Mullen CA, Snitzer K, Blaese RM. Long term in vivo expression of retrovirally transferred ADA genes in lymphocyte clones from an ADA-SCID patient treated with gene therapy. J Cell Biochem 1994;(Suppl 18A):240.
11. Ferrari G, Notarangelo L, Servida P, et al. The role of peripheral blood lymphocytes and bone marrow cells in the development of a functional immune system after gene therapy for ADA deficient SCID. J Cell Biochem 1992;(Suppl 17E):187.
12. Hoogerbrugge PM, Van Busechem V, Valerio D, et al. Gene therapy of 3 children with adenosine deaminase deficiency. Blood 1993;(Suppl 1)82:315a.
13. Kohn DB, Weinberg KI, Parkman, et al. Gene therapy for neonates with ADA-deficient SCID by retroviral-mediated transfer of the human ADA cDNA into umbilical cord CD34+ cells. Blood 1993;(Suppl 1)82:315a.
14. Minami Y, Kono T, Muiyazaki T, Taniguchi T. The IL-2 receptor complex: Its structure, function, and target genes. Ann Rev Immunol 1993;11:245-68.
15. Russell SM, Keegan AD, Harada N, et al. Interleukin-2 receptor γ chain: A functional component of the interleukin-4 receptor. Science 1993;262:1880-83.
16. Noguchi M, Nakamura Y, Russell SM, Ziegler SF, Tsang S, Cao X, Leonard WJ. Interleukin-2 receptor γ chain: A functional component of the interleukin-7 receptor. Science 1993;262:1877-80.
17. Puck JM, Kraus CM, Puck SM, Buckley RH, Conley ME. Prenatal test for X-linked severe combined immunodeficiency by analysis of maternal X-chromosome inactivation and linkage analysis. N Engl J Med 1990;322:1063-66.
18. Bolotin E, Smogorewska EM, Annett G, Widmer M, Weinberg KI. Enhancement of immune reconstitution by IL-7 after bone marrow transplant (BMT). Exp Haematol 1994;22:803.

DISCUSSION

R.A. Sacher, E Vellenga – moderators

E. Briët (Leiden, NL): Dr. Sacher, you have made a statement I think from Duke university where one is trying to do bone marrow transplantation on an outpatient basis. That in my mind, should either be science fiction or these patients get transplants they do not need. Maybe you could elaborate a little on that.

R.A. Sacher (Washington, DC, USA): Bill Peters is very provocative and energetic and he was talking about peripheral blood stem cell transplantation[1]. Combining both blood stem cells and autologous bone marrow or peripheral blood stem cells alone could indeed decrease the period of obligatory cytopenia. He sees a role for these strategies as an emerging trend to outpatient transplantation. Whether he has done it or not I do not know, but he certainly talks about that very vigorously at meetings.

J.A. Zwiebel (Washington, DC, USA): Dr. Davies, any thoughts about how you might increase topo II expression clinically?

S. Davies (Oxford, UK): Promotor and phosphorylation studies may identify some means of increasing topo II expression. We have characterised a CHO (Chinese hamster ovary) mutant cell line that is hypersensitive to topo II inhibitors and cross-sensitive to cAMP analogues. It has been shown to overexpress the PKA (protein kinase A) regulatory subunit RIα. Transfection of this regulatory subunit into parental CHO cells results in increased sensitivity to topo II targeting drugs.

J.A. Zwiebel: Any thoughts about how you could do this clinically, I mean to get over the problem of drug resistance. It sounds like you do that with gene transfer, but it is very difficult to get that gene into all the tumour cells.

S. Davies: Clinical trials are underway using cAMP analogues to upregulate expression of the R1α subunit of PKA prior to treatment with topo II antagonistic drugs.

---

1. Personal communication.

E. Vellenga (Groningen, NL): Can you further speculate about the role of growth factors in treatment of AML, because growth factors can enhance the cyclic states of the AML cells and perhaps also upregulate the topo II.

S. Davies: From cell line studies it seems that topo IIα levels fluctuate during the cell cycle and that actively dividing cells, with high levels of topo IIα are more sensitive to topo II targeting drugs.

P.F.W. Strengers (Amsterdam, NL): Dr. Sacher, you told us about the study of Lane, who gave CSF to donors to stimulate stem cell function[1]. Do you think that, apart from the ethical point of view, you can also enhance an oncogenic stimulation in such a person of which you do not know his full physical condition, because your application is *in vivo*.

R.A. Sacher: That is certainly a theoretical and ethical question. I have heard that discussed in terms of whether there is stem cell exhaustion. Is this what you are referring to? Maybe at some point in time when these people need chemotherapy or some other medication, you may limit the ability of their marrows to respond. I think this is all theoretical at this point. I will say that prior to Lane's presentation there was a publication by Bensinger in Blood[2], that also alluded to this, namely that people are now looking at the use of growth factors to stimulate allogeneic donors and harvest their peripheral blood in contradistinction to the donor marrow. Now again, to what extent are we imparting some damaging influence by harvesting a litre of marrow? It certainly appears to recover, but in terms of the long term effects on stem cells in marrow I have no evidence that there is a damaging or deleterious effect. But I also of course do not know any evidence in terms of the peripheral blood stem cell harvesting causing stem cell exhaustion. I guess it is a question of what would you prefer to do: Donate your marrow under anaesthesia or donate your peripheral blood and be primed by a growth factor. I have heard donors express both points of views. Some would say: "Rather put me under and harvest my marrow" I think you are dealing with special people here anyway. Others would say: "I much prefer to have my peripheral blood harvested".

R.Y.J. Tamminga (Groningen, NL): You mentioned stem cell exhaustion. What do you think about the stem cell exhaustion in patients whom you give stem cell support after expansion of stem cells in culture?

---

1. Lane TA, Law P, Maruyama M, et al. Harvesting and enrichment of hematopoietic progenitor cells mobilized into the peripheral blood of normal donors by granulocyte-macrophage colony-stimulating factor (GM-CSF) or G-CSF: potential role in allogeneic marrow transplantation. Blood 1995;85:275-82.
2. Bensinger WI, Price TH, Dale DC, et al. The effects of daily recombinant human granulocyte colony-stimulating factor administration on normal granulocyte donors undergoing leukapheresis. Blood 1993;81:1883-8.

R.A. Sacher: Well, I think we are clearly on a rapid learning curve. It is a theoretical consideration. Looking back perhaps to the use of differentiated growth factors and their potential effect on the stem cell that you are priming, I think there is no evidence in reality that you get stem cell exhaustion if you for example are priming an individual with erythropoietin or G- or GM-CSF. To try to answer your question; basically I do not think anyone knows. Extrapolating from other information in terms of whether you in reality get stem cell exhaustion there does not seem to be evidence that you do, when you are priming with differentiation growth factors. I think that clearly we are quite far from widely using CD34 enriched populations that have been expanded *ex vivo* presently. Most of them have been enriched such as in the one study I showed you from Shpall[1]. Of course as I pointed out in some of the other data many of those cells are differentiated, yet they still engraft. So it is presumably apparent that there is a sufficient self-renewal population. I think time is going to tell, though.

M. El-Ekiaby (Cairo, Egypt): Can I ask about the cord blood cells? If the expression of the HLA antigens is low, this may help compromise HLA matching in allogeneic transplantation.

R.A. Sacher: You actually have a small population of cells that are not expressing HLA-DR. Of course, the larger population of cells do. I did not show any of the data in terms of relative sub-populations of lymphocytes in cord compared to adult blood. There are substantial differences. CD45RA is much more enriched than CD45RO; these cells are presumably earlier unprimed precursors and this may be a benefit. But in terms of HLA matching I do not know that this really limits the ability to the HLA match. Certainly in the unrelated registry they were able to HLA match for at least 50 transplants.

E. Vellenga: Can you tell us something about the organisation of the peripheral stem cell isolation procedure which you have in your hospital, because you mentioned several times that peripheral stem cell isolation is indeed transfusion medicine, is an affair which can only be supported by the blood bank. In my view when you talk about peripheral stem cell isolation and transplantation it is not voluntary, but has to be used for the transplantation, demonstrating the involvement of the clinic. I think the organisation for the peripheral stem cell transplantation is a very important issue and perhaps you can tell something about how it is organised in your hospital. Perhaps dr. Smit Sibinga can tell something about the organisation in our hospital.

---

1. Shpall EJ, Jones RB, Bearman SI, et al. Transplantation of enriched CD34-positive autologous marrow into breast cancer patients following high-dose chemotherapy: influence of CD34-positive peripheral-blood progenitors and growth factors on engraftment. J Clin Oncol 1994;12:28-36.

R.A. Sacher: From my point of view being both a clinician and a laboratorian, I treat patients as well as harvest and process the cells. I do not want to minimize the complexities of the interrelationships between the blood bank and the clinician. I think that, however, the blood banks' experience with GMP, labelling and processing and certainly regulatory requirements is preferentially beneficial in terms of controlling the product component. Clearly a lot of the cells are harvested from the marrow or peripheral blood from patients. The blood banks have experience with harvesting platelets and leukapheresis products from donors. I believe it should be a co-operative type of arrangement. However, I feel very strongly that this should be at least in part influenced very actively by the blood bank. That is my own personal opinion. I know that in fact in our centre the blood bank and transfusion medicine discipline is heavily involved. There are other centres where it is primarily the oncology or haematology/ oncology programme – Johns Hopkins is an example. They collect, they in fact are involved in the apheresis instruments, they process, harvest the cells and they use them. The blood bank is not involved there. I see the potential for some tough protection here and in tough interactions; what is mine is mine, what is yours is yours. However, I think that in this evolving area it should really be a cooperation and I think that the blood banks should take an active, pro-active stand. That is my opinion.

C.Th. Smit Sibinga (Groningen, NL): Probably, I would phrase it differently. I understand what you say in the comment you made in what is mine is mine and what is yours is yours. Our basic philosophy is what is yours is mine and mine is yours and actually is ours. It brings me back to the definition which was discussed a few years ago in 1991, when we discussed the theme of Transfusion Medicine: Facts and Fiction[1], where the WHO definition of transfusion medicine came up to the floor: It actually deals with that part of the health care system as we define it, which is involved in both the provision as well as the use of human blood and blood components including the stem cells and related cell lines. So that brings you actually to that 'ours' type of approach. In the set up which we have created over the years here in Groningen, there is a very strong cross-fertilisation in a close cooperative type of system between the clinic and the blood bank. Of course, the laboratory is important, but it happens at the bed-side and that is where you should be if you really want to develop. Therefore we formed a team of clinical haematology, clinical oncology and blood bank with some related other disciplines to that as well. But the nucleus is these three. It is a very good and cross-fertilising type of approach to our opinion.

But I have a few questions. First of all the beautiful presentation of dr. Goodenow based on the initial work of the Nobel price winner, dr. Philip Sharp, whom I had the fortune to meet at the ceremonies in Stockholm, a delightful person. Dr. Goodenow, you came by the end of your presentation to some of the therapeutic prospects and you compared the drug versus the gene approaches in

1. Transfusion medicine: Fact and fiction. Smit Sibinga CTh, Das PC, Cash JD (eds). Kluwer Academic Publ. Boston/Dordrecht/London, 1992.

the induction of apoptosis in the reversal of differentiation and in the effect on genomic instability. Now, how do you see that implemented in practice.

B. Goodenow (Santa Ana, CA, USA): I think the challenge to using a genetic approach to reverse the chemogenesis will reside on being able to target specific genes within the body. Clearly that is the challenge at hands. So vector delivery systems that can operate *in vivo* will be critical. Jack Roth at M.D. Anderson has been inserting wild type p53 genes into tumours[1] and there have been approaches that involve both direct injections into the tumour as well as *ex vivo* delivery of p53 and then reintroduction into the patient. Even though theoretically one would want to target each within every tumour cell within the body, there does appear to be a bystander effect that if you induce apoptosis in a large enough number of tumour cells you seem to alarm the immune system into generating an immune response to those tumours. So, even though you may have to target a large number of tumours it may open the door for other therapeutic responses in patients.

C.Th. Smit Sibinga: What kind of delivery system are you thinking of?

B. Goodenow: More than likely we are talking about either vectors that are clearly safe to be used *in vivo* in patients. There have been studies involving retroviruses, the next generation may be something like AAV vectors. Alternatively there may be chemicals, liposomes that can be used to whatever change.

C.Th. Smit Sibinga: Dr. Freeman, I have listened carefully to your presentation on gene transfection and the role the blood bank could play in the future in setting up human gene therapy trials. One of the messages in between the lines is, do we need also to get involved in virology to get access to viral vectors, is that correct?

S.M. Freeman (New Orleans, LA, USA): I think basically understanding how it works is probably the point I am trying to make. I think the virology is fairly complex. There will be worked out as I showed many vectors and many vector systems. I think at some point one will sort of emerge into what is going to be used or a number will emerge into what is being most effective in a different situation. I think understanding the system so, that when the technology becomes available and comes into the blood bank we can then put it in place; I think that is the important part. I am not sure within the blood bank we are going to figure out what the virology is and what is the best to do, but I think part of our role is implementation.

C.Th. Smit Sibinga: So kind of an assemblage institution in cooperation with other (including virology oriented) institutions that prepare the vectors and then put them in place. Such kind of an approach.

---

1. Roth JA. Clinical protocol for modification of oncogene and tumor suppressor gene expression in small cell lung cancer. Cancer 1993;4:383-86.

S.M. Freeman: Yes, there are going to be two ways that the vectors are coming down the line, from companies eventually when it becomes more commercialized. Companies will have these vectors and either send supernatants for transduction or packing cell lines. Either each blood bank or hospital will have a sort of GMP to do the transductions or in some way get the reagents or the cells and then have to manipulate to be implanted.

C.Th. Smit Sibinga: Then a question to dr. Sacher. In the mentioning of various growth factors important for the *ex vivo* expansion you did not mention the role of stem cell factor. Was that deliberately or could you give us some further ideas on the role of stem cell factor in the ultimate expansion?

R.A. Sacher: No, I actually did not mention other specific factors except of course G-CSF in terms of mobilising. However, there was information I showed on cord CD34 enriched populations using interleukin-1, IL3 and stem cell factor plus erythropoietin. If you look at the recipe du jour which seems to be the best, they all contain stem cell factor with IL-3 plus or minus other factors either IL-1 or IL-6.

C.Th. Smit Sibinga: How about shifting away from the foetal calf serum to human serum or even to non-serum or non-plasma mixtures.

R.A. Sacher: Well, I think there is this sort of interesting political debate in the United States, especially regarding foetal calf sera, which is used of course in the US. Yet, it is not licensed for human use, but it has been used since 1970. Now whether this is going to be grandfathered or grandmothered I do not know. Clearly the fact is switching to try and find alternative sources. In our laboratory we have found that at least in IL-2 activation we do not need xenogeneic serum, we can use AB plasma. I think others are looking at alternative sources and some of the commercial companies – I know Gibco is an example – is looking at serum-free media. Yes, I am aware of a move towards finding alternative serum-free systems.

C.Th. Smit Sibinga: Don't you think that the presence of factors like fibronectin might be of importance to increase the cell-cell contact?

R.A. Sacher: Yes, that is possible in *ex vivo* expansion. As I said I do not want to minimise the serum or recombinant factors that could be used in a variety of recipes. I think that conceivably to really effectively expand *ex vivo* you may well need stroma. I might have mentioned there was an interesting communication from Bordeaux[1]. They essentially were looking at growth factors and cell propagation in marrow material that is thrown away with the harvest. In other words that filtered material rather than the filtrate. Of course, we filter and we throw away the bone particles and stroma and adipous tissue and all the other things. In reality

1. Personal communication.

that creates more, that produces more stem cells than the marrow that we harvest and they talk about that as a haematron or haematon. It was a very interesting abstract.

D.E. Onions (Glasgow, UK): I have a specific question, but I just like to make a comment on the point about using foetal calf serum. One should certainly get away from it. I think what is often missed by many audiences is that 70% of foetal calf serum batches that are used commercially can be contaminated by a virus called bovine polyoma virus. This virus infects human cells, it is a potentially zoonotic virus. It belongs to a group of potentially oncogenic viruses and many people are not even aware of the existence of this virus let alone about screening for this virus. So I would strongly endorse getting away from calf serum.

But my question was actually directed to dr. Goodenow, who gave a really excellent talk. I do have a problem with the concept of trying to deliver p53. I really feel it is going to be extremely difficult to deliver p53, with an efficiency that is going to be therapeutically beneficial. In addition, I understand that a number of human tumours also have involvement with MDM2 which is a downstream gene from p53 so that your therapeutic effect would not necessarily be operative. However, the transcriptional activation sites for p53 have been identified. For solid tumours one could think of linking prodrugs activation genes to those sites and using that as a method.

B. Goodenow: I would agree with that. I cited the p53 as the first experiments to be done with genes that address the whole issue of inducing apoptosis, but I would agree with you that there are better strategies that have yet to be tried.

IV. GENE TECHNOLOGY, ETHICS AND THE FUTURE

ETHICS AND GENETIC MANIPULATION

V. Boulyjenkov

Introduction

Rapid advances in genetic technology and human genome research make it almost certain that the majority of genes will be localized within the next few years. It is proposed that the application of new genetic knowledge will provide possibilities for the diagnosis and treatment of a wide spectrum of diseases including communicable and noncommunicable ones, as well as to reveal the predisposition before the appearance of the disease. However, social and ethical issues concerned with improving genetic-testing techniques, which evolve faster than advances in treatment, are raised. These ethical issues are not linked with the technology itself but with its proper use. Such progress in DNA technology often evokes fears of control of peoples' reproductive behaviour for political ends. Scientific, medical and lay communities should ensure that information and technology will be used to preserve the dignity of the individual. One of the ways to avoid the misuse of information is to convene discussions at different levels (health car professionals, policy makers, mass-media, schools, etc.) in order to establish a firm understanding of actual and potential applications of new genetic technology.

It is also important to recognize that these issues involve the majority of human rights. Ethical questions in connection with genetic approaches should be viewed in the light of their general objective, which is to help people with a genetic disadvantage to live and reproduce as normal and as responsible as possible.

The World Health Organization (WHO) has long asserted the principle that health is a fundamental human right. As we further enter the decade of the 1990s, human rights, social justice and ethical issues will become more and more important. Human rights in health and medicine must be seen within the wider framework of basic human rights, for the rights of the patient are the rights of man. They involve three related issues: freedom of expression and the right to be informed; respect for the integrity of the individual, including freedom to decide; and, prohibition of discrimination of any kind. In the 1990s, WHO will emphasize the human rights aspect of health in all programme activities [1].

Some ethical issues in medical genetics.

The guiding principles of medical geneticists, that are included in profressional teaching and adhered to in practice, have been studied empirically and summarized in a set of "guidelines". Core principles are the autonomy of the individual or the couple, their right to adequate and complete information, and the maintenance of the highest standards of confidentially.

The ethical issues connected with new genetic technology are very broad. They can be approached here only in a selective manner, with emphasis on a few outstanding topics.

For example, there is increasing awareness that genes of the normal range of genetic variation, which may confer a predisposition of resistance to common disorders, do not themselves cause disease. In fact, most bearers may be completely healthy. Every measure should be taken to ensure that individuals can have tests for such characteristics, without fear that the results could be used to their disadvantage, for instance, in limiting choice of employment or life insurance. Information concerning a healthy person's genes should be generally considered as the property of the person.

The possibility of predisposition testing for monogenic diseases has opened up "new" populations for such testing. No longer is the presence of disease confirmed by the first appearance of symptoms in adults. The young adult, the child, the fetus and even the embryo can now be tested for actual presence of the gene which usually will be expressed much later in life (e.g., Huntington) or has great variability of expression (e.g., myotonic dystrophy). Autonomy, non-directive counselling and freedom of choice have long been the hallmarks of genetic testing. Cultural and attitudinal differences as well as the availability of services and care for the disabled also influence such decisions. It is recommended that the medical genetic service should not be used for non-medical purposes, such as sex selection, etc.

The combination of informatics and genetic technologies has created fears that the most intimate personal sphere of privacy, that is, genetic decision-making, will be subject to scrutiny. The concept of privacy itself has developed from that of control over one's property, to control over one's person and now, to control over information about oneself. In human genetics, it is closely tied to the right of liberty especially as concerns reproductive choice.

The traditional paradigm of genetic testing and treatment is giving way to that of providing genetic information without accompanying palliative or curative intervention. In the absence of treatment and of public education and understanding of genetic conditions, such information should be kept confidential and subject to individual consent prior to release. The acceptance of collaborative or international research should depend on the assurance of such anonymity. The mechanisms of protection for medical information need to be strengthened and affirmed.

The ethical aspect of genetic counselling is very important. The familial nature of genetic information creates special obligations extending beyond the patient. Contact with affected relatives should be left to the patient. Genetic counselling requires specific knowledge, the ability to communicate and time. This cannot be done without training, proper supervision and without compensation under state health or private insurance schemes. The preservation of autonomy, the assurance of complete information and of confidentiality are essential. Choices are undoubtedly influenced both by personal values with regards to the sanctity of human life, by the wish to avoid human suffering and by cultural, if not socio-economic constrains in the absence of treatment or of complete state support for the disabled or chronically ill. If the objective of medical genetic services is "to help people with a genetic disadvantage to live and to reproduce, as normal as possible" [2], then its realization depends on counselling.

The broadest of the real ethical issues is the limited availability of genetic services. The care of the handicapped and support for their families is universally deficient, and at the same time the services that can now be provided for responsible family planning are not effectively delivered, and are unequally distributed even in developed countries. The limited delivery of these services is partly due to inadequate provision of health education for the community, and technical information for health professionals.

At the same time much of bioethics and bio-law is concerned with conflicts of rights. The transfer of such an adversative approach to human genetics would be extremely detrimental to the well-being of affected persons, their families and to the populations concerned. This is especially important because of the nature of genetic disease and genetic information (personal, familial and social). It is also important because genetic reproductive decision-making speaks not only to present relationships but also to future generations. Individual, professional and collective responsibility for decision-making should be based on public education, on widespread knowledge of exact and precise genetic information and not on an adversative approach or on claims of rights. Public discussion, education and participation in the direction of research, in the development of public health programmes and in decisions concerning priorities and funding is essential. It is proposed that a number of international organizations including the WHO could take a leadership role in the dissemination of such information.

Gene therapy

Most public attention has been accorded to attempts at direct gene therapy where a gene is introduced into a somatic cell in order to correct a pathological problem. Gene therapy is the introduction of a gene sequence into a cell so that it can modify the behaviour of the cell in a clinically relevant fashion. It is an enabling technology which may be exploited in several ways – to treat a genetic mutation (as for cystic fibrosis), to kill a cell (as for cancer), or to modify susceptibility (as for coronary artery disease). The gene may be introduced using a virus (usually a retrovirus or adenovirus) or lipid or receptor targeting. There are disadvantages to all these approaches, e.g., with viral vectors there may be pathogenicity and the size of the DNA that can be introduced is limited, while lipid and receptor systems are as yet relatively inefficient in promoting uptake and expression of

DNA. However, there seems little doubt that in several years' time new gene delivery systems will be developed which combine the advantages of all existing systems, without their disadvantages.

There is now universal legal, scientific and medical agreement that somatic gene therapy poses no new ethical problems. It is considered that gene delivery to somatic cells to treat a disease is ethical, and that is in the community interest for gene therapy to take its place alongside other forms of medical treatment. It is useful to think of gene therapy as a way of using genes pharmaceutically, comparable to any other pharmaceutical delivery system. Like all other new therapies, gene therapy should be properly tested for safety before its wide application in clinical practice.

At present, clinical trials are proceeding in two areas. Several hundred cancer patients are in gene therapy research programmes, mostly using genes to enhance toxicity of chemotherapeutic agents, or tumour suppressor genes. A small number of patients with single gene disorders that seem particularly suitable candidates for study are taking part in clinical trials. They include patients with immune deficiency due to adenosine deaminase (ADA) deficiency, cystic fibrosis, and familial hypercholesterolaemia. At present all trials are at a very early stage, mainly monitoring toxicity, dosage and efficacy rather than definitive treatment. Trials are foreseen for many other inherited disorders, including thalassaemia, sickle cell disease and haemophilia. While single gene disorders are important in their own right, they are also models for wider applications in future. There is much interest in the possibility of using somatic gene therapy for common disorders including diabetes, coronary heart disease and autoimmune disorders.

Somatic gene therapy does not appear to require a special set of regulations, but does need to be brought clearly into the normal system of licensing of medicines, and approval by ethics committees which govern the introduction of new clinical products. Ethical aspects need to be coordinated internationally to ensure that the same general level of regulation is generally applied, or there is a risk that trials will be carried out only in places with less rigorous regulatory standards.

There is a great commercial interest in gene therapy. Much of the technology is subject to patent protection, and many genes have also been patented. This may raise problems of equitable access to therapy in the future. It is important to ensure that access is not restricted only to those who have the ability to pay, particularly as the underlying technology is basically simple, cheap and applicable in developing countries. Several international organizations have recommended that patenting should be used in a facilitative way, to guarantee a return for a useful invention or application in relation to therapy, rather than in a restrictive way by allowing the patenting of gene sequences for which no use, or only identity, has been established.

Technology transfer

As already mentioned, the broadest of the real ethical issues is the limited availability of genetics services. Inevitably the social and ethical aspects of genetics services differ between developing and developed countries, because economic factors are so critical and genetic disease may be so destructive, when there is no social support system. Social, religious and ethical acceptableness in different countries are not adequate. The acceptability of some genetic testing is decided on general social and medical grounds, rather than in a genetic one only, and a genetic diagnosis service can operate only within the framework of such general decisions. The specific health problems in developing countries often have a genetic basis or genetic component showing that the burden of congenital and genetic disorders is greatest to them. It is important to encourage genetic studies in populations with specific problems to ensure that technology and resources are available to them, and to maintain international collaboration.

Although many countries do not have the resources to perform some sophisticated genetic research, it is important that all of them have the possibility to participate in social and ethical discussions as well as be informed about the transfer of technology. This should be foreseen especially for less-equipped countries. In the future, many diagnostic and screening tests will be developed on the basis of the findings of the modern genetic research. The special needs of each country must be assessed in order to establish genetic services. A number of international organizations could play a catalytic role in assessing countries with a view to equipping them with genetic services in the following ways: to advise the country on the choice of the technology to be transferred through appropriate assessment by in-house expertise or on advice from consultants as well as to facilitate exchange of information and expertise necessary for the implementation of the technology transfer.

Conclusion

A 1989 international survey of ethics in the practice of human genetics revealed several areas of consensus (although cultural differences in the translation of these areas remain). The principles of accessibility, of autonomy, of non-directive counselling, of consent and choice, of respect for confidentiality and for the integrity of the person are widely accepted. The work of the Council of Europe towards a Bioethics Convention as well as UNESCO's (United Nations Educational, Scientific and Cultural Organization) and CIOMS's (Council for International Organizations of Medical Sciences) work on the development of an international instrument for the protection of the human genome are steps in this direction. It is highly recommendedthat international, regional and national instruments affirm these areas of consensus in human genetics and research. An organization such as WHO could have a major role with respect to information, guidance, dissemination and affirmation concerning consensus ethics in medical genetics [3].

Acknowledgements

This article is based on the discussion at WHO Scientific Group held in Geneva from 23-25 November 1993. I thank all participants of the Group for the fruitful discussion.

References

1. WHO document: WHA43/DIV/4. 1990:1-20.
2. WHO document: HDP/WG/85.10. 1985:1-47.
3. Ethics and human genetics. Proc 2nd Symposium CoE on Bioethics. Council of Europe Press, Strassbourg 1994.

IS THERE A ROLE FOR TRANSFUSION MEDICINE IN THE GENETIC CORRECTION OF GENETIC DISORDERS AND OTHER DISEASES?

J.A. Zwiebel

Introduction

Initially viewed principally as a means of treating inherited genetic diseases, gene therapy is now seen as a promising approach for virtually all kinds of disorders, and by disciplines as diverse as oncology, cardiology, endocrinology, and infectious diseases [1, 2]. There has been a rapid growth in the number of clinical trials that utilize gene transfer either for cell marking or therapeutic intent. While the usefulness of the gene transfer for patient care is not yet known, what is emerging is a profusion of different strategies and applications of clinical gene transfer. Its potential impact likened to that of the introduction of antibiotics, gene therapy may very well become part of the standard armamentarium of all clinicians. If gene therapy succeeds in realizing even part of its promise, there will be a need in medical institutions for a facility that can dispense the agents to be administered to patients in a gene therapy procedure. The transfusion laboratory, with its well-established role for the collection, processing and distribution of cells and other blood components, is well-suited to serving this need.

What are the elements that are required to carry out a clinical gene transfer procedure? What would be the role of the transfusion laboratory for carrying out gene therapy? The answers to these questions lie in the approaches that are currently being investigated for inserting new genetic information into cells.

Gene therapy: The ideal

An optimal gene therapy procedure would be easily administered and would allow us to target specific cells in an efficient manner and to express the inserted genes only when required. As yet, efficient gene transfer coupled with the temporal and spatial control of transgene expression has not been accomplished. The vectors suffer from problems of either inefficient gene transfer, loss of gene expression, or concerns about safety [3]. The immediate goal continues to be constitutive gene expression in gene-modified cells in order to produce relevant amounts of protein of interest. Targeted gene delivery and regulated gene expression remain elusive aims. However, newer gene transfer techniques and an emerging understanding of gene regulations undoubtedly will bring us closer to accomplishing these goals.

Table 1. In vivo and *ex vivo* gene transfer for gene therapy: NIH-approved protocols.[1]

Disorder	Cellular target	Gene	Method/Vector
Malignancy	Tumor cells, fibroblasts, tumour infiltrating lymphocytes	IL-2, IL-4, IL-12, HLA-B7, interferon-γ, tumour necrosis factor, herpes simplex virus thymidine kinase (plus ganciclovir), granulocyte-macrophage colony stimulating factor, antisense K-*ras*, antisense c-*myc*, p53, insulin-like growth factor I, multi-drug resistance gene, B7	*Ex vivo, in vivo*/ retrovirus, adenovirus, liposomes
ADA deficiency	Lymphocytes, haematopoietic progenitor cells	ADA	*Ex vivo*/retrovirus
Hypercholesterolaemia	Hepatocytes	Low density lipoprotein receptor	*Ex vivo*/retrovirus
Cystic fribosis	Bronchial epithelium	CFTR	*In vivo*/adenovirus, liposomes
Gaucher disease	Haematopoietic progenitor cells	Glucocerebrosidase	*Ex vivo*/retrovirus
Hunter syndrome (Mucopolysaccharidosis Type II)	Lymphocytes	Iduronate-2-sulfatase	*Ex vivo*/retrovirus
AIDS	Haematopoietic progenitor cells	HIV-IT(V), *Rev*, ribozyme	*Ex vivo*/retrovirus
Alpha-1-antitrypsin deficiency	Respiratory epithelium	Alpha-1-antitrypsin	*Ex vivo*/retrovirus
Rheumatoid arthritis	Synovium	IL-1 receptor antagonist	*Ex vivo*/retrovirus
Fanconi's anaemia	Haematopoietic progenitor cells	Complementation group c	*Ex vivo*/retrovirus

1. Source: National Institutes of Health, Office of Recombinant DNA Activities.

Ex vivo vs. direct *in vivo* gene therapy

The inefficiency of early attempts at introducing new genetic information into cells made it necessary to cultivate cells *in vitro* in order to carry out gene transfer successfully. In addition, the ease of accessing and reimplanting bone marrow cells, the initial targets for gene therapy, was another reason for pursuing the *ex vivo* approach to gene therapy. Carrying out the gene transfer procedure *in vitro*, does have additional advantages. First, by first isolating the target cell, it is possible to achieve tissue specificity of transgene expression. Second, it may be possible to optimize production of the therapeutic agent by selecting for its expression in the gene-modified cell population. Third, one may be better able to ensure the safety of the gene transfer procedure by examining, for example, for the presence of replication-competent virus before administering the gene-modified cell to the patient. On the other hand, the *ex vivo* gene transfer method requires sophisticated tissue culture expertise and is both costly and labour-intensive. Moreover, the introduction of the gene-modified cells may be complicated by the inability of those cells to become efficiently reincorporated into the tissues of the recipient.

Being able to introduce new genetic information directly into tissues *in vivo* is certainly appealing. This approach is simple and does not require cell isolation and cultivation. Thus, it would ultimately facilitate the widespread availability of gene therapy, even in the local community setting. However, direct *in vivo* gene transfer as yet cannot be used to target a specific tissue or cell type. Hence, transgene expression by non-target tissues, particularly the germ line, may be an undesired consequence of the *in vivo* gene transfer procedure.

Currently, both *ex vivo* and *in vivo* gene transfer methods are being used for gene therapy. For example, cystic fibrosis is being treated using an adenoviral vector to deliver the cystic fibrosis transmembrane regulator gene directly to bronchial epithelial cells *in situ*. In contrast, for the treatment of severe combined immunodeficiency due to adenosine deaminase (ADA) deficiency, lymphocytes or bone marrow progenitor cells are removed from the patient, transduced with a retroviral vector containing the ADA gene, and then reinfused. The diseases currently under study with approved clinical protocols are listed in Table 1. Genetic diseases that are being evaluated experimentally for gene therapy are listed in Table 2.

How genes are inserted into cells.

While great strides have been made over the last decade in vector development, gene transfer and stable gene expression remain the greatest limitations to achieving successful gene therapy. To address these issues, there are ongoing efforts towards modifying vector design as well as the introduction of novel methods of gene transfer, such as the use of cell surface receptor ligands conjugated to the DNA of interest [4].

The currently available methods for introducing new genetic information into cells are listed in Table 3. Until now, retroviruses have been the most popular means of transducing cells because of their ability to integrate into the cellular genome in a stable fashion and to permit efficient gene expression. However, they suffer from a number of shortcomings, including the need for cell division in order for gene integration to occur, a limit in the size of the gene that can be transferred, and the potential risk of insertional mutagenesis with neoplastic transformation [5].

Due to their stability, adenoviral vectors can be concentrated to titers that are several logs higher than is achievable with retroviral vectors. The high viral titre allows efficient *in vivo* gene transfer to occur. Moreover, adenoviruses can infect non-dividing cells [6-11]. On the other hand, following adenoviral infection the transgene exists as an episome that is eventually lost from the cell. Expression of adenoviral proteins by infected cells may also result in an immune response that may result in toxicity and may also interfere with subsequent attempts to introduce a therapeutic gene. Adenoviral vectors may be cytopathic and have been observed to be fatal in animals when administered in large quantities.

Adeno-associated virus (AAV) can also be concentrated tc high titre. AAV integrates into host DNA at a site on chromosome 19 [12, 13]. While AAV can be used as a viral vector [14-16], it appears to be prone to rearrangement.

Table 2. Candidate genetic disorders for gene therapy.[1]

Disease	Gene	Reference
Haemoglobinopathies	α globin β globin	[94] [15, 95-97]
Primary immunodeficiency	1. Adenosine deaminase 2. Purine nucleoside phosphorylase	[98-101]
Von Willebrand disease	Von Willebrand factor	[102, 103]
Haemophilia A and B	Factors VIII and IX	[52, 69, 104-106]
Duchenne muscular dystrophy	Dystrophin	[107-110]
Leukocyte adhesion deficiency	CD18	[111-113]
Chronic granulomatous disease	1. Cytochrome b-245 β subunit 2. p47 and p67 neutrophil oxidase	[114] [115, 116]
Familial hypercholesterolaemia	Low density lipoprotein receptor	[49, 57, 117-120]
Alpha-1-antitrypsin deficiency	Alpha-1-antitrypsin	[121-125]
Ornithine transcarbamylase deficiency (urea cycle)	Ornithine transcarbamylase	[107, 126]
Alpha propionyl CoA carboxylase deficiency (amino acid metabolism)	Alpha propionyl CoA carboxylase deficiency	[127]
Methylmalonyl-CoA mutase defi ciency (amino acid metabolism)	Methylmalonyl-Coa mutase	[54, 128]
Lesch-Nyhan syndrome	Hypoxanthine-guanine phosphoribosyltransferase	[129, 130]
Niemann-Pick disease (lysosomal)	Acid sphingomyelinase	[20, 53]
Gaucher's disease (lysosomal)	Glucocerebrosidase	[131-134]
Mucopoysaccharidosis VII (lysosomal)	β-glycuronidase	[32]
Alpha-L-fucosidase deficiency (lysosomal)	Alpha-L-fucosidase	[55]

1. From [135], used with permission of the publisher.

Table 3. Gene transfer methods.

Method	Stable integration?
Viral:	
– Murine retrovirus	Yes
– Adenovirus	No
– Adeno-associated virus	Yes
– Herpes virus	No
– Vaccinia virus	No
– Poliovirus	No
Nonviral:	
– Calcium phosphate	Possibly
– Liposomes	Possibly
– DNA-ligand complexes	Possibly
– Bioballistics	Possibly

Modified herpes viruses are being studied for their ability to target neuronal cells and express recombinant genes [17, 18]. Although expression of foreign genes in neuronal cells has been successful with herpes virus vectors, the viral stocks that are used for gene transfer are heavily contaminated with helper virus and are associated with significant cytotoxicity *in vivo*.

Of the non-viral methods of gene transfer, ligand-conjugated DNA complexes are the most promising for clinical gene transfer [4, 19]. While most physical methods suffer from low efficiency gene transfer, receptor-mediated gene uptake by cells has been shown to be efficient and may also permit selective targeting of cells that display a particular cell surface receptor. The addition of adenoviral components to the DNA-protein complex improves gene transfer by facilitating the release of the gene from endosomes in the cell. However, DNA integration may not be as stable, nor result in the high level gene expression, as found with retroviral integration, a process that is accomplished by the formation of a nucleoprotein integration complex. However, the simplicity, safety, and potential for direct *in vivo* injection account for the appeal of receptor-mediated DNA gene transfer.

Liposomes are another potentially useful vehicle, with impressive reports of efficient gene transfer *in vivo* into diverse cells such as lung epithelium, vascular smooth muscle and endothelial cells, and myoblasts [20-25]. The intralesional administration of the HLA-B7 gene in patients with melanoma is currently being evaluated for its ability to stimulate an antitumour immune response [26].

Gene transfer into haematopoietic progenitor cells

Bone marrow cells have always been viewed as ideal targets for gene transfer for a number of reasons (see Karlsson for a review [27]). Bone marrow is readily obtained and manipulated *ex vivo*. Moreover, by genetically modifying (i.e., transducing) haematopoietic stem cells, one would be able to repopulate the bone marrow and provide a lifetime supply of gene corrected cells. Indeed, early studies in mice, using retroviral-mediated gene transfer (see below) demonstrated the feasibility of this approach, with efficient transfer of marker genes into cells that were capable of repopulating the bone marrow of lethally-irradiated animals [28, 29]. Long term expression of transgenes was seen occasionally as well [30-33]. However, in subsequent primate studies, there was a loss of expression that was associated with the disappearance of the transgene animals that underwent an autologous bone marrow transplant (ABMT) gene transfer procedure [34]. The results suggested that only committed progenitor cells actually took up the transgene.

More recently, a number of groups have demonstrated prolonged recombinant gene expression both in human bone marrow in long-term bone marrow culture [35] an *in vivo* in a primate ABMT gene transfer model, albeit at a low frequency of ~2% [36, 37]. These encouraging results, suggesting haemopoietic stem cell transduction appear to be due to two factors. First, retroviral integration may be promoted by stimulating bone marrow stem cells to cycle with a number of recombinant cytokine molecules (including combinations of IL-1α, IL-3, IL-6, and stem cell factor) [38]. Second, as a result of bone marrow enrichment of pluripotential cells, such as with antibodies to CD34, there is an increased likelihood of infecting the desired target cell [39, 40]. It also has been suggested that purifying the small population of cycling stem cells that are capable of being transduced may also facilitate their engraftment [3]. In a clinical test of this approach in patients, investigators in Italy, Holland an at the NIH are treating children with severe combined immunodeficiency secondary to adenosine deaminase (ADA) deficiency.

Autologous CD34-expressing peripheral blood of bone marrow progenitor cells are transduced with an ADA-containing retroviral vector and reinfused into patients [41]. Since SCID patients have virtually no detectable T cells, the genetically-corrected lymphocytes will have a survival advantage that will allow them to expand *in vivo* and repopulate the immune system.

The treatment of ADA deficiency with gene therapy has a number of features that are illustrative of what now constitutes an attractive gene therapy candidate. First, normal ADA gene expression is under simple regulation (i.e., there is no complex feedback control of expression), and, second, a wide range of expression is associated with normal cellular function. Similarly, correction of haemophilia may also be possible with gene therapy, since only a small increase in factor VIII or IX production may significantly ameliorate the disease. Unfortunately, this is not true for some of the other haematologic diseases that are potentially curable with allogeneic bone marrow transplantation. For example, while thalassaemia potentially could be treated by inserting a normal globin gene into erythroid progenitor cells, balanced alpha and beta globin chain synthesis is required to fully correct the cellular abnormality. Such closely regulated gene expression is not yet possible.

Greater attention is now being focused on the potential for correcting genetic abnormalities in the foetus. *In utero* gene transfer is attractive both as a means of preempting irreparable injury as well as affording a period of immune tolerance that may permit allogeneic implants of gene corrected cells. An *in utero* sheep bone marrow transplant-gene transfer model has provided encouraging results [42] and surgical manipulation of the human foetus is now possible [43, 44].

The transfusion medicine unit – with its expertise in the processing of homeopathic cells – has already a key component in the application of clinical gene transfer. Current applications of haematopoietic cell gene transfer include gene marking – the insertion of gene sequence to permit tracking the fate of cells *in vivo* – and gene therapy. Some examples of therapeutic gene transfer are listed in Table 1.

Gene transfer into different cell types

The past several years has seen a rapid increase in gene therapy strategies under development in nearly all medical specialities. Gene augmentation therapy – the insertion of genes into cells to augment an existing function or, alternatively, to confer upon the cell a new function – allows virtually every cell and tissue to be a potential target for gene transfer. In addition, exploiting the biological characteristics of particular cell types may facilitate local or systemic gene delivery. Some of the cell types under study are highlighted below.

Lymphocytes

Lymphocytes have a number of attributes which make them attractive vehicles for delivery of recombinant molecules. First, these cells will respond to antigen or cytokines stimulation by expanding their numbers by many orders of magnitude. Second, since lymphocytes exist within the circulation and migrate throughout the body, they are attractive vehicles for systemic drug delivery. Third, since lymphocytes are sequestered within the circulatory system, they do not require the provision of a vascular supply that is necessary for implants of non-haematopoietic cells. These characteristics, coupled with their ability to express foreign genes [45, 46], make lymphocytes appealing targets for gene therapy.

Fibroblasts

Despite their ease of cultivation and promising *in vitro* transgene expression, [20, 47-56] genetically-modified fibroblasts have repeatedly failed to sustain transgene expression *in vivo*. Studies to investigate this problem have revealed that there is a shut-off of gene expression of implanted cells [48, 50]. However, these cells may still be useful where only short-term gene expression is desired, as for the treatment of cancer. For example, Lotze and colleagues are inoculating melanoma patients with interleukin-4 or interleukin-12-expressing autologous fibroblasts, plus irradiated autologous tumour cells, in order to activate an anti-tumour immune response. Short term cytokine expression may be sufficient for immune activation and, moreover, the eventual loss of cytokine gene expression may avoid the potential toxicity of sustained cytokine production.

Hepatocytes

Because of their importance for both synthetic and metabolic pathways, hepatocytes are an important target for gene replacement therapy. Using the *ex vivo* gene transfer approach, Wilson et al., successfully expressed the low density lipoprotein receptor (LDLR) in deficient hepatocytes *in vivo* in the Watanabe hereditary hypercholesterolaemic rabbit [57]. In a preliminary report of a clinical trial approved by the NIH recombinant DNA Advisory Committee (RAC), Wilson and colleagues observed a reduction in cholesterol levels in a patient who underwent transplantation of autologous, LDLR-transduced hepatocytes [58].

While promising, the considerable tissue culture support that is required for *ex vivo* hepatocyte gene transfer restricts the application of this procedure to properly equipped centres. Seeking to overcome this limitation, Woo and colleagues have had success using both retroviral and adenoviral vectors for direct *in vivo* hepatocyte transduction. The phenylalanine hydroxylase [59], α-1 anti- trypsin [60], and Factor IX genes [61] have been successfully expressed in animals, although the level of gene expression may be insufficient to be clinically effective.

Respiratory epithelial cells

The respiratory epithelium is easily accessible and has been genetically-modified *ex vivo*, using either retroviral-mediated gene transfer [62] or receptor-mediated endocytosis of transferrin-polylysine-DNA complexes [4], and directly *in vivo*, using liposomes [63], retroviral vectors [64] or adenoviral vectors [8, 9]. Several investigators have already received RAC and Food and Drug Administration (FDA) approval to treat cystic fibrosis with adenoviral vectors that contain the cystic fibrosis transmembrane regulator gene.

Introduction of viral vectors directly into the patient's airway holds promise for the treatment of other respiratory tract disorders, including α1-anti-trypsin deficiency [8] and lung cancer (see "Tumour cells" below).

Vascular cells

The cells of the blood vessel wall, which include endothelial cells and vascular smooth muscle cells, are attractive targets for gene transfer [65] for a number of reasons. First, endothelial cells are strategically located for secretion of therapeutic products into the bloodstream. Second, they are capable of expressing recombinant proteins such as rat growth hormone [66], tissue plasminogen activator [67, 68], and Factor IX [69] in a stable and efficient manner. Third, genetic modification of vascular smooth muscle would be useful for the study and treatment of conditions that affect the vessel wall, including thrombosis and intimal hyperplasia.

Both *ex vivo* and direct *in vivo* gene transfer methods have been used to introduce genetically modified endothelial cells (GMEC) into the vascular compartment. These methods include (i) balloon catheters to seed blood vessels with endothelial cells that had been genetically modified *ex vivo* [70], (ii) *in situ* transduction of vascular endothelial cells using the specially designed balloon catheters to infuse the vessel with various vectors [71, 72], and (iii) seeding of implantable vascular prostheses, such as grafts and stents [67]. Recombinant genes also have been inserted into vascular smooth muscle using balloon catheters [73]. All these procedures share the common goal of delivering agents to the vicinity of the vascular wall in high local concentrations.

Endothelial cells also exist in the microvasculature that is found in all tissues, where capillary beds form vascular networks with a surface:volume ratio that is much greater than in larger, muscular vessels. My own laboratory is investigating the possibility of incorporating genetically-modified endothelial cells into microvascular networks that are generated in response to angiogenic stimuli. Following development, neoangiogenesis occurs normally during wound healing, placental growth, and pathologically in association with cancer and diabetes. In addition, it is possible to induce the vascularization of an artificial matrix implant that has been impregnated by fibroblast growth factor (FGF) [48, 74]. Thus, there exists the possibility of targeting GMEC into angiogenically active sites [75], such as tumour deposits of "neo-organiods" [76] that have been generated using FGF-matrix implants. Once in place in these sites, GMEC might express transgenes that, in one instance, would interfere with tumour growth (local production of a cytokine, for example), or, alternatively, would replace a missing protein, such as Factor VIII.

Muscle cells

Myogenesis results from the fusion of mononuclear myoblasts, eventually resulting in the formation of multinucleated muscle fibres. Myoblasts exist in muscle tissue as satellite cells along muscle fibres and are amendable to *ex vivo* gene transfer, as has been shown experimentally for dystrophin [10, 77], as well as other genes not ordinarily expressed in muscle cells, such as Factor IX [78] and growth hormone [79, 80]. These gene modified cells can be expanded *in vitro* and then reinjected into muscle tissue where they may fuse with existing muscle fibres.

Direct *in vivo* gene transfer with viral vectors [11], liposome, or calcium phosphate complexes [81], has been accomplished in animals by injecting directly into striated muscle tissue, resulting in cellular uptake and expression of the transgene. Thus, myoblast gene transfer holds promise for either gene replacement or gene augmentation in the treatment of cardiovascular, muscular, and metabolic disorders.

Cells of the central nervous system

Gene therapy may eventually have a role in the treatment of neurological disorders, including epilepsy, Alzheimer's disease, and Parkinson's disease. Gene transfer for the treatment of brain tumours is discussed further below. While neuronal and glial cells have been targeted experimentally [17, 18, 82], non-dividing adult neuronal cells are not amenable to retroviral-mediated gene transfer. Instead, as discussed earlier, modified herpes virus vectors have been used successfully to introduce foreign genes into neurones [18, 83]. Proliferating embryonal neuronal elements can be transduced with retroviral vectors, either by direct *in vivo* gene transfer [84, 85] or by *ex vivo* transduction and cell implantations [86]. In addition, retroviral-transduced fibroblasts secreting nerve growth factor have been engrafted successfully into the brain [51].

Tumour cells

Gene transfer for the purpose of inducing antitumour immune responses can be termed transgenic immunotherapy [87]. This approach is based upon the observation that tumour cells, often expressing potentially immunogenic proteins, appear to induce a state of immune tolerance that enables the tumour to evade immune destruction. The underlying hypothesis is that local cytokine delivery may improve tumour antigen presentation and activation of immune effector cells, such as natural killer cells, cytotoxic T lymphocytes, neutrophils and macrophages. In transgenic immunotherapy, this is achieved by inserting immune activation genes into tumour cells themselves or into adjacent stromal cells.

Numerous studies in animals have demonstrated the feasibility of this strategy, with the generation of local or systemic antitumour immunity. Tumour antigenicity may be enhanced, for example, by the introduction of a foreign HLA gene, or by upregulating Class I expression and moving antigen presentation with the interferon-γ gene. Alternatively, the genes for cytokines such as IL-2 and IL-4 may be inserted into tumour cells in order to activate immune effector cells. Since rapidly growing or bulky tumour may overcome the ability of the immune system to mount an effective antitumour response, transgenic immunotherapy may be most useful (i) in an adjuvant setting following cytoreduction with surgery, radiation, and chemotherapy, and (ii) for immunizing individuals at risk for cancer.

Sensitization of tumour cells to chemotherapy is another kind of cancer gene therapy. Following the original observation by Moolten [88, 89] that herpes simplex virus thymidine kinase (HSVTK) gene renders cells susceptible to killing by ganciclovir (which becomes phosphorylated to the active compound), Freeman observed a "bystander effect" whereby non-transduced tumour cells were also killed by ganciclovir [90]. Implants of vector-producing cells was first suggested as means of delivering HSVTK to brain tumours by Martuze and Brakefield [91, 92] and was shown to be effective in an animal brain tumour model by Culver et al., who also observed a bystander effect [93].

Finally, the correction of genetic abnormalities involving either the activation of oncogenes or the loss or mutation of tumour suppressor genes is being investigated as another gene therapy strategy for cancer.

Safety of clinical gene transfer

Retroviral vector safety centres on two concerns: (a) insertional mutagenesis resulting in cellular transformation and tumourigenesis, and (b) gene transfer into germ line cells. The likelihood of these untoward events occurring is very small in the absence of contamination by helper virus that would lead to continued retroviral infection of other cells. The use of retroviral packaging cells and stringent surveillance for the presence of helper virus has ameliorated this problem. However, the concern over the potential for malignant transformation was born out in a study carried out by a group of NIH investigators. They discovered a high frequency of lymphomas in primates that had undergone bone marrow transplantation with progenitor cells that had been exposed to helper virus-containing retroviral stock. Many copies of the integrated helper provirus should prevent this complication from occurring.

As mentioned earlier, adenovirus infection may be cytopathic due to the inflammation that develops in response to viral protein expression. Further modifications to the vector may succeed in reducing or eliminating this problem. Although no significant toxicity has been observed so far with either liposomal or receptor-mediated gene transfer, experience with these vectors is limited. It is certain that the safety of gene transfer will continue to be carefully studies by investigators and federal regulators alike.

The role of transfusion medicine in gene therapy

At the time of this writing, the NIH RAC has approved a total of 90 protocols, of which 24 are for gene marking and 66 for gene therapy. Although most protocols are intended for patients with cancer, as investigators and regulators become increasingly familiar with this novel modality, one can anticipate submission and approval of gene therapy protocols directed at many disorders of lesser severity. Whether for gene marking or gene therapy, medical institutions will require a laboratory processing area for gene transfer vectors and/or the cells that are to be administered to patients. These procedures must be carried out in conditions that are consistent with good manufacturing standards.

Transfusion medicine units are experienced in the collection, processing, and distribution of blood cells and other blood components. Transfusion laboratories already have become involved in clinical protocols that involve gene transfer into haematopoietic cells. No other facilities comparable to the transfusion unit exist in hospitals. Thus, it appears logical that the transfusion service becomes the local processing and distribution site for the cellular and DNA reagents that will be employed in clinical gene transfer procedures. However, in order to take on an expanded role that would encompass both *ex vivo* and *in vivo* gene transfer procedures, transfusion medicine practitioners will have to become proficient in vector technology as well as the cultivation and storage of non-haematopoietic cells. The implementation of these techniques will require an expansion of existing resources, including the acquisition of personnel with the requisite gene transfer and cell culture skills. With the gene therapy field rapidly evolving, it is too early to say which cells and vectors will ultimately lead to regular clinical use. Regulatory issues also must be addressed. However, by staying abreast of new developments, and by seeking participation in the development and execution of clinical protocols, transfusion medicine specialists should be able to define an appropriate role in the burgeoning field of gene therapy.

Acknowledgements

The autor wishes to thank Dr. Marc Lippman of the Lombardi Cancer Center for his continued support and encouragement.

References

1. Miller AD. Human gene therapy comes of age. Nature 1992;357:455-69.
2. Anderson WF. Human gene therapy. Science 1992;256:808-13.
3. Mulligan RC. The basic science of gene therapy. Science 1993;260:926-32.
4. Curiel DT, Agarwal S, Rímer MU, et al. gene transfer to respiratory epithelial cells via the receptor-mediated endocytosis pathway. Am J Respir Cell Mol Biol 1992;6:247-52.
5. Weiss RA, Teich N, Varmus HE, Coffin J (eds). Molecular biology of tumor viruses: RNA tumor viruses Vol. 1 & Vol 2, Cold Spring Harbor, NY: Cold Spring Harbor Laboratory 1985.
6. Stratford-Perricaudet LD, Levrero M, Chasse JF, Perricaudet M, Briand P. Evaluation of the transfer and expression in mice of an enzyme-encoding gene using a human adenovirus vector. Hum Gene Ther 1990;1:241-56.
7. Wang Q, Konan V, Taylor MW. Expression of the APRT gene in an adenovirus vector system as a model for studying gene therapy. Adv Exp Med Biol 1991;309B:61-66.
8. Rosenfeld MA, Siegfried W, Yoshimura K, et al. Adenovirus-mediated transfer of a recombinant alpha 1-antitrypsin gene to the lung epithelium *in vivo* [see comments]. Science 1991;252:431-34.
9. Mastrangeli A, Danel C, Rosenfeld MA, et al. Diversity of airway epithelial cell targets for *in vivo* recombinant adenovirus-mediated gene transfer. J Clin Invest 1993; 91:225-34.
10. Ragot T, Vincent N, Chafey P, et al. Efficient adenovirus-mediated transfer of a human minidystrophin gene to skeletal muscle of mdx mice. Nature 1993;361:647-50.
11. Quantin B, Perricaudet LD, Tajbakhsh S, Mandel JL. Adenovirus as an expression vector in muscle cells *in vivo*. Proc Natl Acad Sci USA 1992;89:2581-84.
12. Samulski RJ, Zhu X, Xiao X, et al. Targeted integration of adeno-associated virus (AAV) into human chromosome 19. EMBO J 1991;10:3941-50.
13. Kotin RM, Siniscalco M, Samulski RJ, et al. Site-specific integration by adeno-associated virus. Proc Natl Acad Sci USA 1990;87:2211-15.
14. Muzyczka N. Use of adeno-associated virus as a general transduction vector for mammalian cells. Curr Top Microbiol Immunol 1992;158:97-129.
15. Dixit M, Webb MS, Smart WC, Ohi S. Construction and expression of a recombinant adeno-associated virus that harbors a human beta-globin-encoding cDNA. Gene 1991; 104:253-57.
16. Flotte TR, Solow R, Owens RA, Afione S, Zeitlin PL, Carter BJ. Gene expression from adeno-associated virus vectors in airway epithelial cells. Am J Respir Cell Mol Biol 1992;7:349-56.
17. Huang Q, VonSattel JP, Schaffer PA, Martuza RL, Breakefield XO, DiFiglia M. Introduction of a foreign gene (Escherichia coli lacZ) into rat neostriatal neurons using herpes simplex virus mutants: A light and electron microscopic study. Exp Neurol 1992;115:303-16.
18. Andersen JK, Garber DA, Meaney CA, Breakefiel XO. Gene transfer into mammalian central nervous system using herpes virus vectors: Extended expression of bacterial

lacZ in neurons using the neuron-specific enolase promoter. Hum Gene Ther 1992; 3:487-99.
19. Zenke M, Steinlein P, Wagner E, Cotten M, Beug H, Birnstiel ML. Receptor-mediated endocytosis of transferrin-polycation conjugates: An efficient way to introduce DNA into hematopoietic cells. Proc Natl Acad Sci USA 1990;87:3655-59.
20. Dinur T, Schuchman EH, Fibach E, et al. Toward gene therapy for Niemann-Pick disease (NPD): Separation of retrovirally corrected and noncorrected NPD fibroblasts using a novel fluorescent sphingomyelin. Hum Gene Ther 1992;3:633-39.
21. Uitto J, Christiano AM. Molecular genetics of the cutaneous basement membrane zone. Perspectives on epidermolysis bullosa and other blistering skin diseases. J Clin Invest 1992;90:687-92.
22. Albert N, Tremblay JP. Evaluation of various gene transfection methods into human myoblast clones. Transplant Proc 1992;24:2784-86.
23. Nabel EG, Yang Z, Liptay S, et al. Recombinant platelet-derived growth factor B gene expression in porcine arteries induce intimal hyperplasia *in vivo*. J Clin Invest 1993;91:1822-29.
24. Nabel EG, Gordon D, Yang ZY, et al. Gene transfer *in vivo* with DNA-liposome complexes: Lack of autoimmunity and gonadal localization. Hum Gene Ther 1992; 3:649-56.
25. Hyde SC, Gill DR, Higgins CF, et al. Correction of the ion transport defect in cystic fibrosis transgenic mice by gene therapy. Nature 1993;362:250-55.
26. Nabel GJ. Principal investigator. Immunotherapy of malignancy by *in vivo* gene transfer into tumors. Hum Gene Ther 1992;3:399-410.
27. Karlsson S. Treatment of genetic defects in hematopoietic cell function by gene transfer. Blood 1991;78:2481-92.
28. Eglitis MA, Kantoff P, Gilboa E, Anderson WF. Gene expression in mice after high efficiency retroviral-mediated gene transfer. Science 1985;230:1395-98.
29. Williams DA, Lemischka IR, Nathan DG, Mulligan RC. Introduction of new genetic material into pluripotent haematopoietic stem cells of the mouse. Nature 1984;310: 476-80.
30. Belmont JW, Henkel-Tigges J, Chang SM, et al. Expression of human adenosine deaminase in murine haematopoietic progenitor cells following retroviral transfer. Nature 1986;322(6077):385-87.
31. Dick JE, Magli MC, Huszar D, Philips RA, Bernstein A. Introduction of a selectable gene into primitive stem cells capable of long term culture reconstitution of the hematopoietic system of W/W^v mice. Cell 1985;42:71-79.
32. Wolfe JH, Sands MS, Barker JE, et al. Reversal of pathology in murine mycopolysaccharidosis type VII by somatic cell gene transfer. Nature 1992;360:749-53.
33. Einerhand MP, Bakx TA, Kukler A, Valerio D. Factor affecting the transduction of pluripotent hematopoietic stem cells: Long-term expression of a human adenosine deaminase gene in mice. Blood 1993;81:254-63.
34. Kantoff PW, Gillio AP, McLachlin JR, et al. Expression of human adenosine deaminase in nonhuman promates after retrovirus-mediated gene transfer. J Exp Med 1987;166:219-34.
35. Bordignon C, Yu SF, Smith CA, et al. Retroviral vector-mediated high-efficiency expression of adenosine deaminase (AD) in hematopoietic long-term cultures of ADA-deficient marrow cells. Proc Natl Acad Sci USA 1989;86:6748-52.
36. Van Beusechem VW, Kukler A, Heidt PJ, Valerio D. Long-term expression of human adenosine deaminase in rhesus monkeys transplanted with retrovirus-infected bone-

marrow cells. Proc Natl Acad Sci USA 1992;89:7640-44.
37. Bodine DM, Moritz T, Donahue RE, et al. Long-term *in vivo* expression of a murine adenosine deaminase gene in rhesus monkey hematopoietic cells of multiple lineages after retroviral mediated gene transfer into CD34+ bone marrow cells. Blood 1993; 82:1975-80.
38. Molta JA, Crooks GM, Overell RW, Williams DE, Kohn DB. Retroviral vector-mediated gene transfer into primitive human hematopoietic progenitor cells: Effects of mast cell growth factor (MGF) combined with other cytokines. Exp Hematol 1992; 20:1065-71.
39. Donahue RE, Kessler SW, Bodine DM, et al. *In vivo* evaluation of gene transfer to priate CD34+ cells. J Cellular Biochem 1992;16F:46.
40. Berenson RJ, Bensinger WI, Hill RS, et al. Engraftment after infusion of CD34+ marrow cells in patients with breast cancer or neuroblastoma. Blood 1991;77:1717-22.
41. Hoogerbrugge PM, Vossen JM, Van Beusechem VW, Valerio D. Treatment of patients with severe combined immunodeficiency due to adenosine deaminase (ADA) deficiency by autologous transplantation of genetically modified bone marrow cells. Hum Gene Ther 1992;3:553-58.
42. Ekhterae D, Crumbleholme T, Karson E, Harrison MR, Anderson WF, Zanjani ED. Retroviral vector-mediated transfer of the bacterial neomycin resistance gene into fetal and adult sheep and human hematopoietic progenitors *in vitro*. Blood 1990;75:365-69.
43. Michejda M, Catz CS. Fetal therapy 1994. Fetal Diagn Ther 1994;9:209-12.
44. Luks FI, Deprest JA, Vandenberghe K, Brosens IA, Lerut T. A model for fetal surgery through intrauterine endoscopy. J Pediatr Surg 1994;29:1007-9.
45. Morecki S, Karson E, Cornetta K, et al. Retrovirus-mediated gene transfer into CD4+ and CD8+ human T cell subsets derived from tumor-infiltrating lymphocytes and peripheral blood mononuclear cells. Cancer Immunol Immunother 1991;32:342-52.
46. Kantoff PW, Kohn DB, Mitsuya H, et al. Correction of adenosine deaminase deficiency in cultured human T and B cell by retrovirus-mediated gene transfer. Proc Natl Acad Sci USA 1986;83:6563-67.
47. Palmer TD, Thompson AR, Miller AD. Production of human factor IX in animals by genetically modified skin fibroblasts: Potential therapy for hemophilia B. Blood 1989;73:438-45.
48. St. Louis DA, Verma IM. An alternative approach to somatic cell gene therapy. Proc Natl Acad Sci USA 1988;85:3150-54.
49. Dichek DA, Bratthauer GL, Beg ZH, et al. Retroviral vector mediated *in vivo* expression of low density lipoprotein receptors in the Watanabe heritable hyperlipidemic rabbit. Somatic Cell Mol Genet 1991;17:287-301.
50. Palmer TD, Rosman GJ, Osborne WRA, Miller AD. Genetically modified skin fibroblasts persist long after transplantation but gradually inactivate introduced genes. Proc Natl Acad Sci USA 1991;88:1330-34.
51. Rosenberg MB, Friedmann T, Robertson RC, et al. Grafting genetically modified cells to the damaged brain: Restorative effects of NGF expression. Science 1988;242:1575-78.
52. Scharfmann R, Axelrod JH, Verma IM. Long-term *in vivo* expression of retrovirus-mediated gene transfer in mouse fibroblast implants. Proc Natl Acad Sci USA 1991;88: 4626-30.
53. Suchi M, Dinur T, Desnick RJ, et al. Retroviral-mediated transfer of the human acid sphingomyelinase cDNA: Correction of the metabolic defect in cultured Niemann-Pick disease cells. Proc Natl Acad Sci USA 1992;89:3227-31.

54. Wilkemeyer M, Stankovics J, Foy T, Ledley FD. Propionate metabolism in cultured human cells after overexpression of recombinant methylmalonyl CoA mutase: Implications for somatic gene therapy. Somat Cell Mol Genet 1992;18:493-505.
55. Occhiodoro T, Hopwood JJ, Morris CP, Anson DS. Correction of alpha-L-fucosidase deficiency in fucosidosis fibroblasts by retroviral vector-mediated gene transfer. Hum Gen Ther 1992;3:365-69.
56. Wilson JM, Grossman M, Thompson AR, et al. Somatic gene transfer in the development of an animal model for primary hyperparathyroidism. Endocrinology 1992; 130:2947-54.
57. Chowdhury JR, Grossman M, Gupta S, Chowdhury NR, Baker JR Jr, Wilson JM. Long-term improvement of hypercholesterolemia after *ex vivo* gene therapy in LDLR-deficient rabbits. Science 1991;254:1802-5.
58. Grossman M, Raper SE, Kozarsky K, et al. Successful *ex vivo* gene therapy directed to liver in a patient with familial hypercholesterolemia. Nat Genet 1994;6:335-41.
59. Peng H, Armentano D, MacKenzie-Graham L, et al. Retroviral-mediated gene transfer and expression of human phenylalanine hydroxylase in primary mouse hepatocytes. Proc Natl Acad Sci USA 1988;85:8146-50.
60. Kay MA, Li Q, Liu TH, et al. Hepatic gene therapy: Persistent expression of human alpha 1-antitrypsin in mice after direct gene delivery *in vivo*. Hum Gene Ther 1992; 3:641-47.
61. Armentano D, Thompson AR, Darlington G, Woo SLC. Expression of human factor IX in rabbit hepatocytes by retrovirus-mediated gene transfer: Potential for gene therapy of hemophilia B. Proc Natl Acad Sci USA 1990;87:6141-45.
62. Engelhardt JF, Allen ED, Wilson JM. Reconstitution of tracheal grafts with a genetically modified epithelium. Proc Natl Acad Sci USA 1991;88:11192-96.
63. Yoshimura K, Rosenfeld MA, Nakamura H, et al. Expression of the human cystic fibrosis transmembrane conductance regulator gene in the mouse lung after *in vivo* intratracheal plasmid-mediated gene transfer. Nucleic Acids Res 1992;20:3233-40.
64. Engelhardt JF, Yankaskas JR, Wilson JM. *In vivo* retroviral gene transfer into human bronchial epithelia of xenografts. J Clin Invest 1992;90:2598-607.
65. Nabel EG, Plautz G, Nabel GJ. Gene transfer into vascular cells. J Am Coll Cardiol 1991;17:189B-94B.
66. Zwiebel JA, Freeman SM, Kantoff PW, Cornetta K, Ryan US, Anderson WF. High-level recombinant gene expression in rabbit endothelial cells transduced by retroviral vectors. Science 1989;243:220-22.
67. Dichek DA, Neville RF, Zwiebel JA, Freeman SM, Leon MB, Anderson WF. Seeding of intravascular stents with genetically engineered endothelial cells [see comments]. Circulation 1989;80:1347-53.
68. Dichek DA, Nussbaum O, Degen SJ, Anderson WF. Enhandement of the fibrinolytic activity of sheep endothelial cells by retroviral vector-mediated gene transfer. Blood 1991;77:533-41.
69. Yao SN, Wilson JM, Nabel EG, Kurachi S, Hachiya HL, Kurachi K. Expression of human factor IX in rat capillary endothelial cells: Toward somatic gene therapy for hemophilia B. Proc Natl Acad Sci USA 1991;88:8101-5.
70. Nabel EG, Plautz G, Boyce FM, Stanley JC, Nabel GJ. Recombinant gene expression *in vivo* within endothelial cells of the arterial wall. Science 1989;244:1342-44.
71. Nabel EG, Plautz G, Nabel GJ. Site-specific gene expression *in vivo* by direct gene transfer into the arterial wall. Science 1990;249:1285-88.

72. Lim CS, Chapman GD, Gammon RS, et al. Direct *in vivo* gene transfer into the coronary and peripheral vasculatures of the intact dog [see comments]. Circulation 1991;83: 2007-11.
73. Lynch CM, Clowes MM, Osborne WR, Clowes AW, Miller AD. Long-term expression of human adenosine deaminase in vascular smooth muscle cells of rats: A model for gene therapy. Proc Natl Acad Sci USA 1992;89:1138-42.
74. Thompson JA, Anderson KD, DiPietro JM, et al. Sit-directed neovessel formation *in vivo*. Science 1988;241:1349-52.
75. Ojeifo JO, Forough R, Maciag T, Zwiebel J. Genetically-modified endothelial cells administered intravenously are incorporated into sites of active angiogenesis. J Cell Biochem 1992;Suppl 16F:50.
76. Thompson JA, Haudenschild CC, Anderson KD, DiPietro JM, Anderson WF, Maciag T. Heparin-binding growth factor 1 induces the formation of organoid neovascular structures *in vivo* [published erratum appears in Proc Natl Acad Sci USA90 1990 Feb;87(4):1625]. Proc Natl Acad Sci USA 1989;86:7928-32.
77. Dickson G, Love DR, Davies KE, Wells KE, Piper TA, Walsh FS. Human dystrophin gene transfer: Production and expression of a functional recombinant DNA-based gene. Hum Genet 1991;88:53-58.
78. Hughes SM, Blau HM. Muscle fiber pattern is independent of cell lineage in postnatal rodent development. Cell 1992;68:659-71.
79. Barr E, Leiden JM. Systemic delivery of recombinant proteins by genetically modified myoblasts [see comments]. Science 1991;254:1507-9.
80. Dhawan J, Pan LC, Pavlath GK, Travis MA, Lanctot AM, Blau HM. Systemic delivery of human growth hormone by injection of genetically engineered myoblasts [see comments]. Science 1991;254:1509-12.
81. Wolff JA, Malone RW, Williams P, et al. Direct gene transfer into mouse muscle *in vivo*. Science 1990;247:1465-68.
82. Short MP, Choi BC, Lee JK, Malick A, Breakefield XO, Martuza RL. Gene delivery to glioma cells in rat brain by grafting of a retrovirus packaging cell line. J Neurosci Res 1990;27:427-39.
83. Geller AI, Keyomarsi K, Bryan J, Pardee AB. An efficient deletion mutant packaging system for defective herpes simplex virus vectors: Potential applications to human gene therapy and neuronal physiology. Proc Natl Acad Sci USA 1990;87:8950-54.
84. Sanes JR, Rubinstein J-LR, Nicolas J-F. The use of recombinant retrovirus to study post-implantation cell lineage in mouse embryos. EMBO 1986;5:3133-42.
85. Price J, Turner D, Cepko C. Lineage analysis in the vertebrate nervous system by retrovirus-mediated gene transfer.Proc Natl Acad Sci USA 1987;84:156-60.
86. Stocker KM, Brown AM, Ciment G, Gene transfer of lacZ into avian neural tube and neural crest cells by retroviral infection of grafted embryonic tissues. J Neurosci Res 1993;34:135-45.
87. Zwiebel JA, Su N, MacPherson A, Davis T, Ojeifo JO. the gene therapy of cancer; Transgenic immunotherapy. Sem Hematol 1994;30:119-29.
88. Moolten FL, Wells JM, Heyman RA, Evans RM. Lymphoma regression induced by ganciclovir in mice bearing a herpes thymidine kinase transgen. Hum Gene Ther 1990; 1:125-34.
89. Moolten FL, Wells JM. Curability of tumors bearing herpes thymidine kinase genes transferred by retroviral vectors. J Natl Cancer Inst 1990;82:297-300.

90. Freeman SM, Whartenby KA, Koeplin DS, Moolten FL, Abboud CN, Abraham GN. Tumor regression when a fraction of the tumor mass contains the HSV-TK gene. J Cell Biol 1992;16F:47.
91. Short MP, Choi BC, Lee JK, Malick A, Breakefield XO, Martuza RL. Gene delivery to glioma cells in rat brain by grafting of a retrovirus packaging cell line. J Neurosci Res 1990;27:427-39.
92. Takamiya Y, Short MP, Ezzeddine ZD, Moolten FL, Breakefield XO, Martuza RL. Gene therapy of malignant brain tumors: A rat glioma line bearing the herpes simplex virus type 1-thymidine kinase gene and wild type retrovirus kills other tumor cells. J Neurosci Res 1992;33:493-503.
93. Culver KW, Ram Z, Wallbridge S, Ishii H, Oldfield EH, Blaese RM. *in vivo* gene transfer with retroviral vector-producer cells for treatment of experimental brain tumors [see comments]. Science 1992;256:1550-52.
94. Li CL, Dwarki VJ, Verma IM. Expression of human alpha-globin and mouse/human hybrid beta-globin genes in murine hemopoietic stem cells transduced by recombinant retroviruses. Proc Natl Acad Sci USA 1990;87:4349-53.
95. Dzierzak EA, Papayannopoulou T, Mulligan RC. Lineage-specific expression of a human beta-globin gene in murine bone marrow transplant recipients reconstituted with retrovirus-transduced stem cells. Nature 1988;331:35-41.
96. Weber-Benarous A, Cone RD, London IM, Mulligan RC. Retroviral-mediated transfer and expression of human beta-globin genes in cultured murine and human erythroid cells. J Biol Chem 1988;263:6142-45.
97. Bender MA, Gelinas RE, Miller AD. A majority of mice show long-term expression of a human beta-globin gene after retrovirus transfer into hematopoietic stem cells. Mol Cell Biol 1989;9:1426-34.
98. Osborne WR, Miller AD. Design of vectors for efficient expression of human purine nucleoside phosphorylase in skin fibroblasts from enzyme-deficient humans. Proc Natl Acad Sci USA 1988;85:6851-55.
99. McIvor RS, Johnson MJ, Miller AD, et al. Human purine nucleoside phosphorylase and adenosine deaminase: Gene transfer into cultured cells and murine hematopoietic stem cells by using recombinant amphotropic retroviruses. Mol Cell Biol 1987;7:838-46.
100. McIvor RS, Goddard JM, Simonsen CC, Martin DW Jr. Expression of a cDNA sequence encoding human purine nucleoside phosphorylase in rodent and human cells. Mol Cell Biol 1985;5:1349-57.
101. Foresman MD, Nelson DM, McIvor RS. Correction of purine nucleoside phosphorylase deficiency by retroviral-mediated gene transfer in mouse S49 T cell lymphoma: A model for gene therapy of T cell immunodeficiency. Hum Gene Ther 1992;3:625-31.
102. Brinkhous KM, Reddick RL, Read MS, Nichols TC, Bellinger DA, Griggs TR. Von Willebrand factor and animal models: Contributions to gene therapy, thrombotic thrombocytopenic purpura, and coronary artery thrombosis. Mayo Clin Proc 1991;66: 73-42.
103. Kaufman RJ, Wasley LC, Davies MV, Wise RJ, Israel DI, Dorner AJ. Effect of von Willebrand factor coexpression on the synthesis and secretion of factor VIII in Chinese hamster ovary cells. Mol Cell Biol 1989;9:1233-42.
104. Dai Y, Roman M, Naviaux RK, Verma IM. Gene therapy via primary myoblasts: Long-term expression of factor IX protein following transplantation *in vivo*. Proc Natl Acad Sci USA 1992;89:10892-95.

105. Brinkhous KM. Gene transfer in the hemophilias: Retrospect and prospect. Thromb Res 1992;67:329-38.
106. Hoeben RC, Einerhand MP, Briët E, van Ormondt H, Valerio D, van der Eb AJ, Toward gene therapy in haemophilia A; Retrovirus-mediated transfer of a factor VIII gene into murine haematopoietic progenitor cells. Thromb Haemost 1992;67:341-45.
107. Grompe M, Mitani K, Lee CC, Jones SN, Caskey CT. Gene therapy in man and mice: Adenosine deaminase deficiency, ornithine transcarbamylase deficiency, and Duchenne muscular dystrophy. Adv Exp Med Biol 1991;309B:51-56.
108. Dubowitz V. The muscular dystrophies. Postgrad Med J 1992;68:500-06.
109. Shrager JB, Naji A, Kelly AM, Stedman HH. A PCR-based assay for the wild-type dystrophin gene transferred into the mdx mouse. Muscle Nerve 1992;15:1133-37.
110. Chamberlain JS. X-linked dystrophies: From gene localization to gene therapy. Curr Opin Neurol Neurosurg 1992;5:610-14.
111. Wilson JM, Ping AJ, Krauss JC, et al. Correction of CD18-deficient lymphocytes by retrovirus-mediated gene transfer. Science 1990;248:1413-16.
112. Krauss JC, Bond LM, Todd RF, Wilson JM. Expression of retroviral transduced human CD18 in murine cells: An *in vivo* model of gene therapy for leukocyte adhesion deficiency. Hum Gene Ther 1991;2:221-28.
113. Krauss JC, Ping AJ, Mayo-Bond L, et al. Complementation of genetic and functional defects in CD18-deficient lymphocytes by retrovirus-mediated gene transfer. Trans Assoc Am Physicians 1990;103:263-70.
114. Thrasher A, Chetty M, Casimir C, Segal AW. Restoration of superoxide generation to a chronic granulomatous disease-derived B-cell line by retrovirus mediated gene transfer. Blood 1992;80:1125-29.
115. Cobbs CS, Malech HL, Leto TL, et al. Retroviral expression of recombinant p47phox protein by Epstein-Barr virus-transformed B lymphocytes from a patient with autosomal chronic granulomatous disease. Blood 1992;79:1829-35.
116. Leto TL, Lomax KJ, Volpp BD, et al. Cloning of a 67-kD neutrophil oxidase factor with similarity to a noncatalytic region of p60c-src. Science 1990;248:727-30.
117. Wilson JM, Chowdhury JR. Prospects for gene therapy of familial hypercholesterolemia. Mol Biol Med 1990;7:223-32.
118. Wilson JM, Grossman M, Wu CH, Chowdhury NR, Wu GY, Chowdhury JR. Hepatocyte-directed gene transfer *in vivo* leads to transient improvement of hypercholesterolemia in low density lipoprotein receptor-deficient rabbits. J Biol Chem 1992; 267:963-67.
119. Wilson JM, Grossman M, Raper SE, Baker JR Jr, Newton RS, Thoene JG. *Ex vivo* gene therapy of familial hypercholesterolemia. Hum Gene Ther 1992;3:179-222.
120. Grossman M, Wilson JM, Raper SE. A novel approach for introducing hepatocytes into the portal circulation. J Lab Clin Med 1993;121:472-78.
121. Garver RI Jr, Chytil A, Karlsson S, et al. Production of glycosylated physiologically "normal" human alpha 1-antitrypsin by mouse fibroblasts modified by insertion of a human alpha 1-antitrypsin cDNA using a retroviral vector. Proc Natl Acad Sci USA 1987;84:1050-54.
122. Garver RI Jr, Chytil A, Courtney M, Crystal RG. Clonal gene therapy: *in vivo* expression of a transplanted monoclonal population of murine fibroblasts containing a retrovirus inserted human alpha 1 antitrypsin gene. Trans Assoc Am Physicians 1987; 100:10-20.

123. Garver RI Jr, Chytil A, Courtney M, Crystal RG. Clonal gene therapy: Transplanted mouse fibroblast clones express human alpha 1-antitrypsin gene *in vivo*. Science 1987; 237:762-64.
124. Kay MA, Baley P, Rothenberg S, et al. Expression of human alpha 1-antitrypsin in dogs after autologous transplantation of retroviral transduced hepatocytes. Proc Natl Acad Sci USA 1992;89:89-93.
125. Crystal RG, Gene therapy strategies for pulmonary disease. Am J Med 1992;92:44S-52S.
126. Grompe M, Jones SN, Loulseged H, Caskey CT. Retroviral-mediated gene transfer of human ornithine transcarbamylase into primary hepatocytes of spf and spf-ash mice. Hum Gene Ther 1992;3:35-44.
127. Stankovics J, Ledley FD. Cloning of functional alpha propionyl CoA carboxylase and correction of enzyme deficiency in pccA fibroblasts. Am J Hum Genet 1993;52:144-51.
128. Sawada T, Ledley FD. Correction of methylmalonyl-CoA mutase deficiency in Mut0 fibroblasts and constitution of gene expression in primary human hepatocytes by retroviral-mediated gene transfer. Somat Cell Mol Genet 1992;18:507-16.
129. Miller AD, Jolly DJ, Friedmann T, Verma IM. A transmissible retrovirus expressing human hypoxanthine phosphoribosyltransferase (HPRT): Gene transfer into cells obtained from humans deficient in HPRT. Proc Natl Acad Sci USA 1983;80:4709-13.
130. Willis RC, Jolly DJ, Miller AD, et al. partial phenotypic correction of human Lesch-Nyhan (hypoxanthine-guanine phosphoribosyltransferase-deficient) lymphoblasts with a transmissible retroviral vector. J Biol Chem 1984;259:7842-49.
131. Choudary PV, Barranger JA, Tsuji S, et al. Retrovirus-mediated transfer of the human glucocerebrosidase gene to Gaucher fibroblasts. Mol Biol Med 1986;3:293-99.
132. Sorge J, Kuhl W, West C, Beutler E. Complete correction of the enzymatic defect of type I Gaucher disease fibroblasts by retroviral-mediated gene transfer. Proc Natl Acad Sci USA 1987;84:906-9.
133. Kohn DB, Nolta JA, Weinthal J, et al. Toward gene therapy for Gaucher disease. Hum Gene Ther 1991;2:101-5.
134. Molta JA, Yu XJ, Bahner I, Kohn DB. Retroviral-mediated transfer of the human glucocerebrosidase gene into cultured Gaucher bone marrow [published erratum appears in J Clin Invest 1992 Oct;90(4):following 1634]. J Clin Invest 1992;90:342-48.
135. Zwiebel JA. Implants of genetically modified cells for gene therapy. In: Hackel E, Aubuchon J (eds). Advances in transplantation. Bethesda, MD: American Association of Blood Banks 1993:113-42.

VECTORS FOR GENE THERAPY: STRATEGIES FOR MAKING GENE THERAPY WORK

D.E. Onions

Introduction

In the last 5 years gene therapy has emerged from laboratory experimentation to clinical reality with the prospect of treating monogenic deficiency diseases, some neoplasias and perhaps ameliorating the effects of persistent virus infections like HIV. It is an axiom in gene therapy that the aim is to deliver a therapeutic gene to as many of the target cells as possible and to ensure the expression of that gene for an extended period. Consequently, gene therapy using haemopoietic stem cell targets is an attractive proposition as transduction of a CD34+ stem cell can lead to the establishment of expression in many progeny cells. However, the delivery of genes and the maintenance of expression in many progeny cells. However, the delivery of genes and the maintenance of expression remain formidable problems. Viral vectors offer the most effective method for gene delivery to haemopoietic cells and out of the first 81 gene therapy applications approved in the United States 63 used retrovirus vectors. While other vectors like adenovirus vectors or adeno-associatedvirus (AAV) vectors may also have a role in transduction of bone marrow cells the retroviruses have a number of advantages. Like AAV they are able to integrate DNA copies of their genomes or proviruses into chromosomal DNA without the complex rearrangements associated with other transduction processes. Nevertheless there are disadvantage with these vectors, in particular there are concerns over their safety and limitations on the insert size that they can carry. Eventually synthetic systems utilising targeting and integration systems derived from viruses may become feasible but in the medium term retrovirus and AAV vectors offer the most useful approach to gene therapy through haemopoietic stem cells.

Retrovirus replication

The retrovirus vectors used in gene therapy have been based on amphotropic murine leukaemia virus, but as discussed below new vectors based on gibbon ape leukaemia virus and feline leukaemia virus hold great promise. These retroviruses all have a similar structure and replication pattern [reviewed in 1]. Each virion carries two copies of an RNA genome within an inner capsid which in turn is

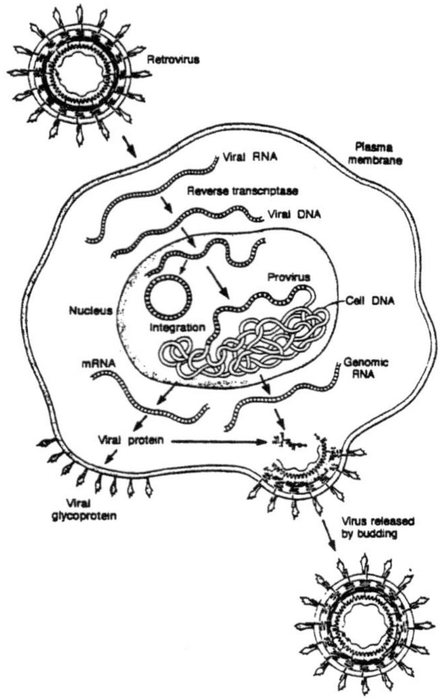

Figure 1.

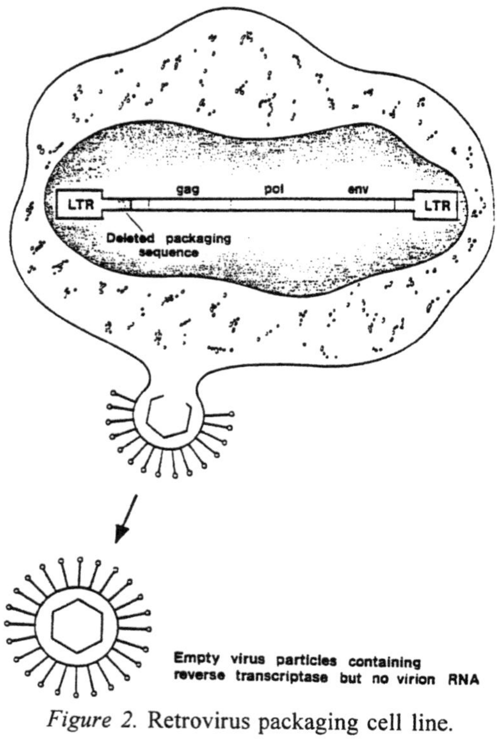

Figure 2. Retrovirus packaging cell line.

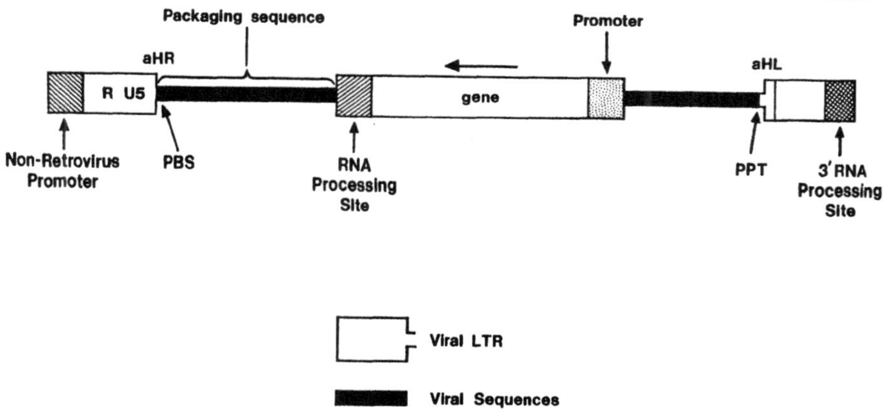

Figure 3. Minimal retrovirus vector.

surrounded by an envelope derived from the host cell membrane that contains two viral envelope proteins. In the simple retroviruses like MuLV there are 3 gene blocks; *gag* encoding the internal structural proteins, *pol* that specifies the reverse transcriptase and *env* encoding the envelope proteins. The major envelope glycoprotein, termed SU binds, to cognate receptors on the cell surface and entry is mediated by fusion of the viral envelope and cell membrane; the latter process being dependant on the activity of a minor transmembrane (TM) envelope protein (Figure 1).

Once the virus core is released into the cytoplasm the genomic RNA is transcribed into double stranded DNA by a virion encoded enzyme, reverse transcriptase which is present in the core of the virus. Reverse transcription is complex and involves two "jumps" during synthesis of the DNA strands. The provirus, migrates to the nucleus as a nucleoprotein complex and becomes covalently integrated into chromosomal DNA through the action of the integrate function of the reverse transcriptase complex. The nucleoprotein complex includes the major capsid protein (CA) as well as the reverse transcriptase integrate and possible the nucleoprotein (NC). The ends of the LTR contain an inverted repeat of 2 to 10 bases that probably forms a recognition site for the integrate as, mutation of this region can reduce the efficiency of integration process. These sequences are referred to as attachment right and left (*att*R, *att*L or aHR and aHL in Figure 3). During the integration a staggered cut is made in the host cell DNA resulting in a duplication of a short stretch of 4 to 6 bases of chromosomal DNA. The viral DNA is shortened, usually by the loss of two bases from each end so that the resulting ends of the viral DNA are always 5′-TG...CA-3′ DNA. All the transcripts of the retroviral genome begin at the 5′R region and all end at the 3′R-U5 border which is the point at which the transcript is polyadenylated. In the commonly used vectors the polyadenylation signal AAUAAA is present within the R region.

In the type C oncoviruses like MuLV and FeLV the splicing patterns are simple. A full length transcript acts as genomic RNA and as mRNA for the *gag* and *pol* genes whereas, a less abundant spliced mRNA is used to express env.

The *env* transcripts originate at the start of R and in most viruses there is a splice donor site (SD) in the leader sequence upstream of gag. The splice acceptor site for this transcript (SA) is in the terminal region of the *pol* gene which is in a different reading frame from env. In selecting expression systems for retrovirus vectors note should be taken of the relative abundance of spliced and unspliced message.

The basis of retrovirus vectors

Retrovirus vector systems consist of two elements a packaging cell line and a vector. The underlying principle of retrovirus vector systems is that sequences necessary for packing viral RNA can be identified. In all retroviruses, the major determinant of RNA packaging is a sequence lying between U5 and *gag* normally referred to as φ (psi). In MuLV a sequence extending downstream from the splice donor to the point immediately preceding the *gag* initiation codon is sufficient to enable packaging of RNAs including non-viral RNAs [2, 3] although efficient packaging requires sequences extending into the *gag* gene.

The size of the φ containing sequence can also act as a constraint on packaging. No lower limit on size has been defined. Recently a piscine retrovirus with a 11.5 kb genome has been sequenced (Hart and Onions unpublished), the largest so far recorded, and transcripts extending beyond the 3'U3 region, up to 11 kb in size, have been packaged into ALV. In most MuLV vectors discussed below an insert of around 6 Kb can be accommodated.

The simplest packaging line consists of a provirus in which the psi sequence has been deleted. When stabley transfected into a cell, virus particles containing reverse transcriptase will be produced but virion RNA should not become packaged within these particles (Figure 2).

The complementing component in a retrovirus vector system is the vector itself. The vector must contain a packaging sequence but much of the structural coding regions can be deleted (Figure 3). Often a selectable marker gene like *neo* is incorporated into the vector. A multiple restriction site may be introduced downstream to facilitate cloning of different genes of interest. The genes can be driven off the LTR as a spliced or unspliced transcript, or alternatively a separate promoter could be incorporated and the gene driven in either transcriptional orientation. When in the opposite orientation to the provirus a separate polyadenylation signal has to be included at the end of the gene.

To produce a packaged vector the vector construct is transfected into the packaging cell line (Figure 4). Cells containing the vector can be selected for by using adding substrate (G418 in this example) that is toxic to cells not containing the marker gene. At this stage it is usual to pick clones and after recloning to screen for those clones releasing the highest titre of virus. This is an important step and when conducted rigorously can considerably improve the titres of vector virions obtained. The resulting clones of cells should release virus particles containing an RNA transcript of the vector including the *cis*-acting sequences necessary for its reverse transcription and integration.

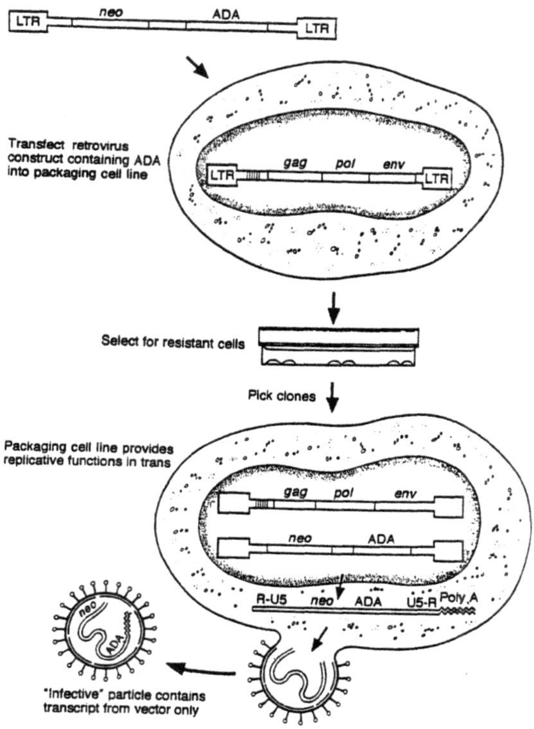

Figure 4. Packaging vector.

Safety and efficacy of retrovirus vectors

Retrovirus vectors are derived from a group of viruses that are capable of activating oncogenes at their sites of integration through promoter insertion, enhancer activation or disruption of cis-acting regulatory sequences [reviewed in Figure 4].

Consequently there are understandable concerns over the safety of such vectors. In general harmful consequences are only associated with the replication competent viruses and therefore rigorous testing of vectors for such viruses under the formal conditions of Good Laboratory Practice (GLP) is the most important feature of safety evaluation.

Recombination between the vector and the packaging sequence can lead to the generation of wild type replication competent virus

Most systems used in gene therapy are based murine amphotropic packaging cells that is, cells containing proviruses derived from wild mouse viruses that have envelope proteins that enable the virus to infect murine and a range of non-murine cells including human cells. In simple retrovirus vector systems described above recombination between the vector and packaging construct occurs rapidly even after transient transfections and leads to replication competent retrovirus (RCR) production.

The consequences of a vector stock containing replication virus cannot be easily predicted. In general the establishment of persistent (non-latent) infection by this

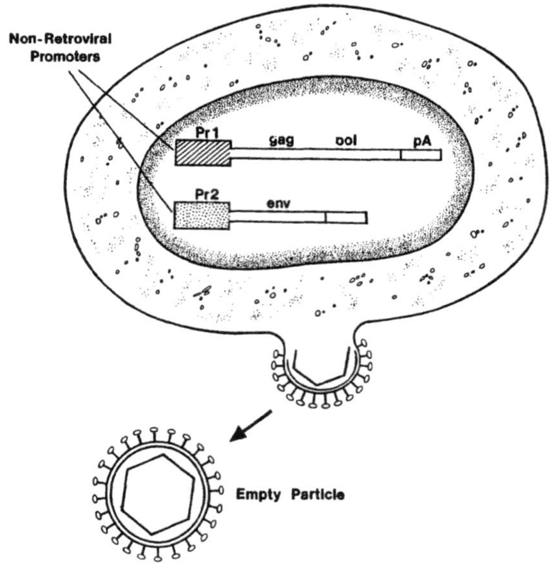

- Non-retroviral promoters
- *Env, gag & pol* genes on separate constructs
- Packaging line non-murine, not expressing retroviral or VL30-like sequences

Figure 5. Second generation packaging line.

class of retroviruses requires quite high levels of virus which is in contrast to many lentivirus infections. For instance to achieve a near 100% infection rate in cats older than 6 months, requires in excess of 10^3ffu of virus.

The studies on the safety of amphotropic MuLV in primates like those reported by Corneta et al. [5] indicate that viraemia is not a common finding even after administration of high titres (7.2 x 10^7ffu) of replication competent virus. However, caution should be exercised in considering these findings. The method of delivery of the virus was different from procedures used in gene therapy of haemopoietic stem cells. Secondly the time scale of the first reported study is still quite short term, just over two years. Some strains of FeLV continue to induce leukaemia for periods in excess of 4 years. Moreover it is clear from studies on cats that latent exogenous retrovirus can be reactivatedand, in immunosuppressed animals, viraemia and disease may result.

The resent report by Donahue et al. [6] of T-cell lymphomas following exposure to high levels of replication competent virus reinforces the need for caution. In Donahue's study, bone marrow cells were infected with a vector preparation known to contain 10^3 to 10^4 infectious particles/m of RCR. The monkeys were severely immunocompromised both by total body irradiation (500Rads × 2) and T-cell depletion from the autologous graft. Three of the 8 monkeys receiving infected CD34+ cells developed T-cell lymphomas within 200 days. Interestingly

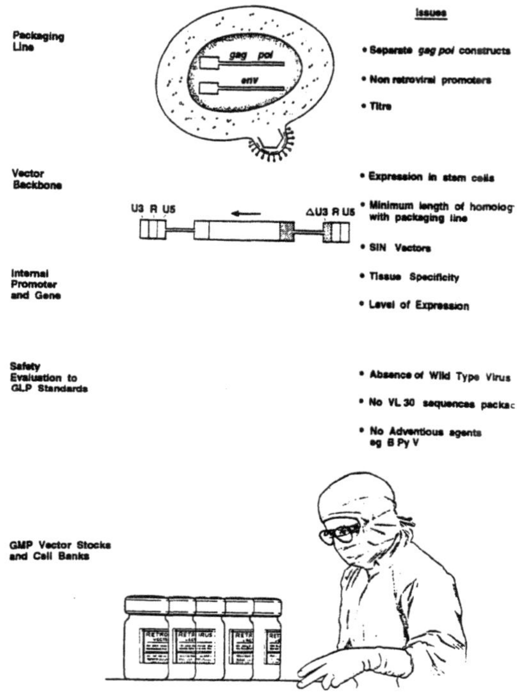

Figure 6. Development of retrovirus vectors for clinical use.

tumour bearing animal had high titre viraemias, a feature that has been suggested to be unlikely consequence of infection by murine viruses as primate complement can inactivate MuLV *in vitro*. However, the latter process may be dependent on the cells used to grow the virus (M. Collins, personal communication).

The creation of a novel retrovirus through recombination of vector sequences with endogenous or exogenous sequences in the target species

The human genome like the genomes of other vertebrates contains several families of retroviral related sequences although these all appear to be defective. Non-homologous recombination between vector sequences and endogenous (genetically inherited) sequences is of the order of 10^{-2} to 10^{-4} where there is some sequence homology between part of the sequences. These events are much less frequent where there is low homology, for instance there is little evidence for recombination between the RD114 endogenous virus of cats and the exogenous FeLV although these can be co-expressed in cell lines.

However, complex recombinations are known. For instance the Kirsten sarcoma was derived by passage of a murine leukaemia virus in rats. The resultant virus contained MuLV sequences, a transduced rat oncogene and VL30 sequences which are related to, but distinct from, infectious retrovirus genomes. These recombinations were dependant on replication competent virus and, for a vector, one can conclude that the risk of producing novel viruses is extremely low.

Mobilisation of vector by human retroviruses

Although gene therapy vectors are defective for replication there are concerns that they could be mobilised and horizontally transmitted to others through superinfection with a human retrovirus like HIV or HTLV. However, HIV and HTLV have a different genetic structure and appear to be unable to rescue defective MuLV proviruses [7]. Moreover in permissive species like cats where defective and non-defective viruses co-exist horizontal transmission of the defective element has not been demonstrated under circumstances where the non-defective component is readily transmitted [8].

The widely used packaging lines used in gene therapy result in the packaging of VL30 retroviral related sequences

Most packaging cell lines releasing amphotropic viral particles are based on NIH/3T3 cells. These express VL30 retroviral related sequences and MCF retroviral sequences that can become packaged into the virions. This is a worrying feature of current vectors since the VL30 sequences have LTRs and could potentially act as insertional mutagens. Moreover VL30 sequences could serve the substrate for further recombinations as occurred in the generation of Kirsten sarcoma virus [9]. In order to improve current gene therapy systems there is a need to rederive packaging constructs into cell lines not expressing retroviral sequences. One reason that murine cells continue to be used is that it enables vector sequences to be introduced into the amphotropic line by infection with an ecotropic MuLV vector. The advantage of introducing the vector sequence by infection rather than by transfection is that in general higher titres of the packaged vector are achieved. Solutions to using amphotropic MuLV vectors in non-murine cells that still permit the introduction of the gene by infection are proposed below.

Design of safe vector systems

Recent developments in vector design have resulted in very much safer systems although there is still room for improvement.

Packaging Cells

In simple packaging lines, wild type virus can even be found in harvests made after transient transfections. Consequently efforts have been directed at improving the safety of packaging cell constructs and while significant improvements have been made there is still scope for further refinement of current packaging lines. Second generation packaging cell lines like PA317 were an improvement in that, in addition to deletion of the packaging sequence, the 3′LTR was also deleted so that two recombinations are necessary to generate a wild type virus. Nevertheless, replication competent virus can be generated in these cells [10].

Third generation packaging lines place the *gag-pol* genes and *env* gene on separate constructs that are sequentially introduced into the packaging cells to prevent recombination during transfection [11, 12]. The two step procedure also has the advantage that the level of *gag-pol* in separate clones can be measured so that the best producers are used in the second transfection. These amphotropic packaging lines φCRIP [11] and GP+envAm12 [12] have become important tools in the development of gene therapy protocols. These workers have made a very significant contribution to the development of safe retrovirus vectors but further improvements can be made. These packaging lines still contain sequences that can form the substrate for recombination. The *env* gene components of φCRIP and its ecotropic equivalent φCRE contain the downstream polypurine tract and inverted repeat at the LTR boundary. When shuttling a vector between PA317 and φCRE recombination was observed after the fourth passage and fifth passage in two separate experiments. Moreover there is a relatively large (>4 kb) overlap in the packaging constructs used to generate φCRE and φCRIP. Codon wobbling can be used to reduce recombination frequency while maintaining the primary protein sequence of the constructs. The ecotropic packaging lines reported by Morgenstem and Land [13] also adopted a split *gag-pol* and *env* construct typical of a third generation packaging line. In this case additional steps were taken to reduce recombination. The region of overlap between the *gag-pol* and *env* expression constructs was reduced to 61bp extending over the common region between *pol* and *env* which are in different reading frames. Transversion mutations were introduced into the final 20 codons of *pol*, retaining the integrity of the coding region of this gene while reducing the homology with *env* to 55% in the overlap region. Similarly wobble mutations were introduced into the 3' of *env* and all sequences downstream of the *env* stop codon were deleted to reduce recombination with ecotropic MuLV sequences present within vectors. A further refinement would be to drive the *gag-pol* and *env* constructs off independent non-retroviral promoters, further reducing the probability of recombination with the vector (Figure 5).

The vectors

A safe retrovirus vector would contain the minimum amount of retroviral sequence consistent with its ability to be packaged, undergo reverse transcription and integrate. The minimum sequence requirement would consist of:

- The R-U5 region including the attachment signals (aHR in Figure 3) required for proviral integration.
- The primer binding site immediately downstream of U5.
- The packaging sequence.
- The polypurine tract.
- The attachment signal left (aHL in Figure 3) and the R region.

This minimal vector is also a self inactivating vector in that it lacks a complete 3'U3 region. Since the U3 region in the virion RNA is derived from the 3' vector U3 region, the progeny vector provirus will lack a functional retroviral enhancer and promoter. Consequently vectors of this form cannot be mobilised by super-infecting virus and are unable to activate cellular genes through the common proviral insertion mechanisms. A minimal vector of this form would only include about 10% of the retroviral sequences found in a replication competent parental virus. However, the main constraint to using SIN vectors is that the titres of virions is usually far lower than for non-SIN vectors.

Efficient vectors usually contain part of *gag* and have deleted splice donor sites. In the simplest case of a vector expressing one gene it is preferable to have part of the *gag* sequence which can increase the titre of packaged infectious virions by tenfold [13]. Unlike the psi sequence which can be in any position within a sequence to effect packaging, the *gag* sequence must be in its native position adjacent to psi to have any effect. Potential recombination problems with this type of vector can be overcome by using *gag* regions from different viruses in the packaging and vector constructs. For instance vectors derived from one virus can be packaged by constructs derived from another virus, (e.g. an FeLV vector could be packaged by MuLV or *vice versa*) so reducing the probability of recombination to an extremely low level.

Design of more effective systems

Producing effective systems requires several elements to be optimised, the ability of the vector to infect the target cell, the titre of the vector stock and the expression of the therapeutic gene in the target cell.

Expression of the therapeutic gene

A key feature of an effective vector is its ability to provide high level expression of the therapeutic gene. Transcription is initiated at the U3-R junction within the 5′LTR of the provirus and requires cellular RNA polymerase II. Several factors affect the level proviral of transcription which can constitute up to 10% of the total cellular mRNA. These factors include:

- The regulatory regions within the U3 region;
- The cell type infected which governs the availability of specific transcription factors;
- The chromosomal location of the provirus. Expression may vary by a factor of 10 fold between clones of infected cells with a similar proviral copy number.

The U3 region contains an enhancer which may be duplicated in particular pathogenic variants of the MuLV and FeLV [14]. In a typical MuLV enhancer of about 75bp there may be binding sites for at least 7 known transcription factors (Figure 3). The central motif within the core of the enhancer is conserved across the mammalian type C oncoviruses and consists of binding sites for LVb, core enhancer binding protein, nuclear factor 1 [15] and glucocorticoid response element [16].

A feature of relevance to the development of vectors is that proviral expression can vary widely in different cell types. Most MuLV strains are inefficient at expressing in early developmental stages including embryonal and haemopoietic stem cells. Proviruses that are not expressed in the stem cell may become permanently downregulated and methylated so that expression does not occur in the differentiated, progeny cells that would normally support retroviral replication [17]. However, mutations within the U3 region and other sites can radically alter expression [18]. Similarly insertion of an enhancer from a polyomavirus capable of replication of locus defining sequences that can target expression to particular tissue compartments like the CD2 control region, used to target transgene expression to T-cells [21, 22].

Targeting of retrovirus vectors

The current retrovirus vectors used in gene therapy are based on amphotropic MuLV but there is current interest in the development of vectors based on related retroviruses like feline (FeLV) and gibbon ape (GaLV) leukaemia virus that infect cells through different cell surface receptors. For instance FeLV of subgroups efficiently infect human cells using receptors distinct from each other and from A-MuLV. The FeLV-B receptor is the same as the GaLV receptor and has been shown to be homologous to a phosphate transporter protein [23, 24]. It is also possible to construct packaging systems using retroviral *gag-pol* genes and envelope genes from other viruses like vesicular stomatitis virus [25] and the possibility of directly engineering the specificity of the vector envelope gene is under active investigation.

There are several advantages of having a combination of murine and feline vectors. Higher titres are generally obtained by infecting a packaging line rather than by transfecting it however it is not possible to infect a packaging line with a vector that uses the same receptor as that vector released from the packaging line. By establishing two packaging lines, one based on MuLV and the other on FeLV one can achieve a number of benefits. First the packaging cells can be non-murine cells that do not package VL30 sequences. Secondly by transferring a murine vector to a feline packaging line or *vice versa* one reduces the homology between the packaging sequence and the vector. In addition by repeatedly infecting the packaging line one can build up the vector copy number which generally increases the titre of vector released.

In the future we may expect to see the development of semi-synthetic vector systems for gene therapy but in the medium term retrovirus vectors offer one of the most attractive systems for gene therapy. Whatever systems evolve our understanding of the biology of viral vectors will play an important role in their development.

References

1. Coffin JM. Retroviridae and their replication. In: Fields BN, Knipe DM (eds). Virology. Vol.2 New York: Raven Press, Ltd 1990:1437-500.
2. Mann RS, Mulligan RC, Baltimore D. Construction of a retrovirus packaging mutant and its use to produce helper-free defective retrovirus. Cell 1983;32:871-79.
3. Mann RS, Baltimore D. Varying the position of a retrovirus packaging sequence results in the encapsidation of both unspliced and spliced RNAs. J Virol 1985;54:401-07.
4. Onions D. Viruses as the aetiological agents of leukaemia and lymphoma. In: Burnett A, Armitage J, Newland A, Keating A (eds). Haematological Oncology. Cambridge: Cambridge University Press 1994:35-72.

5. Corneta K, Moen RC, Culver K, et al. Amphotropic murine leukaemia virus is not an acute pathogen for primates. Hum Gene Ther 1990;1:15-30.
6. Donahue RE, Kessler SW, Bodine D, et al. Helper virus induced T-cell lymphoma in non-human primates after retroviral mediated gene transfer. J Exp Med 1992;176: 1125-35.
7. Takeuchi Y, Simpson G, Vile RG, Weiss RA, Collins MKL. Retroviral pseudotypes produced by rescue of a moloney murine leukaemia virus vector by C-type, but not D-type, retroviruses. Virology 1992;186:792-94.
8. Onions D, Lees G, Forrest D, Neil J. Recombinant viruses containing the myc gene rapidly produce clonal tumours expressing T-cell antigen gene transcripts. Int J Cancer 1987;40:40-44.
9. Itin A, Keshet E. Apparent recombinants between "virus-like" (VL30) and murine leukaemia virus-related sequences in mouse DNA. J Virol 1983;47:178-84.
10. Bosselman RA, Hsu R, Bruszewski J, Hu S, Martin F, Nicolson M. Replication defective chimeric helper proviruses and factors affecting generation of competent virus: Expression of Moloney murine leukemia virusstructural genes via the metallothionein promoter. Mol Cell Biol 1987;7:1797-806.
11. Danos O, Mulligan RC. Safe and efficient generation of recombinant retroviruses with amphotropic and ecotropic host ranges. Proc Natl Acad Sci USA 1988;85:6460-64.
12. Markowitz D, Goff S, Bank A. Construction and use of a safe and efficient amphotropic packaging cell line. Virology 1988;167:400-06.
13. Morgenstern JP, Land H. Advanced mammalian gene transfer: High titre retroviral vectors with multiple drug selection markers and a complementary helper-free packaging line. Nucleic Acids Res 1990;18:3587-96.
14. Fulton R, Plumb M, Shield L, Neil JC. Structural diversity and nuclear protein binding sites in the long terminal repeats of feline leukaemia virus. J Virol 1990; 64:1675-82.
15. Speck NA, Baltimore D. Six distinct nuclear factors interact with the 75-basepair repeat of the Moloney leukaemia virus enhancer. Mol Cell Biol 1987;7:1101-11.
16. Miksicek R, Heber A, Schmid W, et al. Glycocorticoid responsiveness of the transcriptional enhancer of moloney murine sarcoma virus. Cell 1986;46:283-90.
17. Challita P-M, Kohn DB. Lack of expression from a retroviral vector after transduction of murine hemopoietic stem cells is associated with methylation in vivo. Proc Natl Acad Sci USA 1994;91:2567-71.
18. Hilberg F, Stocking C, Ostertag W, Grez M. Functional analysis of a retroviral host range mutant: Altered long terminal repeat sequences allow expression in embryonal carcinoma cells. Proc Natl Acad Sci USA 1987;84:5232-36.
19. Linney E, Davis B, Overhauser J, Chao E, Fan H. Nonfunction of a Moloney murine leukaemia virus regulatory sequence in F9 embryonal carcinoma cells. Nature 1984; 308:470-72.
20. Linney E, Neill SD, Prestridge DS. Retroviral vector gene expression in F9 embryonal carcinoma cells. J Virol 1987;61:3248-53.
21. Greaves DR, Wilson FD, Lang G, Kioussis D. Human CD2 3′-flanking sequences confer, high level, T-cell specific, position independent gene expression in transgenic mice. Cell 1989;56:979-86.
22. Stewart M, Cameron E, Campbell M, et al. Conditional expression and oncogenicity of c-myc linked to a CD2 dominant control region. Int J Cancer 1993;53:1023-30.
23. O'Hara B, Johann SV, Klinger HP, et al. Characterization of a human gene conferring sensitivity to infection by gibbon ape leukemia virus. Cell Growth and Differentiation 1990;1:119-27.

24. Tailor CS, Takeuchi Y, O'Hara B, Johann SV, Weiss RA, Collins MKL. Mutation of amino acids within the gibbon ape leukemia virus (GALV) receptor differentially affects feline leukemia virus subgroup b, simian sarcoma virus, and GALV infections. J Virol 1993;67:6737-41.
25. Emi N, Friedmann T, Yee J-K. Pseudotype formation of murine leukaemia virus with the G protein of vesicular stomatitis virus. J Virol 1991;65:1212-17.

FROM BLOOD STAIN TO PATHOGENESIS STUDY OF HUMAN HEREDITARY DISEASES

C. Férec, B. Mercier, M.P. Audrezet

Introduction

The development of recombinant DNA techniques has permitted in the past years the mapping and cloning of an increasing number of genes responsible for human heriditable diseases. The analysis of the molecular basis of these diseases is now an obligate step to understand the pathophysiology of genes responsible of human inherited disorders. This implicates that the same part of a gene could be examined quickly in a large number of individuals. Several methods, for rapid screening of mutations in a target sequence, have been developed including chemical cleavage [1], RNAse cleavage [2], the systematic sequencing of PCR products, denaturing gradient gel electrophoresis (DGGE) [3, 4], and single strand conformational polymorphism (SSCP) [5]. At this time, SSCP is probably the most commonly used and the most popular of these techniques although its sensitivity is probably situated at 80-90% [6, 7].

In this paper, we illustrate the power of PCR technology which allows the complete analysis of the coding sequence of a gene from a blood stain on a Guthrie card for example. As a model, we have studied the cystic fibrosis gene.

Cystic fibrosis (CF) is the most common autosomal recessive genetic disease in Caucasians, with about 1 in 2500 newborns affected, and a carrier frequency of 1 in 25 [8]. The classical clinical profile includes pancreatic insufficiency and recurrent respiratory infections. However, a subset of patients have milder phenotypes and cannot be identified until they become adults. The gene responsible for CF – called the Cystic Fibrosis Transmembrane conductance Regulator gene (CFTR) – has been cloned in 1989 using a positional cloning strategy [9-11]. The CFTR gene is composed of 27 exons which span 230 kb of the long arm of chromosome 7. It encodes a polypeptide of 1480 amino acids called CFTR, a cAMP-dependent chloride channel. The most common mutation, the deletion of a phenylalanine at position 508 of the protein (ΔF508), was found as soon as the gene was discovered and accounts for about 70 per cent of CF chromosomes throughout the world [12].

The Cystic Fibrosis Genetic Analysis Consortium was created in 1989 to coordinate the identification of other mutations. Since then, over 400 mutations have been reported [13].

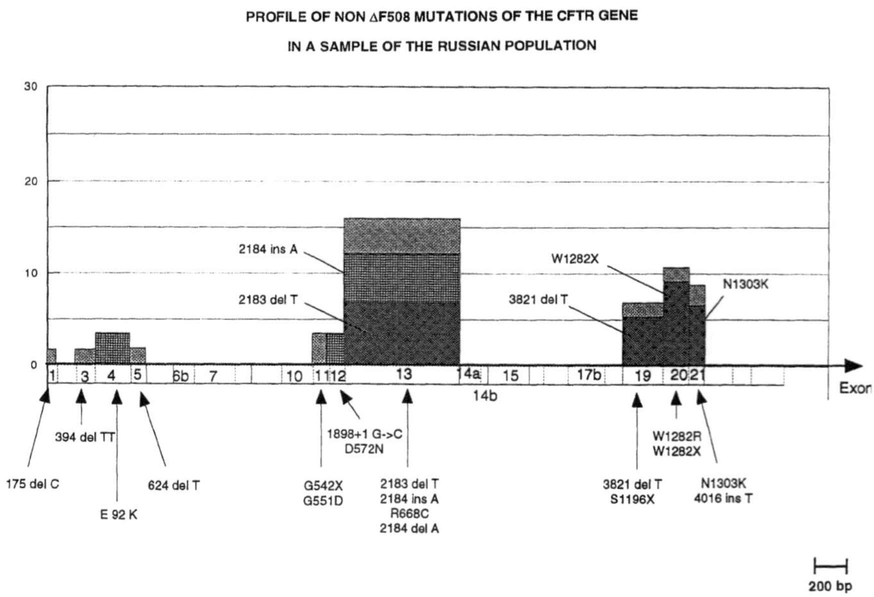

Figure 1. Profile of non Δ508 mutations of the CFTR gene in a sample of the Russian population.

The results we have obtained in studying the CF gene in many patients of various ethnic origin have permitted to improve our knowledge of the distribution of CFTR mutations, the type of molecular abnormalities, the relationship between the genotype and the phenotype and the clinical expression of the disease.

Materials and methods

Patients

The diagnosis of CF was confirmed by at least one positive sweat test and typical clinical findings.

DNA extraction

The retrospective analysis for genetic screening was performed on dried blood specimens. A disk (25 mm^2) of the blood spot was cut out and put into an Eppendorf tube. Red blood cells are eliminated by two washes with NaCl 0,9% and, after 8 min of centrifugation at 8000 rpm the white blood cells are lysed by incubation at 96°C in 150 μl of NaOH 10mM, SDS 0.05%, NaCl 200mM for 5 minutes. Amplifications were performed from an aliquot of 2 μl of the supernatant.

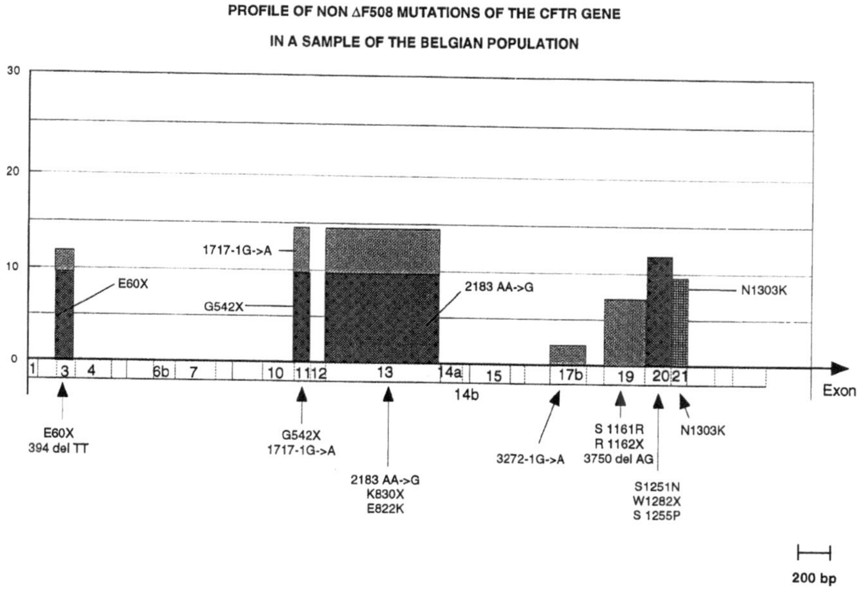

Figure 2. Profile of non Δ508 mutations of the CFTR gene in a sample of the Belgian population.

Amplification

Exon 10 of the CFTR gene was amplified alone, whereas the exons 7 and 11 were coamplified. 2 μl of the DNA solution are amplified in a 100 μl reaction mixture containing 10mM Tris-HCl pH 8.3, 50mM KCl, 1.5mM $MgCl_2$, 125 μM dNTPs, 50 pmoles of each primer and 2 units of Taq polymerase. The samples were subjected to 35 cycles of PCR in a Perkin Elmer Cetus 9600 (1 min at 94°C followed by 5 cycles of 30 sec at 94°C, 30 sec at 54°C, 30 sec at 72°C and 30 cycles of 30 sec at 95°C, 30 sec at 50°C, 30 sec at 72°C). After these cycles, the samples are denaturated for 2 min at 94°C and hybridized for 15 min at 68°C to create heteroduplexes.

Denaturing gradient gel electrophoresis (DGGE)

Gel apparatus and conditions were described elsewhere [4, 14]. Samples were loaded onto a 6.5% polyacrylamide gel (37.5:1) with a linearly increasing gradient from 20% to 70% (vol/vol) [100% denaturant is 7 M urea/40% (vol/vol) formamide] at 75 V for 6 to 9 hours at constant 60°C depending on the melting map of the amplified DNA. Computer analysis was performed using Melt 87, Melt Map Programmes, generously provided by L. Lerman (Massachusetts Institute of Technology). The optimal gradient conditions and migration time for electrophoresis were determined for each PCR product. Sequences of these primers have been previously described [15]. Gels were stained in ethidium bromide and photographed under UV transillumination.

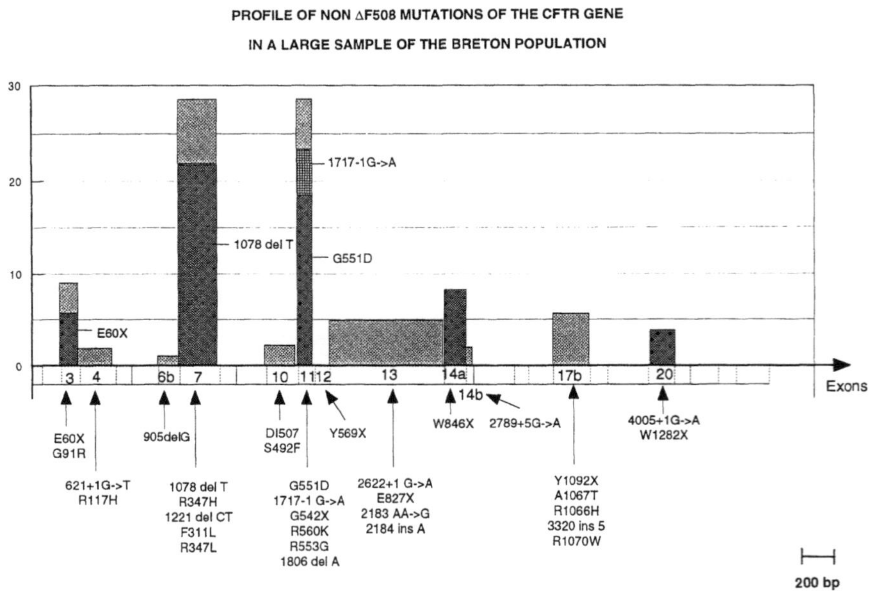

Figure 3. Profile of non Δ508 mutations of the CFTR gene in a sample of the Breton population.

DNA sequencing

Single stranded DNA was obtained in the asymmetric polymerase chain reaction (PCR) [16]. Each single-stranded product was concentrated using Centricon 100 (Amicon, Danvers, Massachusetts) and the reaction product was used for sequencing by the dideoxy nucleotide chain termination method [17]. Each DNA sample was sequenced twice, and each time the mutated allele created or destroyed a restriction site, the mutation was confirmed after amplification and digestion of the PCR product.

Background

The identification of the gene responsible for CF was obtained by a reverse genetic strategy in 1989. This successful approach now called positional cloning represents a major breakthrough in the field of CF research [18]. The gene was first mapped to chromosome 7 and then linkage analysis using DNA polymorphic markers yielded the description and characterization of a 27 exon gene encoding a polypeptide of 1480 amino acids called CFTR protein. The protein is composed of two hydrophobic domains and two nucleotide-binding fold domains which interact with ATP [19].

A large body of evidence indicates the function of CFTR as being itself a chloride channel [20-22]. Shortly after the gene's discovery, it was reported that one particular mutation, corresponding to the loss of a phenylalanine residue at codon 508, occurred at a frequency close to 70% on CF chromosomes world-wide [12]. At least six other mutations have a frequency of over 1% (G542X, G553D, R553X, W1282X, N1303K, 1717-1 G → A) [23].

Most of the other mutations, which occur at extremely low frequencies, are termed private mutations. The accumulation of molecular defects in exons coding for the first and the second nucleotide-binding fold of the molecule has been observed [24]. To look for mutations in the CFTR gene sequence we have developed an approach based on denaturing gradient gel electrophoresis (DGGE). DGGE was described by Lerman and improved first in 1985 with PCR technology development [25] and then with the addition of a GC clamp primer by Sheffield et al. [26]. The technique allows the detection of DNA molecules differing by only a base change whereby each molecule is analysed according to its melting properties. DNA molecules melt in discrete segments, called melting domains varying in length from about 30 to 300 bp. Their migration in a gel gradient of increasing denaturant concentration is dependent on the sequence of these domains. If a mutation or a polymorphism exists in any fragment, its migration is altered compared to that of the wild-type fragment. Direct sequencing of the mutated fragment permits the detection of all possible mutations in a single melting domain of a DNA molecule, e.g. each of 20 mutations reported in exon 11 of the CFTR gene can be excluded for that fragment showing an unaltered mobility. Using this approach, we have analysed the complete CFTR gene sequence, i.e. the 27 exons and their exon/intron boundaries in different populations [27-31].

Results and discussion

The spectrum of mutations in the CFTR gene

Among the 450 mutations reported through the Consortium, only a very small number account for more than 1% and the rare mutations could be a marker of the ethnic origin of patients. For example, the mutation G551D represents about 5% if the CF chromosomes of patients from Celtic origin (Britanny, Ireland). The G542X which leads to a stop codon in exon 11 is common in the Mediterranean area. The W1282X is commonly found in population from Ashkenazi origin in which 60% of CF chromosomes are carrying this defect. [32]. We and others succeeded in analysing the complete sequence of the CFTR in different populations. The different profiles of non Δ508 mutations we have obtained in populations from Russia, Belgium, Britanny are shown in figures 1, 2, 3.

The characterization of these mutations has permitted the assessment of genotype/phenotype correlation and it has been shown that in cystic fibrosis, at least some of the clinical symptoms are genetically determined, e.g. pancreatic status [33]. This has been documented now for a large number of mutations which are missense mutations most of the time located in transmembrane region of the CFTR.

As it was also very probable that the milder form of CF would be associated with certain mutations, we have undertaken a complete analysis of the coding

Table 1. Results of a study.

	Patients genotype	Sex	Age at diagnosis	Professional activity	Age	Sweat test	Pancreatic status	FEV/FV-C	Pseudo-monas age at diagnosis	Sterility	Height weight	Weight*
1	R334W/G542X Exon 7/Exon 11 Arginine → Tryptophan	M	13	Yes Lawyer	42	113	PS	70% 85%	–	Yes	161 cm 67 kg	100%
2	ΔF508/I336K Exon 10/Exon 7 Isoleucine → Lysine	F	13	Yes Trilingual Secretary	35	90	PI (since 5 years)	54% 88%	+ 31 years	Unmarried	162 cm 47 kg	78%
3	ΔF508/H1054D Exon 10/Exon 17b Histidine → Aspartic Acid	M	27	Yes Secretary	42	116	PS	80% 70%	+ 27 years	Yes	161 cm 67 kg	100%
4	ΔF508 Unknown	M	17	Yes Townhall staff	35	80	PI (since 3 years)	not performed	–	Yes	168 cm 53 kg	76%
5	ΔF508/2789+5 G → A Exon 10/Exon 14b Splice mutation	F	39	Yes Secretary	43	90	PI (since 4 years)	89% 99%	–	Unknown	156 cm 56 kg	100%

* Weight expressed as a percentage of ideal weight for height.

	Patients genotype	Sex	Age at diagnosis	Professional activity	Age	Sweat test	Pancreatic status	FEV/FV-C	Pseudo-monas age at diagnosis	Sterility	Height weight	Weight*
6	ΔF508/2789 G → A Exon 10/Exon 14b Splice mutation	F	32	Yes Secretary	36	110	PI (since 5 years)	70% 79%	+ 32 years	2 children	158 cm 52 kg	86%
7	ΔF508/R117H Exon 10/Exon 4 Arginine → Histidine	F	30	No	35	90	PS	40% 45%	–	3 children	160 cm 49 kg	79%
8	ΔF508/I336K Exon 10/Exon 7 Isoleucine → Lysine	M	17	Yes Systems analyst	40	90	PS	90% 70%	–	Yes	168 cm 50 kg	71%

* Weight expressed as a percentage of ideal weight for height.

sequence of the CFTR gene of 8 adult CF patients older than 35 years, manifesting less severe phenotypes of the disease. We have fully identified the genotype of seven of these patients. Several different types of mutations have been found in this group, a splice mutation being present in two patients (2789+5 G → A), a missense mutation located in exons coding for transmembrane region in five patients (R334W, I336K, R117H, H1054D). In this group of patients, we have shown that pancreatic sufficient patients bearing these mild alleles have less severe symptoms with a lower and more delayed Pseudomonas aeruginosa colonization and a well conserved pulmonary function (Table 1) [34].

Conclusion

More than 400 different mutations have been reported in the CFTR gene. All these molecular abnormalities could be identified by scanning the entire sequence of the CFTR gene using different techniques, as SSCP, DGGE or direct DNA sequencing. All this mutations could be detected directly from a blood stain. This allows genetic diagnosis to be performed but also genotype/phenotype correlation could be more precisely established and retrospective studies from deceased patients could be done.

The identification of these mutated alleles had precisely defined the molecular basis of this inherited disorder opening now the field toward the development of an effective gene therapy for cystic fibrosis.

At this time, protocols using adenoviral vectors or liposomes have been used to demonstrate, using animal models, that the molecular defect in cystic fibrosis (cl^- channel defect) can be repaired by gene therapy in vivo. This is really a paradigm in molecular genetics illustrating the progress of the DNA technology in the recent years which allows the definition of the molecular basis of a genetic disease from a simple blood stain, opening the avenue for a specific therapy of cystic fibrosis in a next future.

References

1. Cotton RGH, Rodriquez NR, Campbell RD. Reactivity of cytosine and thymine in single-base-pair mismatches with hydroxylamine and osmium tetroxide and its application to the study of mutations. Proc Natl Acad Sci USA 1988;85:4397-401.
2. Myers RM, Larin Z, Maniatis T. Detection of single base substitutions by ribonuclease cleavage at mismatches in RNA:DNA duplexes. Science 1985;230:1242-49.
3. Fischer SC, Lerman LS. Separation of random fragments of DNA according to properties of their sequences. Proc Natl Acad Sci USA 1980;77:4420-24.
4. Lerman LS, Silverstein K. Computational simulation of DNA melting and its application to denaturing gradient gel electrophoresis. Methods Enzymol 1987;155: 482-501.
5. Orita M, Suzuki Y, Sekiya T, Hayashi K. Rapid and sensitive detection of point mutations and DNA polymorphisms using the polymerase chain reaction. Genomics 1989;5:874-79.
6. Hayashi K. PCR-SSCP: A simple and sensitive method for detection of mutations in the genomid DNA. PCR Methods Appl 1991;1:34-38.

7. Hayashi K, Yandell DW. How sensitive is PCR-SSCP? Hum Mutat 1993;2:338-46.
8. Boat TF, Welsh MJ, Beaudet AL. In: Scriver CR, Beaudet AL, Sly WS, Valle D (eds). The metabolic basis of inherited disease. New York: McGraw Hill 1989:2649-80.
9. Kerem BS, Rommens JM, Buchanan JA, et al. Identification of the cystic fibrosis gene: Genetic analysis. Science 1989;245:1073-80.
10. Riordan JR, Rommens JM, Kerem BS, et al. Identification of the cystic fibrosis gene: Cloning and characterization of complementary DNA. Science 1989;245:1066-73.
11. Rommens JM, Iannuzzi MC, Kerem BS, et al. Identification of cystic fibrosis gene: Chromosome walking and jumping. Science 1989;245:1059-64.
12. The Cystic Fibrosis Genetic Analysis Consortium. Worldwide survey of the delta F508 mutation. Report. Am J Hum Genet 1990;47:354-59.
13. The Cystic Fibrosis Genetic Analysis Consortium. Population variation of common cystic fibrosis mutations. Hum Mutat 1994;4:167-77.
14. Myers RM, Maniatis T, Lerman LS. Detection and localization of single base changes by denaturing gradient gel electrophoresis. Methods Enzymol 1987;155:501-27.
15. Audrézet MP, Mercier B, Guillermit H, et al. Identification of 12 novel mutations in the CFTR gene. Hum Molec Genet 1993;2:51-54.
16. Gyllensten UB, Erlich HA. Generation of single-stranded DNA by the polymerase chain reaction and its application to direct sequencing of the HLA-DQA locus. Proc Natl Acad Sci USA 1988;85:7652-56.
17. Sanger F, Nickler S, Coulson AR. DNA sequencing with chain terminating inhibitors. Proc Natl Acad Sci USA 1977;74:5463-67.
18. Collins FS. Positional cloning: Let's not call it reverse anymore. Nature Genetics 1992; 1:3-6.
19. Collins FS. Cystic fibrosis: Molecular biology and therapeutic implications. Science 1992;256:774-79.
20. Bear CE, Li C, Kartner N, et al. Purification and functional reconstitution of the cystic fibrosis transmembrane conductance regulator (CFTR). Cell 1992;68:809-18.
21. Cheng SH, Rich DP, Marshall J, Gregory RJ, Welsh MJ, Smith AE. Phosphorylation in the R domain by cAMP-dependant protein kinase regulates the CFTR chloride channel. Cell 1991;66:1027-36.
22. Drumm ML, Pope HA, Cliff WH, et al. Correction of cystic fibrosis defect in vitro by retrovirus-mediated gene transfer. Cell 1990;62:1227-33.
23. Tsui LC. Mutations and sequence variations detected in the cystic fibrosis transmembrae conductance regulator (CFTR) gene: A report from the Cystic Fibrosis Genetic Analysis Consortium. Hum Mutat 1992;1:197-203.
24. Tsui LC. Probing the basic defect in cystic fibrosis. Current Opinion in Genetics and Development 1991;1:4-10.
25. Saiki RK, Gefland DH, Stoffel S. Primer directed enzymatic amplification of DNA with a thermostable DNA polymerase. Science 1988;239:487-91.
26. Sheffield VC, Cox DR, Lerman LS, Myers RM. Attachment of a 40-base pair G + C-rich sequence (GC-clamp) to genomic DNA fragments by the polymerase chain reaction results in improved detection of single-base changes. Proc Natl Acad Sci USA 1989;86:232-36.
27. Férec C, Audrézet MP, Mercier B, et al. Detection of over 98% cystic fibrosis mutations in a Celtic population. Nature Genet 1992;1:188-91.
28. Mercier B, Lissens W, Audrézet MP, Bonduelle M, Liebaers I, Férec C. Detection of more than 94% cystic fibrosis mutations in a sample of Belgian population and identification of four novel mutations. Hum Mutat 1993;2:16-20.

29. Audrézet MP, Novelli G, Mercier B, et al. Identification of three novel cystic fibrosis mutations in a sample of Italian cystic fibrosis patients. Hum Hered 1993;43:295-300.
30. Audrézet MP, Canki Klain N, Mercier B, Bravar D, Verlingue C, Férec C. Identification of three novel mutations (457 TAT → G, D192G, Q685X) in the Slovenian CF patients. Hum Genet 1994;93:659-62.
31. Verlingue C, Kapranov NI, Mercier B, et al. Complete screening of mutations in the coding sequence of the CFTR gene in a sample of CF patients from Russia. Identification of three novel alleles. Hum Mutat 1995;5:205-9.
32. Shoshani T, Augarten A, Gazit E, et al. Association of a nonsense mutation (W1282X), the most common mutation in the Ashkenazi Jewish cystic fibrosis patients in Israel, with presentation of severe disease. Am J Hum Genet 1992;50:222-28.
33. Kristidis P, Bozon D, Corey M, et al. Genetic determination of exocrine pancreatic function in cystic fibrosis. Am J Hum Genet 1992;50:1178-84.
34. Férec C, Verlingue C, Guillermit H, et al. Genotype analysis of adult cystic fibrosis patients. Hum Molec Genet 1993;2:1557-60.

THE POTENTIAL IMPACT OF GENE THERAPY IN BLOOD TRANSFUSION

C.V. Prowse

Introduction

The previous presentations at this symposium have given detailed overviews of the current status of the molecular basis of selected diseases and the potential impact of gene therapy and associated technologies on some of these. What role does Blood Transfusion have in taking forward this developing technology, largely carried out to date in academic institutions or spin-off small biotechnology companies? The answer at present is, not a lot.

However Blood Banks and Transfusion Services have established skills in a number of areas (Table 1) that are potentially applicable to the application of (ex vivo) gene therapy. If gene therapy proves useful then as the provision of such a service moves from an academic base towards a clinical service there is an obvious opportunity to involve Blood Transfusion, even if such therapy (as seems likely) is eventually based in a few specialist centres in each country.

Table 1. Blood transfusion activities.

Cell storage
Quality systems
Good manufacturing practice
Patient assessment
Virus validation

The gene therapy cycle

The process of gene therapy development starts with the identification and isolation of the gene (or genes) associated with a particular disease or deficiency, a process largely accomplished in the academic arena. The gene is then packaged into some form of vector to allow its introduction into the target cell of interest. The efficiency of gene introduction and expression must then be assessed initially in cell culture, and then usually in some form of animal model. If all is well one can then return to the patient and undertake a clinical assessment of the developed therapy. This cycle is illustrated in Figure 1.

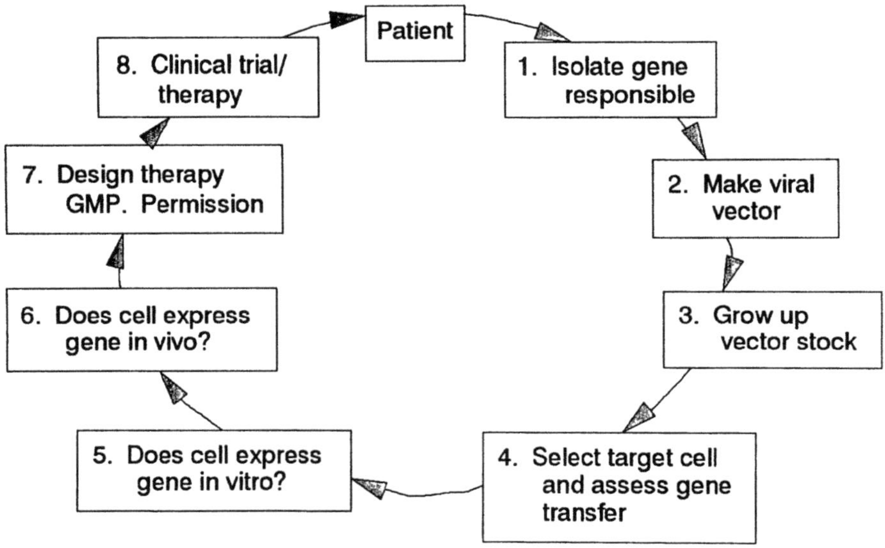

Figure 1. The gene therapy cycle.

Which diseases to treat?

With the current state of technology, gene therapy is currently carried out on somatic cells so as to avoid ethical concerns over passing the induced changes onto future generations, and must be reviewed by a number of ethical, clinical and scientific peer groups before its commencement. Initial studies have concentrated on congenital life threatening deficiency diseases, such as adenine deaminase deficiency and cystic fibrosis, and largely involved disorders of house keeping genes for which low level, unregulated expression is likely to be of benefit. Table 2 lists some such diseases that have been considered for gene therapy. Most of these are rare, as would be expected from their life threatening nature, the most common being cystic fibrosis and antitrypsin deficiency. Technology has only reached a state that allows addition of a normal gene rather than substitution of the defective sequence with a fully functional one. Although progress is being made on methods to allow homologous recombination, the efficiency of such approaches is so low as to make it impractical as yet for clinical assessment.

In recent years applications to undertake gene therapy have become increasingly dominated by those involving treatment of life-threatening acquired diseases, particularly cancer. This, and some other acquired diseases under consideration, are listed in Table 3. In the case of neoplastic disease a number of potential approaches to therapy have been described (Table 4). For patients, researchers and funding bodies such approaches have the obvious attractions that the potential

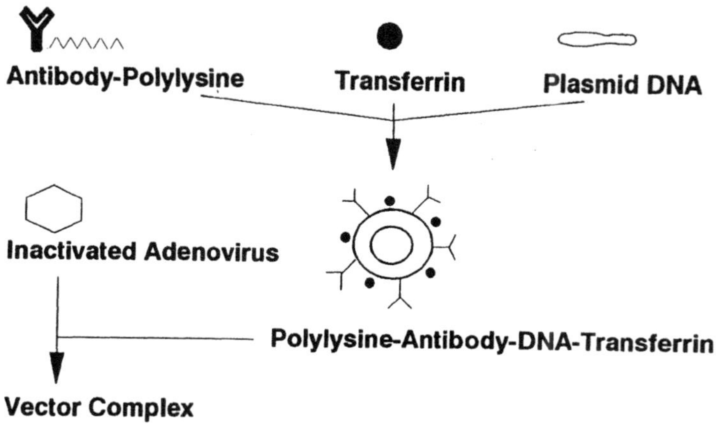

Figure 2. A receptor-targeted non-viral vector.
Polylysine is conjugated to a non-neutralizing monoclonal antibody to adenovirus and to transferrin. Plasmid DNA for the gene of interest is non-covalently complexed to this and inactivated (e.g. by psoralen and ultraviolet light treatment) adenovirus bound via the monoclonal antibody. Transferrin directs the complex to cells bearing the receptor for this protein, while the protein components of adenovirus enable entry of the gene into the cell after lysosomal uptake, bypassing the normal degradation that would otherwise occur.

Table 2. Possible gene therapy: Congenital diseases.

Class	Example	Incidence
Lung disease	Cystic fibrosis	1:2,500
	Antitrypsin deficiency	1:3,500
Lymphocyte deficiency	Adenine deaminase	Rare
Neutrophil deficiency	Chronic granulomatous disease	Rare
Macrophage deficiency	Mucopolysaccharoidosis	1:1,500
Liver deficiency	LDL receptor	1:500
Muscle disease	Duchenne muscular dystrophy	1:10,000
Haemostasis	Coagulation factor VIII/IX	1:10,000
Erythrocyte disorder	Thalassemia	1:600

treatment might be of benefit to far more people than is the case for congenital diseases. However, none of the approaches listen in Table 4 have yet to be clinically established. In addition acquired diseases may often be polygenic, rather than being ascribable to changes in just one gene, and hence it is debatable whether correction of a single gene will or will not offer hope of cure.

Table 3. Possible gene therapy: Acquired or polygenic diseases

Cancer
Thromboembolic disease
Diabetes
Autoimmune disease
Viral disease (HIV)

Table 4. Options for gene therapy of cancer.

Enhanced tumour cell killing (effector or bystander)
Enhanced tumour antigenicity
Change drug sensitivity of normal or cancer cells
Antisense therapy
Ribozymes
Prodrug route (VDEPT)*

* VDEPT: Virus directed enzyme prodrug therapy.

Table 5. Viral vectors.

Class (selectivity)	**Insert size (Kb)**	**Integration**	**Activity on non-dividing cells**	**Titre/ml (log)**
Retrovirus	≤ 7	+	–	6
Adenovirus (epithelium)	7 to 8	–	+	11
Adeno associated virus (+ helper)	< 5	±	?	Low
HSV (neurotrophic)	?		+	?

Gene Vector Development and Assessment

Traditional methods for the introduction of DNA into cells, such as endocytosis of calcium phosphate precipitates, are far too inefficient to enable clinical therapy. As a result a number of virus vectors have been developed (Table 5), particularly those based on retroviruses, to enable high efficiency gene transfer. These differ in their tropism for various cells, the size of inserted DNA they can accommodate, whether cell division is required for their action and whether or not they result in chromosomal integration of the inserted gene. For clinical use it is necessary to ensure that the vector used is not mutagenic, cannot replicate and is of well characterised structure, as well as being available in a suitably high titre. As such the regulations covering production are very similar to that for other pharmaceutical products, involving Good Manufacturing Practices (GMP) and appropriate quality assessment and documentation at multiple stages of production. Such facilities are likely to be beyond the capabilities of all but the larger Blood Banks and Transfusion Centres, and would involve a high risk investment given the low numbers of patients under consideration for any given vector construct.

Alternatives to viral vectors under assessment are listed in Table 6. Of these a current leader is exemplified by the complex of polylysine with the DNA of interest, coupled to a ligand such as transferrin or monoclonal antibody to CD34 enabling targeting to receptors on selected cells, and also to a component, such as inactivated adenovirus, enabling avoidance of the normal intracellular lysosomal destruction (Figure 2). The efficiency of such vectors now approaches that achievable with viral vectors, for gene introduction into cells if not chromosomal integration. While the same regulatory requirements apply as for viral approaches, by their nature such vectors are less restrictive in terms of gene size, potential for self replication, mutagenesis or titre. Even, so, it seems such licensed vectors are more likely to be made available 'over the counter' from pharmaceutical or specialist biotechnology firms, rather than through Blood Transfusion Centres. Exception to this may occur where a large pharmaceutical type unit of a Blood Bank or Transfusion Service forms a close working relationship with a major clinical department with an interest in gene therapy.

Table 6. Non-viral vectors.

Calcium phosphate
Electroporation
Microinjection/bioballistics
Liposomes
DNA-protein conjugates
Dendrimers

Target Cells and Tissues and Pre-Clinical Assessment

The ideal approach for gene therapy involves direct in vivo administration of the vector. While this approach has been pursued in a small number of cases, such as treatment of solid tumours and aerosol administration of adenoviral vectors in cystic fibrosis, most current protocols involve ex vivo introduction of genes into selected cells. In vivo gene therapy will require greater tissue selectivity and/or efficiency of gene transfer than are available with most current vectors, and if achieved would leave little place for any potential involvement of the Blood Transfusion Centre.

In contrast, with ex vivo therapy an opportunity for the involvement of Blood Transfusion exists. The target cell selected should ideally be self renewing such that one treatment would last a lifetime. It should be noted, however, that the initial trials of gene therapy involved transformation of lymphocytes, with a limited in vivo survival, and that this may have advantages in situations where the outcome is not fully delineated. While it may be preferable to select the same tissue as normally expresses the gene of interest, this is not necessary. Thus clinical trials in Chinese patients have shown the feasibility of expressing coagulation factor IX from implanted fibroblasts, whereas this factor is usually expressed by the liver.

Table 7 lists a number of cell types under assessment for gene therapy. Due to histocompatibility considerations there is an obvious preference for use of autologous cells, with blood providing a readily accessible source of such cells.

Table 7. Target cells assessed pre-clinically for gene therapy.

	Ex vivo	***In vivo***
Haematopoietic stem cells	+*	–
Leukocytes	+*	–
Hepatocytes	+*	+
Myoblasts	+	+
Keratinocytes	+	+
Fibroblasts	+	+
Endothelium	+	+
Epithelium (e.g. lung)	–	+*
Neuronal cells	+	+
Chondrocytes	+	+
Cancer cells	+*	+*

* Under clinical assessment.

Although marrow has attracted much study as a source of self renewing haematopoietic stem cells, the recent development of approaches for harvesting stem cells from peripheral blood, following mobilisation with cytokines, has provided an alternative source. In many Blood Transfusion Centres the harvesting of stem cells forms an active area of service development. Enrichment of the self renewing stem cell population from such sources, by positive selection for CD34 expressing cells for example, is equally applicable in the fields of transplantation or gene therapy.

Whichever cell target is selected, prior to clinical studies the transfected cells will need to be assessed for:

- Optimisation of conditions for gene transfection.
- Evidence of adverse changes in the target cells.
- Absence of vector DNA or other virus mobilisation.
- Appropriate gene expression in vitro and in vivo.
- Expansion of the desired cell population for clinical use.

Although some of these assessments are generic, others (for example 5) may be needed on a case-by-case basis, with strict control of the procedures used. It is in this area of close-to-patient activity that the main opportunities and demands may exist for Blood Transfusion Centres. The initial few such studies may well be carried out by academic clinical research departments but, as in the case of

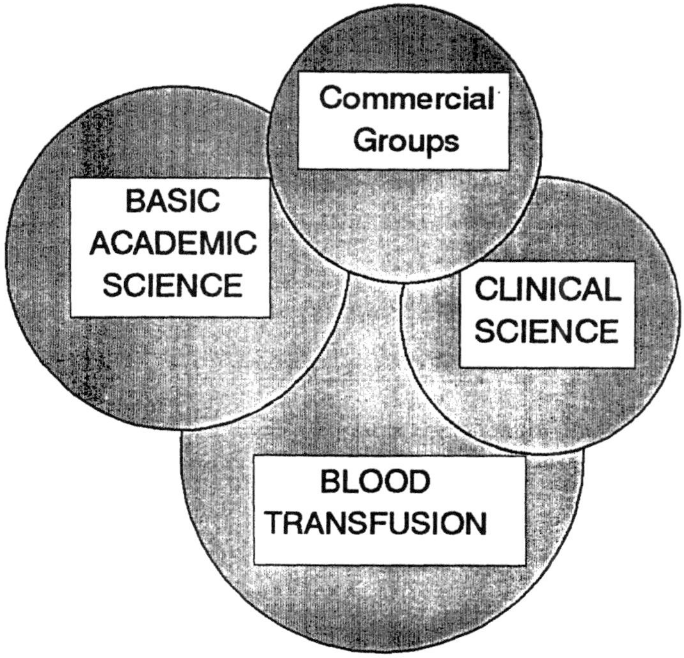

Figure 3. The potential linking role of blood transfusion in gene therapy.

bone marrow transplantations, as such procedures become more routine a service commitment will be sought (Figure 3).

To contribute fully to the above process Blood Transfusion would need to develop its existing expertise in virus assays and in those aspects of cell biology relating to the level and continuing expression of protein synthesis from the foreign genes inserted into the target cells. In addition pre-clinical assessment of transfected cells in vivo will require studies in appropriate animal models, whether these involve normal or naturally deficient models, or 'designer' deficiency models prepared by drug treatment or gene knockout approaches. Alternatively, for these aspects, collaboration could be developed with appropriate academic or commercial institutions.

An interesting development which may provide an intermediate alternative to 'classical' gene therapy is the encapsulation of allogeneic or xenogeneic cells, producing a protein of therapeutic interest, in a semi-permeable membrane. This 'implant' approach differs from such studies as the expression of factor IX from fibroblasts, mentioned above, in that the use of membranes has the potential to allow use of non-autologous cells usable in all patients with a particular deficiency, and also follows for the possible removal and/or replacement of the 'neo-organ' if this is desired. Requirements for the development and validation of cell lines appropriate for this approach would differ little, in principle, from that already outlined.

Clinical Assessment

Early contact with a motivated clinical unit with access to an adequate number of patients is an essential requirement of any clinical assessment. The general approach for such trials would differ little from the standard one for trial of any pharmaceutical product, involving assessment of safety, efficacy and pharmacokinetics. Early drafting of the trial design is required, and full documentation of the method used to prepare gene constructs, its consistency and the outcome of pre-clinical assessment are needed as part of the trial submission to regulatory authorities and ethical committees. Those Transfusion Centres involved in preparation of pooled plasma products have usually development expertise in these fields.

Gene therapy trials differ from those for standard pharmaceuticals in the assays required to assess the safety and efficacy of therapy, many of which will be developed during the pre-clinical phase, in the fact that biodistribution of the products involves transfected cells as well as the novel protein it produces, and the fact that follow-up of patients will be over a considerable time period, if a lifelong cure is the aim.

Conclusions

The potential exists for Blood Transfusion to contribute to the development of gene therapy for the treatment of congenital, and acquired, diseases by acting as a bridge between academic and clinical departments with an interest in such developments. Development of such a collaborative approach requires early contact with all interested parties. Blood Transfusion is unlikely to contribute much to the isolation of genes of interest, in the packaging of these in appropriate vectors and validation of such vectors. However, once such tools are to hand the requirement to isolate and manipulate the target cells of interest, validate their function and assess their function in vivo, in animal models and patients, in accordance with the principles of Good Manufacturing Laboratory and Clinical Practice, may be seen as a natural extension of procedures already undertaken in some Blood Transfusion Centres. Given the comparative rarity of life threatening congenital deficiencies a decision to become involved in gene therapy at present needs to be based on a considered judgement that such an approach will eventually be applicable, and valuable, in acquired disorders, such as cancer, and/or in those congenital deficiencies, such as haemophilia where alternative life saving therapies already exist.

As an example of a potential development one may consider a situation in which the potential of transplanting haemophiliacs with inhibitors with lymphocytes expressing an anti-idiotype antibody gene capable of neutralising the coagulation factor inhibitor. Such a project would involve initial isolation of an appropriate antibody gene and development of an appropriate vector for introducing this into lymphocytes, probably undertaken in an academic research department. The demonstration that such a vector could introduce and express the gene in lymphocytes could be undertaken jointly between the academic department and a Blood Transfusion Centre. Isolation of individual patients cells and application of the developed technology to these, and clinical assessment would involve joint work between Blood Transfusion and an expert Haemophilia Centre.

In the United States the role described here for Blood Transfusion is being taken on in some areas by specialist small biotechnology companies, a trend that is less evident in Europe. If Blood Transfusion groups wish to make a contribution in this field they need to make the commitment and seek out appropriate collaborators.

References

General

1. Verma IM. Gene Therapy. Sci Am 1990;nov.:31-41.
2. Anderson WF. Human gene therapy. Science 1992;256:808-13.
3. Friedman T. A brief history of gene therapy. Nat Genet 1992;2:93-98.
4. Miller AD. Progress towards human gene therapy. Blood 1990;76:271-78.
5. Morgan RA, Anderson WF. Human gene therapy. Ann Rev Biochem 1993;62:191-217.

Regulatory and safety aspects

6. Cornetta K. Annotation: Safety aspects of gene therapy. Br J Haematol 1992;80:421-26.
7. Kessler DA, Sieget JP, Noguchi PhD, Zoon KC, Feiden KL, Woodcock J. Regulation of somatic cell therapy and gene therapy by the food and drug administration. N Engl J Med 1993;329:1169-73.

Haematopoietic stem cells

8. Anderson KC. The rol of the blood bank in haematopoietic stem cell transplantation. Transfusion 1992;32:272-85.
9. The BCSH Blood Transfusion Task Force. Guidelines for the collection, processing and storage of human bone marrow and peripheral stem cells for transplantation. Transfusion Med 1994;4:165-72.
10. Egeland T, Tjonnford G, Steen R, Gaudemeck G, Thorsby E. Positive selection of bone marrow-derived CD34 positive cells for possible stem cell transplantation. Transplant Proc 1993;25:1261-63.

Vectors

11. Miller AD. Retrovirus packaging cells. Hum Gene Ther 1990;1:5-14.
12. Findeis, Aerwin JR, Spitalny GL, Chiou HC. Targeted delivery of DNA for gene therapy via receptors. Trends in Biotechnology 1993;11:202-05.
13. Curie DT, Wagner E, Cotten M, et al. High efficiency gene transfer mediated by adenovirus coupled to DNA-polylysine complexes. Hum Gene Ther 1992;3:147-54.
14. Tai IT, Sun AM. Microencapsulation of recombinant cells: A new delivery system for gene therapy. FASEB 1993;7:1061-69.

Specific aspects

15. Cournoyer D, Caskey CT. Gene therapy of the immune system. Ann Rev Immunol 1993;11:297-329.
16. Karlsson S. Treatment of genetic defects in haematopoietic cell function by gene transfer. Blood 1991;78:2481-92.
17. Lozier J, Brinkhous KM. Gene therapy and the haemophilias. JAMA 1994;271:47-51.
18. Zwiebel JA, Su N, MacPherson A, Davis T, Ojeifo JO. The gene therapy of cancer: Transgenic immunotherapy. Sem in Haematol 1993;30(suppl 4):119-29.

DISCUSSION

E. Briët, C.Th. Smit Sibinga – moderators

E. Briët (Leiden, NL): I would like to ask dr. Boulyjenkov about the use of genetic tests in the field of insurance. It has been always a focus of much interest in the debate between proponents and those who are very scared of the new biology, the new genetics. Could you say something from the point of view of the World Health Organization on how insurance companies should be or would not be allowed to use this type of information?

V. Boulyjenkov (Geneva, CH): This point was considered at the WHO Scientific Group of Hereditary Diseases in Geneva, November 1993, and it was agreed that genetic information should remain the property of individuals and should be considered as private and confidential information. It should be the right of the individual to choose whether to share such information with a third party. People should not suffer if this information is obtained by an insurance company or interested organization. The dignity of the individual should be preserved first and foremost and the means for storing information in the medical services should be strictly confidential and not be shared without the approval of the individual concerned. Information should not be divulged by genetic counselling services. In this regard, administrative recording systems should be reconsidered and evaluated. Health legislations could be reviewed and adapted to the above-mentioned points.

R.A. Sacher, Washington, DC, USA: I like to echo dr. Boulyjenkov's comments. For those of us who are involved in making available molecular diagnostic tests for cancer screening, there is a tremendous race in the United States to try and do this. I think not only at the points relevant with regard to insurance companies and their ability to restrict insurance. One of the key issues is also making available counselling systems such that when tests for example for colon cancer screening or whatever are available. In our laboratory and my department we are looking at setting up molecular diagnostics more from the point of view of making decisions about cancer diagnosis and infectious disease diagnosis. Cancer screening and these screening tests are very difficult and need many social issues to address. The concerns of patients who are suddenly landed with a gene that may or may not express itself yet has a lot of implications. So I wanted to agree and make the statement with regard to counselling. I think that is very important not so much from the blood bank point of view but of course from the WHO's point of view.

E. Briët: Maybe I am a bit more sceptical in the sense that I envisage insurance companies offer very attractive rates for those people willing to take a number of tests on oncogenes or things like that. Is that something one should object to or is that a thing that is just going to happen anyway.

R.A. Sacher: I think you are too optimistic. I think it is going to go in the reverse direction. People are going to be restricted from insurance rather than offering people who in fact have passed and certainly this is applicable to blood donors. These days blood donors are the preeminent insurance risks that if you are a blood donor you probably should be getting preferential rates because you are screened up. But I think the key problem is going to be restriction of insurance rather than offering a better insurance.

E. Briët: I would consider that two sides of the same coin.

C.Th. Smit Sibinga (Groningen, NL): May I ask a question to dr. Boulyjenkov. We have been listening to various aspects in relation to cord blood collection and the application of stem cells and their potential from cord blood. We are dealing then with a situation where either the foetus is not yet born or with newborn infants, where I think there are two issues which I would like you to comment on. First, the newborn individual's rights and the destination of cells for certain purposes is one aspect where others have to define what actually will happen. But the other point is the question coming up to the family to create a new individual. So it will interfere, therefore, with other aspects of life including family planning to which WHO has a particular idea as well. How would you see that in terms of the ethics.

V. Boulyjenkov: You are absolutely correct that there is a strong ethical component in blood collection and family planning. Ethics have always been a fundamental concern of the medical profession. The World Health Organization has set technical standards and proposed guidelines for such widely publicised issues as organ transplants and, more recently, reproductive health expert advisory panels on different WHO programmes assist in reviewing current problems in medicine. As the problem of ethics and health has been given priority in WHO, several programmes, including Blood Safety and Human Reproduction, can provide more specific and appropriate information upon request.

J.F. Harrison (Brentwood, UK): I think there is another very interesting question that we have to ask about cord blood, because if you imagine in the future that blood transfusion services are going to collect and store cord blood, may be expand the stem cells to provide material for transplantation, perhaps for adults.

We have to consider what happens to the foetus. I mean is the foetus perhaps normal or will the foetus that we have taken the cord blood from the placenta going to turn out to have some genetic disease itself. So should we have to follow up the fate of that child from whom we have taken that cord blood before we use it.

R.A. Sacher: I like to comment on that. I think that that theoretical question is not a problem. Why? Because we really are not collecting cord blood, we collect discarded placental blood and in reality in most of the instances where this is collected it is after the foetus, the child has been born. The usual strategy is to try and collect the cord blood or at least the placental blood from the placenta initially *in utero* and then allow it to drip into a receptaculum and then after the placenta is delivered it is aspirated in a sterile way from the vessels at the insertion of the cord. Now, I do not believe this is going to make any difference in terms of effects of the foetus. I guess the other question you raise is the potential for banking the cord blood or the child's cord blood for a catastrophic event in the future. There are strategies and there are commercial entrepreneurs in America that have made this available at a significant price. There I think is perhaps a little bit of over-exploitation.

C.V. Prowse (Edinburgh, UK): I do not think that is the question. I think you are asking if I bank this child's cord blood today, could he be a carrier for cystic fibrosis for example. Should I then be screening for inherited diseases (you can make the list as long as you like) when I bank it. That would make it very expensive.

D.J. Anstee (Bristol, UK): We have heard a lot of discussion about the role of transfusion services in the development of gene therapy, but one question that occurs to me is how are you going to make this happen? Are there any coordinated national strategies for transfusion services to get involved in these kind of procedures or is the assumption made that inspired individuals will somehow make it happen? It would be interesting to hear from dr. Zwiebel whether there is any kind of coordinated strategy within the transfusion service in the US?

J.A. Zwiebel (Washington, DC, USA): In a word no. I think it clearly depends upon like-minded individuals to get together and hammer out these types of protocols. I suspect that will be the way it continues to occur for at least for the foreseeable future. On the other hand a symposium like this one bringing together gene therapists, if you will, with transfusion specialists is a way to begin to bring the two areas together and start to plan along those lines.

E. Briët: Dr. Prowse, could you comment on the situation in the United Kingdom?

C. V. Prowse: In the United Kingdom there was a document produced by a government advisory body, which gave a pointer. They recommended the blood transfusion organisation be involved, but in effect has not picked up on that and has left it to, as you say, the inspired individual to pick up. In the UK there is a National Scottish Service which hopefully can develop a coordinated plan. I think that kind of coordinated approach to research seems to becoming the case in the Netherlands as well. Dr. Smit Sibinga probably knows better than I do.

C.Th. Smit Sibinga: There is to my knowledge not a specific document available in the Netherlands. I know from the discussion with dr. de Koning from the Health Inspection that there are some initial thoughts at governmental level to explore the consequences of these developments which are natural, which are upcoming and to see what regulatory mechanism then should be put in place to avoid a wild growth of situations in our country. There is also within the European community in Brussels not a specific regulation to my knowledge, which deals with gene therapy and the preparative approaches to that. There is a regulation which deals with monoclonal antibody production for human application but no more than that unless I am mistaken.

D.E. Onions (Glasgow, UK): May I comment on that general principle? I do not quite agree with dr. Prowse. There are actually now four companies in Europe that I am aware of.

They are banking vector systems under GMP conditions for use by clinicians. That is what is already happening. It does seem to me that we really have got to look that this is a kind of partnership. There will be academic groups who will become involved with these companies, developing new vector systems whether they be viral or non-viral. It seems to me that they will have to go to expert groups or expert companies that will understand how to GMP bank these, how to GLP test these. We clearly get to the fact that the use of these systems is going to require the blood transfusion services; no doubt about that. It seems to me that we have got to get this interface right. It would seem to me that there are three arms to this; that is the clinicians, innovative companies of various sorts and the blood transfusion services. It would seem inappropriate to me that the blood transfusion service will think that it will get into developing new vector systems in a big way and GLP testing these vectors. I mean that is an enormous piece of work. Where the blood transfusion service does have the skills and the expertise par excellence is in developing the stem cell technology. It seems to me that the company should be delivering the vector systems and that you will be optimising the use of those vector systems with an appropriate stem cell technology. Those are where the interactions are going to be. The regulation in Europe I think is in a bit of a mess. Here in the Netherlands as I understand it, if you use a retrovirus vector it goes to the committee that is involved with the release of recombinant organisms into the environment based on EEC directives. In Britain we do not use that same regulatory route. We use the genetic therapy advisory committee and the medicines control agency. So already in Europe despite the fact that we are a European Union we are actually using different regulatory bodies to approve gene therapy applications. But clearly there will be a united view when there is going to be marketing, because marketing authorization will require DG3 and there is already a draft guideline out for marketing.

D.J. Anstee: I agree exactly with what prof. Onions said is the potential role for the transfusion service in the whole process. So I agree completely with that strategy. My question is how do you make it happen. Are the companies going to come to the transfusion service and say will you do this and if so how are they going to know where to go within the transfusion service to do that. How do you set up a mechanism which creates that network or should there be a national transfusion approach to the companies. How do you make it happen? I agree that that is how it fits together.

C.V. Prowse: Two comments. One, maybe my message was not clear enough: I agree fully with what you say. Vectors are not for transfusionists to develop, the cell engineering maybe. The answer to your question is that I hope there will be a national policy. You do not want to develop expertise in putting cystic fibrosis gene in endothelium and stem cells in five different places in Scotland. I think the answer will be through the lead clinicians initially. If you have a cystic fibrosis group the point of contact between any potential, commercial company, the academic institute, the blood transfusion is the person who has got the patient, so if your blood transfusion service is seeking to develop that kind of service what you should be doing is looking for where the lead clinicians are and begin to talk to them. It is the patient that matters.

D.E. Onions: Maybe I can illustrate this is already happening. For instance the treatment of ADA deficiency here in Europe involved an innovative group based in the Netherlands which is now formed as a company. The GLP testing of that product was done in Scotland in another company that specialises in GLP. That product was then supplied to clinicians widely here in Europe. So already those connections are coming. I would agree with dr. Prowse they are driven largely by the clinicians. These networks are already forming. I do not think you really need to do a great deal to push them. I think what we do need is more interaction between these elements by just talking, that helps a great deal.

C.Th. Smit Sibinga: I fully agree on that. On top of that we have experienced that industry, commercial companies not only in the field of production of vectors but also in the supportive technology are exploring the scenery to look for expert centres where they could cooperate with. So, it is a kind of cross-fertilising mechanism which falls in place in this point in time. The only thing at least in our country is that there is not yet a firm movement noticeable in terms of the regulatory affairs and for that point we have a little freedom for the moment.

J.A. Zwiebel: Bone marrow clearly is getting wide application now in gene therapy as I mentioned earlier. Clearly there is a burgeoning number of applications in other cell types. I would like to hear from the blood bank community what your thoughts are about expanding transfusion medicine into the culture of other cells, whether hepatocytes or fibroblasts or endothelial cells.

C.V. Prowse: I cannot answer for the whole blood banking community. In our own centre we have begun work on endothelial cells and on fibroblasts. On hepatocytes we have not done any work, nor muscle. I suspect we should begin to look at hepatocytes, but that is a difficult one unless you can get actually access to foetal liver, which has its own problems. The problem with that is you then need to think about whether you are dealing with autologous or allogeneic forms of each of those tissues. We tried that and going the autologous route is a difficult organisational problem. There is that delay between harvesting, the time taken for expansion and getting back to the patient. So any technology that enables you to go the allogeneic route for these other tissues is of interest, but I am not sure it exists yet.

J.A. van der Does ('s-Gravenhage, NL): May I add something for the development in the Netherlands. I think that the expertise of blood banks is knowing the needs of the clinic, dealing with samples, identifying them, quality control them, store them. We should use that expertise. If we are not experts in for instance virus genomes etc. let us work together with firms, with university departments who know that. The moment it becomes more volume then the strength, the expertise of the blood banks come in. I agree with dr. Prowse on the four partners he mentioned.

C.V. Prowse: That is one thing that is worth emphasising. The involvement does not necessarily have to be terribly high technology. If somebody can grow hepatocytes in serum free medium, that is a valuable contribution to that kind of process. It is not high-tech, it is basic cell culture. But as far as I am aware it does not exist yet.

C.Th. Smit Sibinga: Dr. Zwiebel, to add to your question, as dr. Van der Does already said the question is that the blood banking community has an extreme experience over decades in handling a very specific tissue, in harvesting that tissue, in preparing the various components out of that tissue, in purification of the tissue, in preservation of the tissue. The next step obviously is in the propagation, the culture of the tissue and the enrichment, that is quite obvious. Not only that needs to be restricted to human blood as such, it could extend naturally to other target cells, which we need for this new development within the field of transfusion medicine, definitely so.

C.V. Prowse: One further comment, and then a specific question. To some extent we are talking to ourselves and to the self-converted here. Be aware that there are other groups promoting themselves within the health providing community as well. So it is slightly competitive.

My specific question is to prof. Onions. You mentioned something that I had not heard before which is that you begin to isolate nuclear targeting sequences from, I think you said, semiviruses. But I am not so quite sure that should enable you to use retroviral vectors in non-dividing cells. Is that approach something that will enable targeted integration using viral, or even non-viral, vectors. Is that an option for the future?

D.E. Onions: The sequences are based, first of all, on an observation of Mario Stevenson in the United States[1] and also from others, where matrix proteins of lentiviruses influence nuclear transport of retroviral sequences into the nucleus of non-dividing cells. If you take a retrovirus like MuLV, the block in getting the provirus into the cell is it does not go into the nucleus of a non-dividing cell. But if you put the nucleic targeting sequence in, it will get in there. So, at the moment the experiments that have been done by a number of groups are either to put these leader sequence from retroviruses, from HIV and in our own case from the feline immuno-deficiency virus. We now are seeing whether we get those proviruses into the nucleus. What we do not yet know is whether they will integrate unless the cell actually divides or that they just hang around until that cell divides. But we can get expression of non-integrated Ig levels. So we do not yet know the full story just as we do not yet know whether we get full integration or whether we just get persistence of the genome in the non-integrated form. But we will get expression, I think.

C.V. Prowse: I understand that the adeno-associated viruses, the wild type virus, tends to integrate at a specific side on chromosome 19. In the modified 'vector' forms of the virus you do not get as good a specific integration. Is that kind of thing telling us an alternative route that may address the question? Can you target integration size?

D.E. Onions: Well, nobody can tell you the integration size yet. Of course, homologous recombination with large pieces of DNA can be done in cell systems but not yet with virus systems. There are a number of us, who are interested in ways of trying to do that. AAV is very interesting as it integrates into chromosome 19, a process that depends on a gene called rep. Ironically that gene has been captured by quite a different virus HHV-6 and occasionally it does integrate but in this case into chromosome 17. So what we do not understand at the moment is the specificity of that integration. We do not understand how it occurs. The problem is that as soon as you take the rep gene out as you have to do with these AAV vectors, usually you get random integration. It is also clear that we do not

1. Gendleman HE, Ratner L, Stevenson M, Emerman M. The vpr protein of human immunodeficiency virus influences nuclear localisation of viral nucleic acids in non-dividing host cells. Proc Natl Acad Sci USA 1994;91:7311-5.

know the consequences of that random integration. So one should be careful to assume that AAV is somehow more intrinsically safe than a modified retrovirus vector. I do not think that necessarily is going to be the case.

E. Briët: I am sure that we could continue this discussion for a long time since there are very many issues of interest that excite us and that we could talk about for many hours to come.

Three years ago I was on the plane with Cees Smit Sibinga from the ISTH congress in Tokyo to Schiphol in Amsterdam and he asked me whether I would be willing to be chairman of his symposium in 1994. Of course I said no, that seems an awful lot of work. He told me then that it would not be very much work; the only thing I needed to do is sum up at the end of the symposium. And now I am afraid I have to deliver. I have made quite a number of pages of notes during this symposium, which would take me very long to tell to you. So, subsequently I condensed that into five statements. After reading the statements I found them horribly banal generalisations, so I am not going to deliver.

But what I would like to say is that we have heard about 20 speakers, who have proven to be excellent teachers whom I have learned very much from. Above all we had a relaxed and very informal meeting, where we got to know new people and where we had plenty of time to exchange ideas and to have stimulating discussions. Cees, your equation for this meeting has evolved during the 19 years that you have organised this and it has condensed into a highly effective formula that has been an example for me. I would like to suggest that we thank Cees Smit Sibinga and his staff for this and to do so by giving a show of hands. Thank you very much.

INDEX

DEVELOPMENTS IN HEMATOLOGY AND IMMUNOLOGY

1. H.R. Lijnen, D. Collen and M. Verstraete (eds.): *Synthetic Substrates in Clinic Blood Coagulation Assays*. 1980 ISBN 90-247-2409-
2. C.Th. Smit Sibinga, P.C. Das and J.O. Forfar (eds.): *Paediatrics and Blood Transfu sion*. Proceedings of the 5th Annual Symposium on Blood Transfusion, organized b the Red Cross Bloodbank Groningen-Drenthe, The Netherlands (1980). 1982 ISBN 90-247-2619-
3. N. Fabris (ed.): *Immunology and Ageing*. 1982 ISBN 90-247-2640-
4. G. Hornstra: *Dietary Fats, Prostanoids and Arterial Thrombosis*. With an Introdu tory Chapter by A. Bleakley Chandler. 1982 ISBN 90-247-2667-
5. C.Th. Smit Sibinga, P.C. Das and J.J. van Loghem (eds.): *Blood Transfusion an Problems of Bleeding*. Proceedings of the 6th Annual Symposium on Blood Transfu sion, organized by the Red Cross Bloodbank Groningen-Drenthe (1981). 1982 ISBN 90-247-3058-
6. J. Dormandy (ed.): *Red Cell Deformability and Filterability*. 1983 ISBN 0-89838-578-
7. C.Th. Smit Sibinga, P.C. Das and H.F. Taswell (eds.): *Quality Assurance in Bloc Banking and Its Clinical Impact*. Proceedings of the 7th Annual Symposium on Bloc Transfusion, organized by the Red Cross Bloodbank Groningen-Drenthe (1982). 198 ISBN 0-89838-618-
8. A.M.H.P. van den Besselaar, H.R. Gralnick and S.M. Lewis (eds.): *Thromboplast Calibration and Oral Anticoagulant Control*. 1984 ISBN 0-89838-637-
9. P. Fondu and O. Thijs (eds.): *Haemostatic Failure in Liver Disease*. 1984 ISBN 0-89838-640-
10. C.Th. Smit Sibinga, P.C. Das and G. Opelz (eds.): *Transplantation and Bloc Transfusion*. Proceedings of the 8th Annual Symposium on Blood Transfusio organized by the Red Cross Bloodbank Groningen-Drenthe (1983). 1984 ISBN 0-89838-686-
11. H. Schmid-Schönbein, L.J. Wurzinger and R.E. Zimmerman (eds.): *Enzyme Activa tion in Blood-perfused Artificial Organs*. 1985 ISBN 0-89838-704-
12. J. Dormandy (ed.): *Blood Filtration and Blood Cell Deformability*. 1985 ISBN 0-89838-714-
13. C.Th. Smit Sibinga, P.C. Das and E. Seidl (eds.): *Plasma Fractionation and Bloc Transfusion*. Proceedings of the 9th Annual Symposium on Blood Transfusio organized by the Red Cross Bloodbank Groningen-Drenthe (1984). 1985 ISBN 0-89838-761-
14. S. Dawids and A. Bantjes (eds.): *Blood Compatible Materials and their Testing*. 198 ISBN 0-89838-813-
15. C.Th. Smit Sibinga, P.C. Das and T.J. Greenwalt (eds.): *Future Developments Blood Banking*. Proceedings of the 10th Annual Symposium on Blood Transfusio organized by the Red Cross Bloodbank Groningen-Drenthe (1985). 1986 ISBN 0-89838-824-
16. A. Berlin, J. Dean, M.H. Draper, E.M.B. Smith and F. Spreafico (eds. *Immunotoxicology*. Proceedings of the International Seminar on the Immunologic System as a Target for Toxic Damage – Present Status, Open Problems and Futu Perspectives, in collaboration with the UNEP-ILO-WHO IPCS and the Commissic of the European Communities. 1987 ISBN 0-89838-843-

DEVELOPMENTS IN HEMATOLOGY AND IMMUNOLOGY

17. T. Ottenhoff and R. de Vries: *Recognition of M. leprae Antigens*. 1987
ISBN 0-89838-887-
18. J.-L. Touraine, R.P. Gale and V. Kochupillai (eds.): *Fetal Liver Transplantation*. 198
ISBN 0-89838-975-
19. C.Th. Smit Sibinga P.C. Das and C.P. Engelfriet (eds.): *White Cells and Platelets i Blood Transfusion*. Proceedings of the 11th Annual Symposium on Blood Transfu sion, organized by the Red Cross Bloodbank Groningen-Drenthe (1986). 1987
ISBN 0-89838-976-
20. C.F.M. Hendriksen: *Laboratory Animals in Vaccine Production and Control*. 1988
ISBN 0-89838-398-
21. C.Th. Smit Sibinga, P.C. Das and L.R. Overby (eds.): *Biotechnology in Bloo Transfusion*. Proceedings of the 12th Annual Symposium on Blood Transfusio organized by the Red Cross Bloodbank Groningen-Drenthe (1987). 1988
ISBN 0-89838-404-
22. C.Th. Smit Sibinga, P.C. Das and C.F. Högman (eds.): *Automation in Bloo Transfusion*. Proceedings of the 13th Annual Symposium on Blood Transfusio organized by the Red Cross Bloodbank Groningen-Drenthe (1988). 1989
ISBN 0-7923-0488-
23. S. Dawids (ed.): *Polymers: Their Properties and Blood Compatibility*. 1989
ISBN 0-7923-0491-
24. C.Th. Smit Sibinga, P.C. Das and H.T. Meryman (eds.): *Cryopreservation and Lo Temperature Biology in Blood Transfusion*. Proceedings of the 14th Annual Sym posium on Blood Transfusion, organized by the Red Cross Bloodbank Groninge Drenthe (1989). 1990 ISBN 0-7923-0908-
25. C.Th. Smit Sibinga and L. Kater (eds.): *Advances in Haemapheresis*. Proceedings c the 3rd International Congress of the World Apheresis Association (Amsterdam, Th Netherlands, 1990). 1991 ISBN 0-7923-1312-
26. C.Th. Smit Sibinga, P.C. Das and P.M. Mannucci (eds.): *Coagulation and Bloo Transfusion*. Proceedings of the 15th Annual Symposium on Blood Transfusio organized by the Red Cross Bloodbank Groningen-Drenthe (1990). 1991
ISBN 0-7923-1331-
27. C.Th. Smit Sibinga, P.C. Das and J.D. Cash (eds.): *Transfusion Medicine: Fact an Fiction*. Proceedings of the 16th International Symposium on Blood Transfusio organized by the Red Cross Bloodbank Groningen-Drenthe (1991). 1992
ISBN 0-7923-1732-
28. C.Th. Smit Sibinga, P.C. Das and T.H. The (eds.): *Immunology and Blood Transfu sion*. Proceedings of the 17th International Symposium on Blood Transfusio organized by the Red Cross Bloodbank Groningen-Drenthe (1992). 1993
ISBN 0-7923-2380-
29. C.Th. Smit Sibinga, P.C. Das and H.J. Heiniger (eds.): *Good Manufacturing Practic in Transfusion Medicine*. Proceedings of the 18th International Symposium on Bloo Transfusion, organized by the Red Cross Blood Bank Groningen-Drenthe. (199 1994 ISBN 0-7923-3009-

DEVELOPMENTS IN HEMATOLOGY AND IMMUNOLOGY

30. C.Th. Smit Sibinga, P.C. Das and E. Briët (eds.): *Hereditary Diseases and Bloc Transfusion.* Proceedings of the 19th International Symposium on Blood Transfusioı organized by the Red Cross Blood Bank Groningen-Drenthe (1994). 1995
ISBN 0-7923-3694-

KLUWER ACADEMIC PUBLISHERS – DORDRECHT / BOSTON / LONDON

www.ingramcontent.com/pod-product-compliance
Ingram Content Group UK Ltd.
Pitfield, Milton Keynes, MK11 3LW, UK
UKHW020250290926
15470UKWH00002B/849
* 9 7 8 0 7 9 2 3 3 6 9 4 5 *